TRANSFORMING THE WORLD

STUART ROSE

TRANSFORMING THE WORLD

BRINGING THE NEW AGE INTO FOCUS

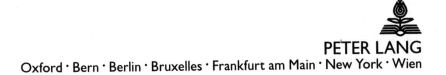

PETER LANG

Oxford · Bern · Berlin · Bruxelles · Frankfurt am Main · New York · Wien

Bibliographic information published by Die Deutsche Bibliothek
Die Deutsche Bibliothek lists this publication in the Deutsche Nationalbibliografie;
detailed bibliographic data is available on the Internet at ‹http://dnb.ddb.de›.

British Library and Library of Congress Cataloguing-in-Publication Data:
A catalogue record for this book is available from The British Library, Great Britain,
and from The Library of Congress, USA

Cover design: Thomas Jaberg, Peter Lang AG

ISBN 3-03910-316-4
US-ISBN 0-8204-7241-7

© Peter Lang AG, European Academic Publishers, Bern 2005
Hochfeldstrasse 32, Postfach 746, CH-3000 Bern 9, Switzerland
info@peterlang.com, www.peterlang.com, www.peterlang.net

Printed in Germany

To Sally, Maggie, and Shaun

Contents

Tables   8
Preface   9

Part One: Main Features of the New Age
1. Bringing the New Age into Focus   15
2. Recent History   43
3. Characteristics of Association   81
4. Getting Involved   107
5. Essential Concepts   131

Part Two: Encountering New Age Domains of Interest
Introduction   159
6. Spiritual Empowerment   163
7. Healing Practices   183
8. Community Activity   213
9. The New Age Experience   233

Part Three: Critical Response
Introduction   263
10. The Christian Response   265
11. Social and Cultural Responses   291
12. Transforming the World   323

Appendix   341
Bibliography   345
Index   363

Tables

1. The rise of channelled teachings in the 1970s   69
2. The age profile of UK New Age and national populations   86
3. The age profile of US New Age and national populations   86
4. Length of association with the New Age by age   88
5. Income levels of New Age participants   91
6. Length of time associated with the New Age by age   95
7. New Age activities 'ever' and 'currently' practised   96
8. Frequency of attending New Age events in a 12-month period   98
9. Proliferation of specialist New Age magazines   115
10. New Age networking in *Kindred Spirit*, Issue 28   117
11. Most influential New Age teachers in 1977 and 1994   177

Preface

All life is comprised of a multitude of passageways along which we choose to travel, and most of us, myself included, do not know where the passages started or where they will end. Perhaps the notion of beginnings and ends is an attempt to rationalize the seemingly non-rational. The New Age is one of the passageways to choose and many people have tried to rationalize what it is generally, without conspicuously successful results. When my opportunity to research the New Age arose it was an attractive prospect and was realized in the submission of a successful doctoral thesis, the genesis of this book. Since that time I have updated, reorganized, and rewritten much of the work in an attempt to create a comprehensive and balanced yet readable study. My prime objective has been to put a finger directly on the pulse of what the New Age is all about.

The strategy I have used to reach this objective is based on a combination of fairness and facts. It incorporates three routes: a thorough study of all the major writings both by commentators and by those involved, an ethnographic sampling of the 'fare' through attendance at many New Age events and workshops, and listening to what participants themselves have to say about the New Age by means of a substantial survey. This method is what gives my study its comprehensiveness and its solid foundations. As a result, *Transforming the World* presents many distinctions and categorizations that bring order to an unwieldy topic, and portrays the New Age as a concrete, living enterprise, not merely a philosophy.

A few words need to be said about the survey of participants. From the outset, I decided to mount a quantitative study. My understanding all along has been that the New Age is not amorphous but composed of many individuals, each following a unique transformational path. This meant that reaching and surveying participants in any significant number would not be an easy task. Various routes aimed at reaching a robust sample of participants were reviewed. I concluded that the most accurate route, which had the potential of reaching the widest spectrum of 'high quality' individuals (that is, long-term participants in the New Age), was via the media. A media search showed that *Kindred Spirit* was the widest-selling New Age magazine in the UK. With the agreement of the publishers, 5,350 questionnaires were inserted in the magazine and mailed to the home addresses of individuals who had committed themselves to at least one year's subscription.

The final questionnaire contained forty-three questions – many of which included a number of subquestions – together with a further six unnumbered questions covering personal details. The questionnaires were to be answered anonymously, although the first part of the respondent's postcode was requested to enable the geographic spread to be checked. In all, the total number of questions and subquestions was 205, in addition to which five hand-counted analyses were made. The questions are provided as an Appendix.

The questionnaire was designed as a four-page A4 leaflet with questions on three pages, the fourth being a fold-up (not prepaid) return postal envelope. The title of the survey – *Survey of New Age Ideas* – was followed by text which described the purpose of the survey, how valuable each respondent's contribution was, instructions on how to complete the questionnaire and, finally, a rider which described the use of the term 'New Age'.

Of the total number of questions, nine were open-ended and in these space was allocated for respondents to give a full descriptive answer. The remaining questions were of the tick-box type with preset answers, but space was often allowed for respondents to insert an answer different from the preset variables if they wished. The majority of questions were conceived by the author but seven were directly influenced by Marilyn Ferguson's study *The Aquarian Conspiracy* in order to see what changes may have occurred since the mid-1970s. The minimum completion time was estimated to be twenty minutes, although the actual time could have stretched considerably longer as some of the open-ended questions required considered opinions or further explanation.

I set the minimum target response level at 200. By the survey cut-off date, 908 questionnaires had been received. Several more questionnaires arrived after this date, but they were not included in the analysis. This total figure represents a 17% response which, as a result, has allowed a substantial amount of statistically valid subgroup analysis to be carried out.

Only one spoiled questionnaire was received. In fact, many respondents wrote unsolicited congratulatory messages reporting how participating in the survey had been a pleasurable and educative experience. A number had included letters or pages of notes of expanded answers to some questions or had given anecdotal reports.

The information received through the questionnaire was translated into a tailor-made coding system that allowed significant scope for variable answers, especially in the case of open-ended questions. The method of analysis employed here was a qualitative interpretation of each answer, which was then coded for statistical analysis. While the statistical results were vital, verbatim records of descriptions which were representative of each identified type gave an additional insight to respondents' views, and these were transcribed for use in the book. Additionally, a random subset of 300 questionnaires was compiled to assess the extent of respondents' use of key words and phrases.

The three routes – the writings, ethnography and survey – are combined in *Transforming the World* to provide a comprehensive description of the New Age. This unfolds in three parts: five chapters examining the main features, four illuminating the principal domains and practices, and two discussing critical responses. The concluding chapter recapitulates and brings to light consistencies and inconsistencies. The summation of what I have found in these studies is encapsulated in the book's title: participating in the New Age entails a transformation of the world – both private and public.

Stuart Rose,
Camlad House, Powys, Wales.
stuart.rose@britishlibrary.net

February 2005

PART ONE

MAIN FEATURES OF THE NEW AGE

1. Bringing the New Age into Focus

The named is the mother of ten thousand things.
Lao Tsu[1]

What is the New Age? To some it is a religion, to others a means to develop their potential in business or life skills, and to yet others the New Age revolves around healing the body, mind, spirit, and planet. There are many interpretations. The New Age is continually evolving, and discussions of what it encompasses and what its component parts might be constitute some of the most controversial and disputed questions that are raised. Is the New Age amorphous, as one American academic suggests,[2] or is there, in fact, some structure or definitive shape to its ideas and activities? In this chapter we try to answer this and other questions by identifying the principal concepts which comprise its parts: what its scope might be, its newness, whether it can be called a movement, its cause, its central ideas, and, finally, looking at what some believe are its main qualities; but first the principal connections are laid bare.

1   Lao Tsu, 1976: One.
2   James Lewis, 1992: 6.

15

Principal connections

There is precious little which ties the disparate elements of the New Age together. The connection between, say, an ecologist and a channeller may, on the face of it, appear to be nil. This is one of the reasons why it is difficult to get a complete picture of what the New Age entails and also why several aspects which are included in this study may not be thought of by some as being part of the New Age. Nevertheless, there appear to be two principal connections which link all the elements – one more obvious and one more subtle, the latter perhaps being the stronger or more deeply rooted of the two. These two connections are, first, what is signified when the word 'new' is used in the title 'New Age' and, second, that the same heightened embodiment of love undergirds each element that the New Age encompasses.

The word 'new' in New Age identifies a change from one way of being or doing[3] to another. This change is often radical. There now exists new spirituality, new economics, new health, new ecology, new politics, new parenting, new community; and there is nothing much on the surface to link many of these together except the fact that they represent a movement away from an old way to a new way. Particularly, although not exclusively, this is seen as a move away from a capitalistically grounded society, which is deemed to be unsustainable for a variety of reasons, to a more sustainable and cooperative way of being and doing for which, as yet, there is no clearly identifiable single nomenclature other than the term 'New Age'. At the outset, it has to be said that the principal characteristic of this newness is that it is not a newness simply for the sake of being new. The perception of this newness, across practically every aspect of Western society, is that this society has been travelling down a road which is doomed to failure in one way or another: not least in business, agriculture, health, religion, and education. This newness is not an all-change, brand-new newness – it involves much more of a change in the way in which

---

3   I use the terms 'being' and 'doing' together in order to indicate that the New Age can be either a lived philosophy, or particular forms of activity, or both. This point will be elaborated in this and later chapters.

people think about their lives: a new mindset, as it were, which also involves bringing back many ideas that have been supplanted by the rapid onset of a technological society.

The second connection, which is suggested here as the motivating 'energy' that drives the onset of the new, is love. This love is manifest in many different ways, although it is nothing whatsoever to do with the romantic love found in relationships between people. In fact, it is often not thought of as love at all but as compassion, care, kindness, or sharing; in this book it is called 'spiritual love' in order to clarify further what is involved.[4] What separates the New Age from the rest of society is an increased injection of love into all aspects of life: loving the environment, loving the body, loving the customer, loving the planet, loving the spirit. By loving more (or being more compassionate, caring, kind, or sharing) a whole new way of being or doing is brought about. This new loving way is called the New Age.

On the surface, it can be seen that what links the New Age farmer to the New Age businessperson or New Age health practitioner, to name but a few of its recognizable manifestations, can be very little, although at a much subtler or deeper level a great deal can be identified that links them; and it is the purpose of this study to explore these seemingly disparate elements. This is not to say that the conclusion to be drawn at the end of the book is that the New Age is a cohesive movement: the New Age is far from this, although the connections between the elements are stronger than might appear from a more cursory glimpse.

Scope

Because the New Age incorporates an extremely broad spectrum of ideas, each person who comes into contact with it seems to have her or his own view of what it entails. Those actually involved are most of-

4   In using the term 'spiritual love', no religious inferences are necessarily implied.

ten interested only partially, that is, in elements which particularly attract them, which means that from within the New Age it is likely that there cannot be found a single idea of its scope; and those looking in from the outside are likely not to be able to see the complete spread of all that is going on, as not all ideas and activities can be made public or visible. The New Age is very much an experiential way of living: knowledge, from books and other people, is seen by those involved to be useful but limited, experience is seen as being more useful, and intuitive insights are deemed essential. A combination of all three makes the whole of what the New Age is about.

Reading through any New Age guide or encyclopaedia[5] it quickly becomes apparent that few, if any, aspects in Western culture and society remain untouched by a New Age approach. Many commentators have provided lists to demonstrate the scope of the New Age. For example, the American thinker on transpersonal psychology Ken Wilber suggests:

> The [term] 'new age' has been used to refer to everyone and everything from so-called channeled material (like *Seth Speaks* or *A Course in Miracles*) to healing by quartz crystals, to pyramid power, to mysticism, Zen, yoga, est, gestalt, Bach flower remedies, Shirley MacLaine, *The Tao of Physics*, *The Aquarian Conspiracy*, psychedelics, designer drugs, East/West studies, new paradigms, the Findhorn community, Lindesfarne, Edgar Cayce, holistic medicine, belief in Atlantis, acupuncture, Ramtha, Lazaris, ESP, Wind Star, paranormal realities, altered states of consciousness, and – this might seem incongruous, but it really isn't – hi-tech anything, computers, lasers, and so on.[6]

Other similar – although in some cases even broader – lists have been compiled by, for example, a cultural historian[7] and an Australian New Age commentator.[8]

At the outset, an important question to ask, therefore, is whether there is any limit to the scope of the New Age. The simple answer is that there appears to be a New Age view on – and a way of transform-

---

5   For instance, those compiled by John Button and William Bloom, 1992, Gerry Maguire Thompson, 1999, or Paul Roland, 2000.
6   Ken Wilber, 1987: 11, italics added.
7   Christopher Lasch, 1987: 80f.
8   Nevill Drury, 1989: 103f.

ing – every issue in society and culture, although within this view, commentators and those involved may have differing ideas as to what can be classified as 'New Age' and what cannot. According to one of its leading 'players', the New Age

> is like a diamond, possessing many facets, [occurring] in all professions, in all walks of life, in a wide variety of situations and cultural circumstances. It is the jewel that contains them all. However, the very vastness and variety of activities, services, products, places, teachings, and events that claim to be new age can be bewildering.[9]

In characterizing what its scope might comprise, perhaps one of the best indicators can be found by reviewing the range in contents of several volumes of essays and collections of writings about the New Age. For example, two anthologies of New Age writings[10] are divided into sections which discuss such subjects as inner voice, holistic health and healing, Gaia, psychology, new science, feminism and the Goddess, shamanism, mystical religion, and practical implications of the New Age (which includes political and social issues). Alternatively, a guide to the New Age offers health and well-being, therapy and self-help, esoteric or spiritual traditions, concern for humanity and the environment, and particular respect for Nature and feminine wisdom.[11] From academe a collection of essays[12] includes, among other topics, healing, community, channelling, business training, neopaganism, women's issues, and astrology. Finally, a collection of critical essays[13] covers such areas as science, various paranormal subjects including UFOs and astral travelling, psychotherapeutic techniques, Eastern spirituality, music and television, and economics. From these representative volumes, while there exist many common themes, it

9   David Spangler, 1984: 77.
10   Compiled by one of Britain's champions of the New Age, William Bloom, 1991, 2000. See also Paul Roland, 2000.
11   Eileen Campbell and J. H. Brennan, 1990: 7.
12   James Lewis and J. Gordon Melton, 1992.
13   Robert Basil, 1988. There are several other collections of essays about the New Age covering similar subjects and these include Duncan Ferguson, 1993, and Steven Sutcliffe and Marion Bowman, 2000.

can also be seen that there are many variations in the scope and interpretation of the New Age.

Analysis of the New Age press provides no further clarification. For example, a typical issue of *Kindred Spirit: The Guide to Personal and Planetary Healing* from Britain contains articles on architecture, death, ecomusic, health, shamanism, group therapy, parenting, and Carlos Castaneda. Alternatively, a regular issue of *New Age*, the American journal for holistic living, has features on astrology, Tibet's ancient healing tradition, and natural beauty, together with routine articles on health, nutrition, mind/body, spirit, and transformative arts.

From all this, there seems to be an almost limitless scope to the New Age. Its activities concern, on the one hand, the most inner and private realms of an individual's psyche and, on the other hand, the most public realms of society. Some might say that environmental issues are important; others, that they are not. The same goes for aspects of traditional religions and of communities, the design of the home, and so on. Searching for one formal and accurate definition of what the New Age might represent is therefore not a very productive exercise. Other avenues need to be explored to enable us to reach a satisfactory characterization of its scope.

Is it new?

Extending what has already been said above, there is no doubt that a new wave of change felt by some has been unfolding since the 1960s, although whether it is new or not remains debatable; and perhaps the momentum of this change can be traced more to the development of mass communication systems – starting with the proliferation or broadcasting of information through books, magazines, and tape cassettes, and continuing through the more individual and narrowcast access via the Internet – which has enabled many more people to find out and get involved. Prior to the 1960s, as will be shown in more detail in the following chapter, a great many – if not most – of New Age ideas already existed or were being developed. For example, many forms of what is now called complementary medicine existed before – and were displaced by – the advent of allopathic medicine, not least of which might be acupuncture from ancient China and the use of herbs and essences which were documented in ancient Egypt. Rather than regarding it as something new, it is more profitable to perceive the New Age as a reaction to what those involved now see as a reductionistic and mechanistic society, a reaction which appears to be overturning many of the established 'tables' – for example, as more and more complementary and alternative therapies are proved to be efficacious they are being brought back into the medical mainstream. Many other examples can be given where such a reversal is taking place: the use of money, what we eat, how we educate our children and, not least, in the realms of spirituality.

The New Age is not millennialistic: its ideas go back through history and are expected to travel well into the future. The change, for most participants, from the second to the third millennium is anticipated to be a gentle occurrence. One commentator from academe, however, believes that the New Age as a whole 'is at least nominally concerned with the "pursuit of the millennium"'[14] although there is little real evidence to support this claim. A historian of religion, for example, comments, 'I don't think this talk of the new millennium automatically bringing a new consciousness of reality is particularly sensible. I don't buy it. I think it is misleading.'[15] Certainly, a few New Age writers and participants have seen a variety of apocalyptic visions, although these are not millennialistic. The New Age, as most writers describe it, is not about the end of the world: it concerns building a better, 'new', and transformed world.

Nor, as I will show, are many of those involved greatly interested in astrology. By this I do not mean reading horoscopes – most people do this at some point in their lives – but more serious involvement, for example through analysis of birth charts. The astrological change from a Piscean to an Aquarian Age will not, most astrologers agree, occur overnight. The change from one astrological age to another happens

14   Wouter Hanegraaff, 1996: 98.
15   Georg Feuerstein, 1997: n.p.

over three to five hundred years, they say. Hence, in astrological terms, the Age of Aquarius is only now starting to become influential, and in the course of time its characteristics are expected by some to make an increasingly stronger impact. This is not to say that there will not be significant dates for New Age astrologers – for example, the harmonic convergence of planets in 1987 – but the overriding astrological notion regarding the change is thought to be one of slow transition.

One American academic finds that the New Age is part of a new coalescence of both the traditional and the modern: what he calls the 'transmodern'. From his research, he concludes that 'we are seeing the emergence of a new cultural form, Integral Culture – a new constructive synthesis of Modernism and its antithesis, Traditionalism – a synthesis which moves beyond both while not rejecting either.'[16] He finds, in his *American Lives* survey, that while the idea of a new Integral Culture was identified fifty years ago by a Russian-American sociologist,[17] it has only substantially arisen since the 1970s, yet its roots, as I will show in more detail in the following chapter, go back further. According to this view, transmodernism's contemporary roots are

> found worldwide in the writings of various intellectuals of the mid-twentieth century, in the New Age movement, in the humanistic psychology and transpersonal psychology movements, in the ecology movement, and in the women's movement, which all date from the 1960s on. All find major elements of the Modern worldview unacceptable, with a growing loss of faith in it. This worldview is the 'leading edge and subject to change', and incorporates the personal into the social and political: they [transmodernists] reinvent themselves, so why could society not be reinvented too?[18]

There is much to be said in support of these findings that a new synthesis seems to be evolving, although, in the description given, the New Age is separated from elements such as humanistic and transper-

16   Paul Ray, 1996: n.p.
17   See Pitirim Sorokin, 1941.
18   Paul Ray, 1996: n. p.

sonal psychologies and ecology, which many writers, including myself, see as part and parcel of the same wave of change.

The many hundreds who participated in my survey believed overwhelmingly that there has been a general rise in New Age ideas and activities; and, over two-thirds of respondents believed that Western society is entering a new era. Furthermore, and supporting the *American Lives* findings, my survey shows that the New Age is not seen as something entirely new. In fact, very few of those involved see the New Age in this way. On the one hand, those few who did see it as entirely new comprised primarily older people, while, on the other hand, almost one-fifth viewed the New Age as predominantly a resurgence of ancient influences: a view, it can be added, that is held least by younger participants. Yet the majority of participants – almost 80% – (again as in the American survey) see the New Age to be a synthesis of both ancient influences and the new.

Where is it?

Simply put, there does not seem to be a geographic area which is completely untouched by the influence of New Age ideas. It may well be strongest in the English-speaking world – and strongest of all in California – as many of its most important teachers (I use this word in its broadest sense) are English-speaking and hold workshops in the US, Canada, the UK, Australia, and New Zealand. However, New Age ideas and activities seem to occur in most democratic states – in South America, Africa, the Far East, Continental Europe, and many other countries, and are probably least represented in Muslim and Communist countries.[19]

---

19 Colleagues in Brazil and Poland have undertaken studies into the growing effect of the New Age in their countries; see James Lewis and Gordon Melton, 1992 for its impact in Nigeria, Japan, and Italy; and Chrissie Steyn, 1995 for a South African study.

With the same teachers travelling the world, together with the flow of books (many of which are translated into different languages), cassettes, and videos, there exists a global element in the New Age message. Of course, cultural differences exist but these do not seem to affect the central ideas and activities. Moreover, in comparing the findings of my survey with other surveys carried out in the US, again no real difference seems to exist, which means that the evidence I have gathered is likely to be widely applicable. This globalization is wholly in tune with one of the principal core ideas of the New Age, as I will discuss below.

Is the New Age a movement?

The term 'movement' can be used either as a means of identifying particular groups and institutions (usually spelt with a capital M) or in the sense of a more general progression towards some end purpose. Movements in the former sense have been described anthropologically as having a decentralized, segmented, and reticulated structure, and examples can be seen in the International Humanist and Ethical Union or the Human Potential Movement. Accordingly, such movements, are 'neither an amorphous collectivity nor a highly centralized autocracy'.[20] One sociologist with a particular interest in the New Age believes that this description represents 'perhaps the most accurate sociological construct applicable to the New Age, Neo-pagan and similar non-institutional, boundary-indeterminate movements'.[21] However, while the New Age may be seen to contain some aspects of the three characteristics described, use of the term 'movement' in this case can be misleading because a Movement (institution) normally requires at least some form of overarching structure together with some special objective or function and 'authority', none of which the

20   Luther Gerlach and Virginia Hine, 1979: 78.
21   Michael York, 1995: 326.

24

New Age has to any marked degree. This is not to say that there is no unity in the New Age; there is, but it is not particularly structured.

The New Age need not be seen as an institution but as a dynamic flow into a new age described, for example, in Marilyn Ferguson's influential book *The Aquarian Conspiracy*,[22] in terms of a paradigm shift. This shift is claimed to be towards a new period of time, a new epoch – astrologers might say even a new aeon – wherein, over the course of time, many, if not all, aspects of the 'old' life will be transformed. Examples of these changes are outlined by Ferguson and include areas which would have an increased importance in such a transformed society, such as conservation, cooperation, intuition, and holism.[23] As can be imagined, the concept of a new age in these terms appears to be substantially more pervasive and complex than might be suggested by the concept of it being a single structured Movement. Furthermore, study shows that within the New Age separate streams of ideas and activities exist, some of which have more clearly defined structures, as might be seen in areas of ecology and psychotherapy, for example. One Christian critic recognizes this diversity, as he has subtitled his study *The Cosmic Self* 'a penetrating look at today's New Age Movements',[24] thereby recognising the plurality of the New Age.

The New Age, then, cannot be accurately described as a single structured Movement. It might be more apt to describe it as a network – or, indeed, a network of networks – comprising individuals each following one or several ideas and activities and sharing certain core values. In this context, the New Age has been described as 'a not-mainstream, local phenomenon, manifesting relatively holistic cosmological ideas and relatively individualistic social practice'.[25]

The fact that the New Age contains few organizational structures – a feature which corresponds with remarkable accuracy to the basic principles of anarchistic thought[26] – reflects the New Age view that

22 Marilyn Ferguson, 1982: 26f.
23 Op. cit.: 360ff.
24 Ted Peters, 1991.
25 Ruth Prince and David Riches, 2000: 18.
26 Clifford Harper, in describing the basis of anarchism, argues that 'human beings are at their very best when they are living free of authority, deciding things among themselves rather than being ordered about' (1987: vii); and John Clark

most structures actually suppress the notion of individuality and self-responsibility. Echoing this view, one academic commentator maintains that 'New Agers feel that they – and they alone – are responsible for their lives.'[27] This concept of network negates, or substantially reduces, the role external authority might play in participants' lives and, in turn, has helped give rise to the view that the New Age is amorphous.

It is my experience that those involved in the New Age do not see that they are participating in a Movement, although they might accept the term 'movement' as that of a flow or pathway of ideas and activities; many think of it in terms of a network. Moreover, participants generally do not use the term 'New Age'. One of the reasons for this has been that the media use the term freely – often to denigrate – particularly in connection with travellers and the like (who do not necessarily follow the ideas and activities of the New Age). Among those involved in the New Age, terms such as 'new consciousness' are sometimes used in its place.

What is more, the sheer number of people who are involved in some degree with the diversity of New Age ideas and activities seems to preclude use of the term 'movement' in any substantive way, except in the broadest of terms – as 'flow' or 'pathway' mentioned above. No agreed estimate of how many people are involved has been established. One guesstimate,[28] influenced by a 1993 telephone survey into 'self-described religious adherences' in America, suggests no more than ten million people, although this figure excluded important areas of New Age interest such as ecology and complementary health. An-

defines four characteristics which the 'true' anarchist needs to have, which include: '(1) a view of an ideal, non-coercive, non-authoritarian society; (2) a criticism of existing society and its institutions, based on this anti-authoritarian ideal; (3) a view of human nature that justifies the hope for significant progress toward the ideal; and (4) a strategy for change, involving immediate institution of non-coercive, non-authoritarian, and decentralist alternatives' (1986: 126f).

27   Paul Heelas, 1996a: 25.
28   Op. cit.: 107ff.

other,[29] perhaps more comprehensive, finds that over ten per cent of American adults, or twenty million people, have values and life patterns that are broadly consistent with the wide span of New Age ideas and activities described here. Worldwide, the New Age is becoming a very substantial voice indeed, although whether this voice can be described as a movement remains doubtful.

On this point, it is revealing to look at which words some of the principal academic commentators use to describe the New Age. Paul Heelas describes it as the 'New Age Movement' (this is the title of his book on the subject), as do James Lewis and Gordon Melton (who see the New Age as 'a synthesis of many different preexisting movements and strands of thought') and Michael York; Wouter Hanegraaff uses the word 'movement' sparingly; and another sociologist, Steve Bruce, appears not to use the word 'movement' at all: instead he talks of 'New Age religion', 'New Age thought', 'the New Age cultic milieu', or simply 'the New Age', and observes that 'many of its key ideas are widely diffused throughout the culture.'[30] There is little continuity. In the present study, I tend not to use the word 'movement' because it implies at least some form of structure. There is none, and describing the New Age as such can be misleading.

What is its cause?

I want to look at finding an answer to this question not from commentators outside the New Age but from the views of those actually participating in its ideas and activities. A more complete look into social and cultural views is given in later chapters.

---

29 Paul Ray, 1996. Ray called these people 'core cultural creatives'. Yet another sociologist, Robert Wuthnow, reports that 15% of Americans hold some New Age beliefs, while a further 12% want to know more (1998: 123).
30 Paul Heelas, 1996a; Michael York, 1995; James Lewis and Gordon Melton, 1992: xi; Wouter Hanegraaff, 1996; Steve Bruce, 1996: 197.

From questions asked in my survey, two distinct yet related views on what has caused the current New Age were given by almost two-thirds of those involved. These are that the New Age has been brought about either by the momentum created by an overall dissatisfaction with, or despair of, existing materialist society (38%), or by the influx to the planet of positive external influences – described principally as increasing vibrations or energy and external forces at work (21%). These views are not separate but interrelated, the latter sometimes being thought to result from the occurrence of the former.

The first view was expressed in three ways. Some mentioned a general dissatisfaction. A middle-aged nurse and masseur, for example, described the cause as 'dissatisfaction with traditional answers whether from church, law, or medicine. A belief that there is more', and a charity executive of similar age wrote of the 'realization that humanity has been duped by the churches, governments, and social conditioning. Realization that we are on course for self-destruction.' Others used stronger language. A masseur and aromatherapist saw that it was 'the rape of the Planet. If it is to survive at all the so-called "New Age" ideas of ecology etc. are essential to redress the balance,' and a ninety-three-year-old woman believed the New Age was 'inevitable. Two world wars in one generation; enemies praying to the same God for victory; widespread disbelief; hopelessness; above all, increasing belief in man's cleverness in re-making the world to fit into his new scientific knowledge which will destroy all if continued. It may be too late now.' Others expressed a reaction against materialism and the Church. Here, a male management consultant wrote of 'repressed spirituality from Thatcher-type capitalism and increasingly meaningless Western Christian religions', and another man, this time a public relations consultant to the computer industry, saw that 'people are bored with consumerism and "The Church". They appear to be returning to spiritual and cultural roots and are more open to esoteric ideas.'

The second view, relating to the influx of positive external forces, was also given primarily in three forms. First was the view that current growth in New Age activity was being caused by increasing

Cosmic[31] vibrations, and here a younger[32] natural beauty therapist gave the cause as being 'probably through channelling, which is bringing the wisdom, though backed by inadequacy of existing religions', and a middle-aged osteopath believed that there has been 'a speeding up of the cosmic vibrations because the darkness in man has allowed the vibration to slow down too much'. The idea that more particular external forces were at work was also given. For instance, a middle-aged mother wrote about 'the incarnation of more spiritually advanced beings here to guide mankind and give new direction to those trapped in materialism', and a younger businesswoman pointed to 'the reincarnation of souls – Higher Souls – to the Planet to "rescue" mankind from its self-destructiveness'. The final view, although numerically small, was that astrological influences were causing change and, in this regard, a typical view was given by a male student who saw 'an alignment of the planets that will bring about a new cycle – a raising of the level of human consciousness to a higher plane of love and creativity'.

The idea that an influx of positive external forces is creating the change begs the question: why now? As can be seen in many of these examples, people in the New Age appear to believe, in the same way as those who are dissatisfied with materialistic society, that society has gone astray. Benevolent Cosmic forces, they say, are having to intervene now to put the situation back on to what is seen as a more even – or harmonious – footing.

Apart from these two related ideas given by the majority of participants, two further ideas that were given about the cause of the New Age are worthy of note. The first broadly concerns education and was given by six per cent of those involved; they wrote of increasing opportunities for education facilitated by more publicity, better communications, travel, and the wider availability of books which, in turn, they believed enabled more people to have greater insight with regard

---

31 'Cosmic' is spelt with a capital 'C' because in the New Age it can refer to the Cosmic Christ.

32 The ages of survey participants were given in ten-year bands, for example, 25–34 years old, and these have been subsequently grouped into 'younger' (under 35 years old), 'middle-aged' (35–54 years old), and 'older' (over 55 years old).

to personal and social change. The second idea, given by five per cent, was described as contagion in terms of the infectious spread of New Age ideas through, for example, the pyramid effect, the 'hundredth monkey' principle, the domino effect, and synchronicity. In this regard, a middle-aged trainer described what is happening as 'a seeding of ideas that is spreading outwards like the drop of a pebble into a pool'.

Overall, from within the diversity of views given, what can be learnt from participants is that there exists significant agreement on the cause of the New Age at this time. For these people, the New Age represents a substantial change to a more spiritually imbued and more meaningful quality of life, one where the best of both older and newer ideas for personal fulfilment and peaceful social coexistence are actively sought and practised. Moreover, participants tend to have optimistic and positive attitudes to the problems of change. It would appear that their underlying theme is that society has become 'dis-eased' and requires the healing attributes of what is contained within the New Age to assist in enacting radical curative change.

Central ideas of the New Age

There have been many attempts to define the central ideas or beliefs incorporated in the New Age. For example, from the outside and from American commentators comes a ten-part definition, while another gives twelve 'enduring and constructive themes'. Two British anthropologists have given five criteria. From within the New Age, David Spangler identifies four 'criteria for recognising the new age spirit at work' as he has encountered it.[33] As in the assessment of the scope of

33 Lowell Streiker, 1991: 51ff; Glenn A. Olds, 1993: 69ff; Ruth Prince and David Riches, 2000: 55f; David Spangler, 1984: 82ff. A number of other authors from various countries have also compiled such statements including, from the US, Gordon Melton *et al.* 1990: xvff; from the UK, Stuart Wilson, 1989: 17ff, who gives twenty-one definitions of the New Age; and, from Japan, Shimazono Su-

the New Age surveyed above, in each case the definitions given appear closely related although each contains varying degrees of difference. However, one of the most comprehensive and succinct statements summarizing the central concepts incorporated in the New Age is given by William Bloom,[34] co-founder of Alternatives in Piccadilly, London, one of the leading New Age centres in England. The reason why I suggest Bloom's statement is the most comprehensive is that, although compiled by Bloom, it was subsequently circulated for comments and criticism and, therefore, is the result of the considered opinion by many who are active in the New Age. By and large, it has to be said that not all participants or commentators might agree with Bloom or, at least, would accept that all of Bloom's concepts are necessarily involved in the New Age.

Bloom puts forward what I have reduced to six ideas which he sees are 'not meant to be a box of beliefs – [to] get in and stay in. They are meant as an open-ended scaffolding on to which we can hang our experiences, wisdom and intuition.' Bloom is not suggesting that there is any set structure to the ideas involved; collectively, he says, these ideas do not comprise a belief system. In its place, he uses the analogy of a scaffolding onto which each participant can add whatever ideas she or he may wish, and in any direction. There is no specific structure to anchor the scaffolding or to determine its shape. Each of these ideas is now studied as an introduction to what amounts to a composite of the main convictions held by many – if not most – New Age individuals.

First, Bloom asserts that 'All life – all existence – is the manifestation of Spirit.' In this instance, Bloom suggests that all life forms – for example, from plants to people – are part of God (or whatever name is applied to what is claimed to be the Supreme Consciousness or Absolute Being). On this point, there seems to be a divergence of views regarding the interpretation of the term 'spirit' in the New Age. On the one hand, Bloom gives a supra-mundane interpretation and

sumu presents five characteristics of new spirituality movements which can be seen to have many similarities to the New Age, (cited in Haga and Kisala, 1995: 239).

34   The following citations are all from William Bloom, 1990: 12ff.

31

suggests that the same spirit is also found in all religions, whereas, on the other hand, at least one commentator interprets the notion of spirit to denote a humanistic state of ultimate human consciousness, summed up as 'a highly optimistic, celebratory, utopian and spiritual form of humanism'.[35] As will be shown below, Bloom's ideas appear to incorporate the notion of a transcendence of the humanistic state – which he describes as being confined to 'the chemistry of the brain'[36] – which, in my experience, is also the view of the majority of participants. As can be imagined, the difference between these two views is substantial.

Bloom's second idea is that 'All life, in all its different forms and states, is interconnected energy,' which entails the assumption that there is no division or separation between, for example, people and God. This idea runs counter to mainstream Christian, Judaic, and Islamic doctrines, which are dualistic in nature, but not to some Eastern religious traditions, which, on the whole, are monistic.

Two further points can be seen to emerge from the idea of interconnectedness. First, on a spiritual plane, through the idea that there is no separation between God and people, Bloom does not necessarily claim that people themselves can become God – a state which has been asserted by some New Age teachers[37] and by humanists.[38] However, what Bloom does imply is that individuals can have a direct experience of God.

Second, on a more mundane level, the concept of interconnectedness suggests that all life forms are intimately connected. As a consequence, there exist ideas of codependency,[39] coresponsibility, and cooperation between New Age individuals (as well as all individuals

---

35   Paul Heelas, 1996a: 28.
36   John Button and William Bloom, 1992: 44.
37   Cited in Paul Heelas, 1996a: 5. The actress and New Age personality Shirley MacLaine seems to have amended this assertion. In a later work than that cited by Paul Heelas she appears to agree with William Bloom when she argues that 'The most controversial concept of the New Age philosophy [is] the belief that God lies within, and therefore we are each part of God. Since there is no separateness, we are each Godlike, and God is in each of us' (1991: 100).
38   Joel Kovel, 1978: 154.
39   In the term's literal sense, not specifically psychotherapeutic.

and other life forms), for whom the concept of interconnectedness appears to form an essential unifying basis and *raison d'être* in their lives.

In his third idea, Bloom suggests there are two levels of consciousness that each individual possesses. On the one hand, Bloom describes 'an outer temporary personality [which] is limited and tends towards materialism'. This outer personality, according to Bloom, is driven by the ego, can often be self-centred, and may not be of the level of interconnected consciousness. On the other hand, he suggests that people have a 'multi-dimensional inner being (soul or higher self) [which] is infinite and tends towards love'. This Higher Self, it is argued, is accessible to all, although not without effort. Moreover, the effort required is reported to often result in a transformation of an individual's life away from egocentric ways of being, towards ways of being which are driven more by unconditional love and compassion. This transformation is reported to affect both the Higher Self and the way in which the transformed individual approaches the growth, health, and well-being of her or his community.

Fourthly, Bloom argues that 'All souls in incarnation are free to choose their own spiritual path.' Two important points arise from this idea. First, according to Bloom's description, the Higher Self is a spiritual incarnation; and his (repeated) use of this word suggests that a central feature of the New Age is the concept of reincarnation.[40] In this view, the higher element within each person may have had many previous incarnations and could well incarnate again at future times. Bloom describes the outer personality as being 'temporary', which implies that he believes in the possibility of a more permanent reality.

---

40   While there are various ideas about reincarnation in the New Age, two are more prevalent. In the first of these, reincarnation follows the traditional Eastern religious view that we continually incarnate in this world in order to develop and improve our spiritual lives and, at some future point, perhaps become enlightened and halt the process. The second idea is that we are spirit beings who have incarnated at this point in space and time for a specific purpose. We have chosen this particular 'stage' to play out whatever purpose we, as spirit beings, have chosen, which entails choosing our parents and our life events prior to incarnation. From this view, we have the choice of where (in the Cosmos), when, and how frequently this might take place.

Moreover, a large number of individuals active in the New Age report paranormal experiences, and many of these are claimed to entail contact from spiritual beings – that is, channelled contact – and recollections from past lives. Here, again, there is a divergence of views because at least one commentator's ideas about the New Age do not incorporate such features.[41] Conversely, others suggest that belief in reincarnation is one of the ideas that help to identify participants in the New Age, another contending that such belief is prevalent in both the New Age and the Neo Pagan movement.[42]

The second important point arising from Bloom's fourth idea is that each person is wholly free to choose her or his own spiritual path. Bloom's idea suggests that there is no one 'right' spiritual path in the New Age, and that all such paths are seen to be equally good. Indeed, Bloom suggests that 'All religions are the expression of [the] same inner reality.' This idea is further illustrated by the American Louise Hay, perhaps the widest-known name in complementary health, who, for example, suggests that

> It is vital that we release foolish, outmoded ideas that do not support us and nourish us. I feel strongly that even our concept of God needs to be one that is for us, not against us. There are so many different religions to choose from. If you have one now that tells you you are a sinner and a lowly worm, get another one.[43]

From Bloom's idea it would appear that there is no requirement for spiritual exclusivity in the New Age, as an eclectic mix of beliefs

---

41 Paul Heelas, for example, does not directly refer to the subject of reincarnation in relation to the New Age as he believes that interests such as 'astrology, reincarnation, past lives, the Holy Grail, the Cathars, the pyramids, Atlantis, corn circles, UFOs, and so on [...] might not be New Age per se' (1996a: 166); and with regard to past-life regression, Melvin Harris suggests that this is not evidence for reincarnation but for cryptomnesia, the unconscious memory of normally learnt information (1988: 133).

42 James Lewis, 1992: 2; Gordon Melton et al., 1990: xvi; Michael York, 1995: 148.

43 Louise Hay, 1988: 136. Hay's teacher was the Christian writer Norman Vincent Peale whose book *The Power of Positive Thinking* published in 1953, has sold 15 million copies and has obviously been widely influential.

or religious traditions could be followed simultaneously if an individual so desired.

The final two ideas that Bloom describes suggest that, first, there are enlightened teachers in our midst and, second, there seems to be a larger influx in the number of such teachers at this time than existed previously. The result of this is that, according to Bloom, 'we are undergoing a fundamental spiritual change in our individual and mass consciousness. This is why we talk of a New Age.'

With regard to the first point, Bloom describes the source of the increased number of teachers as 'souls who are liberated from the need to incarnate'. This seems to be a clear reference to the concept of Karma – that is, the law of cause and effect – which is fundamental to Hindu and Buddhist religions and is implicitly linked with the notion of reincarnation. It would appear from Bloom's descriptions that New Age belief on this point is similar to, but not exactly the same as, Eastern religious traditions. This difference can be seen in that, within many of the Eastern traditions, there exist prescribed moral and ethical codes of conduct governing what an individual might need to achieve within one lifetime in order to be reborn into a higher state or to break free of the cycle of *Samsara* (continual return to earthly life) altogether. However, no such prescribed code appears to be standard to the New Age.

Furthermore, Bloom himself reports that he has acted as a channel[44] for teachings given by discarnate spirit beings.[45] Likewise, many New Age individuals claim to be able to gain access to – or guidance through – channelled sources, although whether this contact is with the spiritual realm or the Higher Self, if either exists, has not been determined. A New Age encyclopedia suggests that 'One positive outgrowth of the channeling phenomenon is the encouragement for individuals to develop their own connections to a source of higher wisdom, especially through intuition. In that regard channeling moves

---

44   Channelled sources are described as including 'nonphysical beings, angels, nature spirits, totem or guardian spirits, deities, demons, extraterrestrials, spirits of the dead, and the Higher Self' (Rosemary Ellen Guiley, 1991: 88).
45   William Bloom, 1995a.

from the theatrical arena of an anointed few to the everyday routine of all people.'[46]

Bloom's last point, that a fundamental spiritual change is occurring, can be viewed in a number of ways. Many individuals involved in the New Age are likely to agree that this change affects both their Higher Selves and what Bloom calls their 'outer personality'. It most visibly involves a shift away from an egocentric and materialistic outlook on life towards one that is more compassionate, cooperative, and holistic. Additionally, the change Bloom identifies is seen as being evolutionary and, as such, he believes it will not be brought about by any sudden shift or revolution. In fact, in the same way as astrologers, Bloom and other commentators suggest the change will take many hundreds of years to take place fully.[47]

Bloom's scaffolding of ideas can be viewed in a number of different ways. For example, it can be seen to form the basis of a non-dualistic and deeply spiritual set of life-defining ideas or, alternatively, it can be seen as the foundation of a paranormal view. There can be many interpretations. New Age ideas, according to one critic, 'are not limited or censored by having to accord with any master principles which shape a coherent identity', leading him to the view that 'the New Age is the embodiment of individualism'.[48] However, this view is contrary to the second of Bloom's ideas, that of interconnectedness, and provides us with a clear example of how many commentators from outside of the New Age, particularly from academe, interpret its ideas from a different perspective – as Bloom indicates, by attempting to turn the scaffolding into an anchored structure. It does not work. Hence any conclusion drawn from this type of view can be inaccurate.

On a different point, it is important to note that none of the ideas that Bloom suggests is completely new. The influences on the New Age are many: from traditional religions (both Western and Eastern), from eighteenth- and nineteenth-century Romanticism in terms of such notions as organic unfolding progress, intuitive reasoning, and

46   Rosemary Ellen Guiley, 1991: 91.
47   Such as Ken Wilber, 1987: 12.
48   Steve Bruce, 1996: 215, 225.

transcendent spirituality – William Blake has been an inspirational figure to many participants – from the surge of interest in parapsychology in the twentieth century, and from many other sources. What is new is the way in which these ideas have come together at this time to form a radical alternative to – or synthesis of, as has been suggested above – to both the traditional and the modern, and this can be described as a re-assertion of the more positive elements (connectedness, love, unity in diversity, nature, etc.) while despatching the more negative aspects (greed, consumerism, separateness, unchecked science, etc.) to history. These topics will be met throughout the course of this book.

Participants in the New Age seek a stronger spiritual basis to their lives as a reaction to what they see as a technocratic, dehumanized, and meaningless existence which has been the result of social and cultural change started by the Industrial Revolution and which is still continuing to evolve. The New Age is also a stand against the blandness seen in mass participation in what is interpreted as an unnatural global culture, along the lines of 'unity in diversity' rather than the sameness and compliance which globalization necessitates. Viewed in this way, the New Age must be seen, at least in part, as a protest movement, albeit mostly a peaceful and harmonious one, and as a movement for a shared individualism. While the notion of a shared individualism might seem contradictory, it succinctly characterises how participants themselves view what has been happening: they are intensely concerned about their individual life paths on all their different levels, while also being deeply concerned about their fellow beings – all beings, that is, not just human – and the planet and universe itself.

Main qualities

This final introductory section looks specifically at what New Age participants themselves see as the principal qualities of their ideas and activities, adding vital ethnographic evidence to what has been said by key New Age individuals and by commentators.

In my survey, participants were asked to rate how important six qualities were to the New Age. These qualities and the degree of their centrality were: spiritual affairs (92%), personal transformation (91%), healing (90%), holism (88%), ecology (81%), and feeling good (73%). My findings show that all of the qualities given were thought by at least around three-quarters of those involved to be always or often involved in their practices. Furthermore, in no instance was there a statistically meaningful number of people who claimed that any of these characteristics were never involved in the New Age. This result demonstrates that those involved seem fairly certain about what some of the main New Age qualities are: that it is a highly spiritual and transformatory way of being which incorporates not only personal concerns but also concerns for the world around them.

Turning to a more in-depth look at these qualities, the survey also asked those involved to describe in a few words what they thought the New Age was all about, and well over 800 answers, many at length, were given. Overall, and consistently with what has been indicated above, particularly with regard to structure, the findings show that the New Age is not viewed as a single idea but that it is made up of a combination of ideas. To some this illustrates its interconnected character, although to others this finding might fuel the argument that the New Age is amorphous.

In searching for which key words were used most of all in the descriptions, three sets – often used in combination – are of note, and here it can be seen that there is a strong correlation between participants' views on what is causing the New Age and its main qualities. The three sets are 'personal transformation', 'greater spirituality', and 'less materialistic'. With regard to 'personal transformation', the words used by participants included: an 'awakening' (or 're-awakening') of consciousness, 'heightened awareness', 'more enlightened', 'raised consciousness', 'new recognition', and 'opening'; whereas 'greater spirituality' produced no such variation, except that participants often referred to both an individual and planetary increase in spirituality. Thirdly, 'less materialistic', apart from relating to a reduced reliance on the material world, also incorporated the notions of a failure of Western culture and religion, and the ending of worn-out industrialized society. Other key descriptive words which were used, albeit to a lesser extent, included: 'ancient wisdoms', 'better environment', 'connectedness', 'harmony', 'Divine Energy', 'healing', and 'holistic'.

Drawing a generalised conclusion from these findings, it appears that those involved see the New Age in terms of a substantial change within themselves, the qualities of which are a heightening of their spirituality, the acknowledgement of a Divine Energy, and the expression of love. It involves a rediscovery of old ways that, they believe, have been devalued in the last few centuries, a reduction in materialistic values and consumption and a concomitant rise in those values concerned with connectedness, harmony, and holism, all this together with concern for the environment. It is significant that these sentiments are remarkably similar to those incorporated in the basic New Age ideas expressed by William Bloom in the previous section. No sentiments were expressed which go beyond Bloom's description – thus suggesting the possibility of a high degree of unanimity among participants, however diverse their interests. There is also little evidence to show that improvements in personal prosperity came to individuals' minds in their descriptions of what they believed the New Age provides.[49]

A deeper analysis of participants' views reveals five principal themes of how they saw that the New Age could be described. The first reflected the idea that the New Age represented 'greater awareness', and was frequently expressed in terms of an expansion or transformation of consciousness, both personal and planetary. Greater awareness, typically, was described by a middle-aged charity worker as being a 'movement towards greater self-awareness and awareness of one's impact on society. An awareness of the Planet and human beings', and other creatures', future upon it. A movement working for

---

49   This is particularly contrary to Paul Heelas's thesis, in which he seems to ignore what he calls the 'counter-cultural wing of the New Age' – which, as I will show, is the more substantial part – while concentrating on what is personal growth, which is more to do with the Human Potential Movement (Paul Heelas, 1999: 55).

positive change.' A second theme related particularly to the idea that the New Age signified a 'growth in spirituality' and was typically seen, as a younger lecturer put it, as the 'beginning of a more spiritual era in human development, emphasizing the need to express spirit creatively and to act intuitively in order to go forward'. Thirdly, participants described the New Age as 'recurrence and renewal'. Thus, a middle-aged therapist talked of the 'rediscovery of old, ancient values but with [a] modern psychological framework, and individual-centred rather than tribe-centred', and a middle-aged marketing consultant succinctly wrote 'rebirth, real-ization, readjustment, relief'. The fourth theme was related to the third, although, in this instance, participants wrote more specifically about a 'reaction against materialism'. Here, one individual, a middle-aged accountant, wrote about 'a desire to reject the orthodoxy of modern life and economic political systems prevailing, believing that such systems cannot/will not be changed due to vested/self interests of those in authority and the apathy of the majority of society'. The final theme suggested that the New Age was very much to do with a more 'holistic outlook' on life combined with the possibility of a more peaceful coexistence for humanity, and, representative of this view, an older (over 75 years of age) retired secretary saw the New Age as 'a new way of BEING. It is based on [...] learning to live side by side with everybody. Sharing and caring. What a wonderful world it will be.'

The overriding sentiment revealed in this assessment of New Age qualities is noticeably not a negative one: rather, it is one which is extremely positive and full of optimism. The main qualities of the New Age are thought by those involved to be achievable, not as some eschatological reward but right here and now through the most important quality: that of spiritual transformation.

Summary

This chapter set out to describe what is encompassed by the New Age and to address the issue of whether it might be correctly described as amorphous or to see if there exists some form of structure or definition at its basis. What we have seen is that there are distinctive features in its range of ideas, that there is no structured Movement, and that there are some broadly agreed basic ideas. It may still be argued that the New Age appears amorphous. Yet, as one American academic points out, with deeper analysis 'the whole phenomenon becomes less amorphous' – although she adds 'this is not to say that it appears less eclectic.'[50]

In the minds of those involved, we have seen that the New Age represents a change to a new paradigm, one which emphasizes a reduction in external forms of authority and a rise in self-responsibility, thus, seemingly, reducing or even doing away with a reliance on hierarchical structures. The principal areas of interest show an emphasis on ideas and activities to do with spirituality and healing. Other areas of interest exist – particularly those concerned with community, the environment, and creative activities – although these do not appear to be as central as the former. And in William Bloom's six basic New Age ideas we can see what amounts to an established spiritual basis, a view that is echoed by participants. Underlying all of this is what can be described as a subtle undercurrent of love, manifesting in many different forms and suffusing all ideas and activities. Without this 'energy' – albeit subtle but not necessarily weak – what we have been discussing cannot be considered to be central to the New Age.

Having brought the New Age into focus in this chapter, it becomes clear, using Bloom's analogy, that no more than a scaffolding of ideas exists which participants adapt and extend – even partially discard – to create their own particular New Age worldview.

---

50   Mary Farrell Bednarowski, 1991: 215.

2. Recent History

Parallels certainly abound between our era and renaissances of the past: the computer and the printing press, LSD and caffeine, the holograph and perspective painting, the wheel and the spaceship, agriculture and the datasphere. But cyberians see this era as more than just a rebirth of classical ideas. They believe the age upon us now might take the form of categorical upscaling of the human experience onto uncharted, hyperdimensional turf.

Douglas Rushkoff[1]

A large number of influences have helped mould the features of the development and expansion of the New Age to where it stands at the beginning of the third millennium; and there is evidence to suggest that during specific periods certain characteristics have become more important than others, although this is not to say that the New Age has grown through clearly defined periods. In the 1960s, for example, counter-cultural activities were predominant; in the 1970s and 1980s, the Human Potential Movement and women's activities were key features; and, in the 1990s, the New Age became characterized by healing concerns and transpersonal spirituality. Commencing by charting important originating influences, this chapter identifies key historical features, concluding with a description of the New Age at the turn of the millennium.

---

1   Douglas Rushkoff, 1994: 18.

Pre-1960s

Concerning timing, a New Age chronology has been proposed[2] which starts with the founding of the Theosophical Society in New York in 1875, thereby suggesting that this was when the New Age began. On the other hand, another idea[3] suggests two roots to the New Age, one theosophical and the other based on the eighteenth-century ideas of Franz Mesmer and Emanuel Swedenborg. It is also clear that late-eighteenth-century Romanticism was, and perhaps still is, influential. According to historian Richard Tarnas, Romanticism was one of the two distinct streams of culture which stemmed from the Renaissance, the other, its opposite, being the Enlightenment. Tarnas traces the course of Romanticism to the present day,[4] and describes the difference between the streams in that

> Whereas the Enlightenment temperament's high valuation of man rested on his unequalled rational intellect and its power to comprehend and exploit the laws of nature, the Romantic valued man rather for his imaginative and spiritual aspirations, his emotional depths, his artistic creativity and powers of individual self-expression and self-creation [...] Whereas for the Enlightenment-scientific mind, nature was an object for observation and experiment, theoretical explanation and technological manipulation, for the Romantic, by contrast, nature was a live vessel of spirit, a translucent source of mystery and revelation [...] In the Enlightenment, scientific vision, modern civilization and its values stood unequivocally above all its predecessors, while [...] Romantics radically questioned the West's belief in its own 'progress,' in its civilization's innate superiority, in rational man's inevitable fulfilment [...] The spirit of the Enlightenment rebelled against the strictures of ignorance and superstition imposed by theological dogma and belief in the supernatural, in favour of straightforward empirical and rational knowledge and a liberating embrace of the secular [...] The Romantic's attitude toward religion was more complex [...] God was rediscovered in Romanticism − not the God of orthodoxy or deism but of mysticism, pantheism, and immanent cosmic process.[5]

---

2   Gordon Melton *et al.*, 1991. See also Gordon Melton, 1988.
3   Kay Alexander, 1992.
4   Richard Tarnas, 1996: 366ff.
5   Op. cit.: 367ff.

What is clear from Tarnas's description is that the dichotomy which existed in the eighteenth century still exists in a similar form between New Age ideas and late-twentieth-century capitalism, a subject which will be referred to again below and in later chapters.

Alternatively, a different view suggests that there is nothing new about the New Age, that its core concepts have existed throughout the last two to three thousand years, and that they are perennial. Here, the suggestion is that there is a form of modern Gnosticism which 'encompasses not only the different underground religious communities, but also key attitudes on the parts of certain intellectuals toward the nature of man, toward society and history';[6] included in this view is the work of Friedrich Nietzsche and Carl Jung. The argument given is based on the idea that, regardless of the historical period, certain cultural and social events cause Gnostic ideas to surface and that these ideas often are about a quest for the eternal. Indeed, it is suggested that 'the Gnostic attitude had its *raison d'être* in the experience of time's utter incoherence by those alienated from traditional modes of temporal symbolism',[7] and the comparison is made between the present New Age and other notable periods including that of the mystics of the Middle Ages and German Romanticism of the late eighteenth century. A Christian critic of the New Age also supports this view.[8]

Yet another commentator similarly suggests that the advent of the New Age is not new 'but a modern revival [...] of a longstanding tradition of what may be called the alternative spirituality of the West [...] going back at least to the Greco-Roman world'.[9] To further complicate attempts at pinpointing originating influences of the New Age, many of its widely used ideas and activities are patently not new but have been drawn from practically all historical periods.

What appears to be a clear feature, however, is that many of these influences were primarily spiritual in character. In fact, it is suggested that the New Age is much more a spiritual appearance – or re-appearance – than anything else; that is, for example, rather than aris-

6   Carl Raschke, 1980: xi.
7   Op. cit.: 20.
8   Ted Peters, 1991: 56.
9   Robert Ellwood, 1992: 59.

ing from appearances such as the rise in leisure and communications, the baby-boom generation, drug use, etc., which I describe below. With regard to its spiritual character, David Spangler notes that

> The idea of the new age as a spiritual phenomenon comes from mystical and psychic revelations and predictions of prophets such as Nostradamus and, more recently, the American psychic Edgar Cayce. It is also discussed and prophesied in the works of metaphysical and esoteric groups such as the Theosophical Society, and the Lucis Trust [...] the teachings of the Austrian mystic and scientist Rudolf Steiner [and] in the spiritual traditions of other cultures.[10]

Important twentieth-century influences on the spiritual content of the New Age must include, firstly, the decline in influence of traditional Western Christianity (more marked in Europe than North America,[11] and more Protestant than Catholic) and, secondly, the introduction to the West of alternative spiritual traditions. Of the two, the influx of Eastern spiritual traditions appears to have had a markedly greater impact than the decline of Christianity.[12]

The British sociologist Colin Campbell has also noted this Easternization of the West. Campbell suggests that

> It is in the heartland of 'the West' itself that 'Westernization' is facing its fiercest challenge, a challenge which is being mounted from a perspective which is, in essence, 'Eastern'. This is happening because the dominant paradigm or 'theodicy' which has served the West so effectively for 2,000 years has finally lost its grip over the majority of the population in Western Europe and North

---

10 David Spangler, 1984: 19.
11 It needs to be pointed out that the New Age has become much more established in the USA – especially in California – where Christianity remains strong, than in Northern Europe where Christianity has shown significant decline.
12 This decline does not presuppose that the propensity to be religious or spiritual has also declined. Thomas Luckmann (1967: passim), for example, suggests that religion became 'invisible', that an individual's religiosity had simply ceased to be a public phenomenon in terms of church attendance. Luckmann's argument is that there exists no hard evidence to substantiate claims that religiosity per se has declined – in fact, research shows that the extent of belief in God or the supernatural has remained high during the same period (see for example, a Gallup poll (1995: 25) in the UK, and as Frederick Levine reports in the US, (1989: 83)).

America. They no longer hold to a view of the world as divided into matter and spirit, and governed by an all-powerful, personal, creator God; one who has set his creatures above the rest of creation. This vision has been cast aside and with it all justification for mankind's domination over nature. In its place has been set the fundamentally Eastern vision of mankind as merely part of a great interconnected web of sentient life.[13]

Campbell identifies many aspects of the Easternization of the West, not simply Eastern spiritual ideas together with medical and cultural ideas, from yoghurt to acupuncture, but what he sees as a paradigm shift, the influence of Eastern ideas on Western thinkers, for example, the theologian Paul Tillich and the philosopher Herbert Marcuse. This difference in styles of thought has been highlighted in psychological research[14] which Campbell uses. These findings produced the following list of categories pertaining to East–West styles of thought:

East	West
synthesis	analysis
totality	generalization
integration	differentiation
deduction	induction
subjective	objective
dogmatic	intellectual
intuition	reason
anti-science	science
personal	impersonal
moralistic	legalistic
non-discursive	assertive
affiliative	power
ecstasis	order
irrational	rational
imaginative	critical[15]

From this list it is clear to see that much of New Age thought incorporates more of Eastern rather than Western influences.

13   Colin Campbell, 1999: 47.
14   David J. Krus and Harold S. Blackman, 1980: 947–55.
15   Op. cit.: 43.

Also of particular influence has been the rise of alternative spiritual movements which evolved during the earlier part of the twentieth century. These include both those that were emerging prior to the advent of the twentieth century and those new to the twentieth century. Of the former, for example, the Rosicrucian order was not officially constituted until 1915 although it had existed in various forms since the late fifteenth century, and Swedenborgism developed in the eighteenth century.

Regarding spiritual movements which were new to the West, one of the most influential has been the Theosophical Society, founded in 1875. It was through the Society's efforts that

> The great philosophies of the East were distilled and marketed en masse to Western civilization to a greater extent than had ever been possible at any previous time in history. The enormous Theosophical publishing machine thus set the stage for the familiar countercultural fascination with these topics, beginning in Ascona, Switzerland and Munich circa 1900, and continuing through the beatniks, hippies, Greens, and New Agers of more recent times.[16]

Other important individuals and movements which arose during this period include George Ivanovitch Gurdjieff, who started to teach before the first World War in Russia, continuing thereafter in France, and Paramahansa Yogananda who founded the Self-Realisation Fellowship in California in 1920. In England, the Buddhist Society was founded in 1929 by Christmas Humphries, and White Eagle Lodge in 1936 by Grace Cooke. In the East, Pak Subuh commenced teaching in Indonesia in the 1930s and Subud was brought to the West with the help of the Gurdjieffian J. G. Bennett in the 1950s; and in India, for example, Sri Sathya Sai Baba's ashram at Prashanthi Nilayam, founded in 1944, has attracted many Western followers.

Moreover, spiritual traditions from around the world have spread to the West, often imported or enlarged by immigrant populations. Additional to the teachings already mentioned are Baha'i, the different forms of Buddhism, Hinduism, Islam, Sikhism, Sufism, and Taoism.

Sympathetic writers, and thinkers too, flourished during this time. Those with an Eastern spiritual influence included Paul Brunton, W. Y. Evans-Wentz, Rene Guenon, Hermann Hesse, Aldous Huxley,

16   Richard Noll, 1994: 67f.

and Thomas Merton, and from the East itself the writings of D. T. Suzuki and Swami Vivekananda became widely read in the West; authors with a Western esoteric or psychic influence included Edgar Cayce and Dion Fortune; and there have been many other highly influential individuals following various interests and including Pierre Teilhard de Chardin, Kahil Gibran, Manly P. Hall, Carl Jung, and Rudolf Steiner. The list is very long indeed.

Coupled with the spiritual, the most notable social influences prior to the 1960s were two world wars and great material scarcity in Europe, contrasted with the following post-WW2 boom and material abundance, epitomized at the end of the 1950s by British Prime Minister Harold Macmillan as 'You've never had it so good'. In the arts and popular culture, Cubism and Dada came and went, the cinema arrived, as did dance music from Charleston to Swing to Jive. The advent of new technology which started with the phonograph and subsequent popularization of recorded music and then, significantly, by the introduction of radio and television, created a new form of 'authority' which, it has been said, spearheaded the invasion of family life by market forces[17] – an authority which continues to hold sway.

Clearly, the contemporary New Age did not start from scratch in the 1960s. What happened at this time was that many different forms of life, including alternative spiritualities, hitherto practised by only a small number of people very quickly became widely known through mass communications and the endorsement of celebrities. Given this credibility, many of these movements soon became accepted by some as having a validity equal – if not greater – than that of traditional Western ideas.

The Counter-Culture

The blossoming of the contemporary New Age occurred during the period of counter-culture; and this time must be considered as its most

17   Christopher Lasch, 1995: 96f.

important historical period, spanning from the late 1950s to early 1970s and bracketed, for example, by the ending of conscription in the UK in 1960 and its ending in the US in 1973. With conscription still in effect in America during the counter-culture, together with the involvement in the Vietnam War, a highly focused protest movement among American youth was created – indeed, much more so than in Britain. Against this background, a minority of mostly young people rebelled against modern society itself. In fact, according to historical accounts, 'the counter-culture was fundamentally anarchistic without being conscious of it.'[18] What this group rebelled against, cultural theorist Theodore Roszak[19] suggests, is what he has called 'the myth of objective consciousness'. Roszak's main thesis about the development of the counter-culture is that society was being led by impersonal technology in the form of a social dynamism which bred a self-perpetuating cycle, endlessly regenerating itself with the same impersonal nature. The counter-culture was, according to Roszak, seen as a bold attempt to break this cycle; the ideas of Herbert Marcuse and social theorist Norman Brown, by the way Allen Ginsberg and Alan Watts, were central in bringing into play mystical, occult, magical, and spiritual elements, together with Paul Goodman's ideas for an anarchic communitarian society. Roszak's principal observation on mainstream Western society is that it was misguidedly based on the myth of the benefits which a technocratic culture could bring. He argues that to counteract this there had to be an increased element of subjectivity – a 'personalist sense of community'[20] – and this is what, at heart, he believes the counter-culture offered.

In social and political terms, the period was filled with traumatic events. It included wars in Vietnam and the Middle East, civil unrest in Cyprus and Northern Ireland, and the near apocalypse brought about by the Cuban missile crisis. The Berlin Wall was built and the Cold War commenced. The USSR invaded Czechoslovakia. President Kennedy, his brother Robert, and Martin Luther King were assassinated. A new political force – the New Left – became established and

18   Peter Marshall, 1993: 544.
19   Theodore Roszak, 1970.
20   Op. cit.: 206.

student protest erupted in America, Spain, and France, culminating in four students being shot dead by the National Guard at Kent State University in the US in 1970. The first man rocketed into space, an achievement followed by space walks and, in 1969, the first manned landing on the moon. The first heart transplant took place in 1967. The Watergate Conspiracy was uncovered in 1972 with the subsequent impeachment of President Nixon; and in the following year Britain joined the European Community.

In terms of culture, the 1960s were filled with the explosion of 'new' forms of alternative (and in the main) youth culture – starting with the Beat Generation in the late 1950s and moving on to the Hippies and their peace-filled notion of 'flower power' in the 1960s. Musically, the period started with a mixture of dance crazes and protest songs and ended with Pink Floyd's seminal *Dark Side of the Moon* album (released in 1973) which, in the lyrics of the song entitled *Money*, foretold the oncoming of a second phase of the New Age which had a pronounced materialist content. In between these times many different music strands developed, epitomized by such recording artists as Bob Dylan, The Beatles, the Beach Boys, The Who, the Rolling Stones, together with Jimmy Hendrix and Janis Joplin (who both died in 1970) – many of whom 'publicly wrestled with the religious questions of where we came from, why we are here, and where we are going'.[21] There were festivals such as those at Woodstock in the US and on the Isle of Wight in the UK, and Yoko Ono and John Lennon had 'bed-ins' for peace. Many of the leading musicians – including David Bowie, John Lennon, and Pete Townsend – were products of art schools. In the arts itself, Minimalism was developed in classical music and notably expounded by Philip Glass and Steve Reich, while Pop Art, led by Andy Warhol and Richard Hamilton, and Op Art, came and went.

Even so, the characteristics of the counter-culture were not unique. Historical similarities have been noted with the Bohemians of Paris in the late nineteenth and early twentieth centuries who were characterized by 'odd dress, long hair, living for the moment, having no stable residence, sexual freedom, radical political enthusiasms,

21   Steve Turner, 1995: 117.

drink, drug taking, irregular work patterns, [and] addiction to night-life'.[22] It is suggested that 'more recent incarnations like the Beat Generation of the 1950s or the hippiedom of the 1960s'[23] reflect the earlier characteristics of the Bohemian lifestyle. And the use of drugs, especially psychedelics (both for pleasure and mind-expansion) is reported to have been widespread among those involved in the counter-culture.[24]

Spiritual enterprises of the counter-culture reflected its eclectic nature. For example, CND was launched in the UK in 1958, and the Maharishi Mahesh Yogi arrived in California the following year, as did the Unification Church. Esalen in California and Findhorn in Scotland were established in 1962. In 1965 ISKCON was founded in the US, and in 1967 The Beatles enjoyed a relationship with the Maharishi Mahesh Yogi and Transcendental Meditation. Samye Ling Tibetan Centre was set up in Scotland by Chogyam Trungpa in the same year, followed by Auroville in South India in 1968.[25] Greenpeace started informally in 1971.

Turning to assess where those involved in the counter-culture might have been found, it is fair to say that activity occurred mostly among the disaffected campus-based American middle-class youth; and primarily in California which has played 'a unique role in the gestation and nurture of what is unusual, and often downright weird, in American life. The variety of psychological flora and fauna here is amazing. Cults and sects grow like weeds. "Gurus" abound.'[26] Another commentator points out that 'the Aquarian Conspiracy, needless to say, is nurtured in California.'[27]

And it was out of California that editions of the *Whole Earth Catalog* originated, in one volume encapsulating the entire substance

22   Jerrold Seigel, 1986: 12.
23   Op. cit.: 5.
24   Marilyn Ferguson, 1982: 93f.
25   During the counter-culture many tens of thousands of young people, myself
      included, travelled overland on the 'Hippie Trail' from Europe to India and be-
      yond and received first-hand experience of different forms of spirituality.
26   Jacob Needleman, 1970: 36.
27   Marilyn Ferguson, 1982: 153.

of the counter-culture. The last catalogue, published in 1971, described its market in the following way:

> We are as gods and might as well get good at it. So far remotely done power and glory – as via government, big business, formal education, church – has succeeded to the point where the gross defects obscure actual gains. In response to this dilemma and to these gains a realm of intimate, personal power is developing – power of the individual to conduct his own education, find his own inspiration, shape his own environment, and share his adventure with whoever is interested.[28]

As a whole, the principal characteristics of counter-cultural activities can be seen as being disparate, anarchic, subjective, and romantic. There appears to have been little order or direction to the events, no central authority, and no overall leadership. This situation changed for the youth generations of the 1970s and 1980s. After 1973 when, with the cessation of American involvement in Vietnam and of conscription and, therefore, with the removal of the prime focus of the youthful anti-war protest activities, a new era came about which was characterized by the increasing importance of material concerns, with counter-culturalists growing older and starting to build families and careers – a transition that resulted in the counter-culture becoming 'the industry for boutiques and pornographic forms of sexual license. Indeed, the mind-expanding "drug culture" of the sixties gave way to the sedating "drug culture" of the seventies.'[29] A similar view, too, sees considerable change in the American transition from the 1960s in that 'The conflict between utilitarian culture and counterculture in the 1960s left *both* sides of the battlefield strewn with expired dreams and ideological wreckage. It resulted in the disillusioned withdrawal of young and old, hip and straight alike, away from active concern with public institutions and back into the refuge of private life.'[30]

---

28   Whole Earth Catalog, 1971: 1.
29   Murray Bookchin, 1990: 149f.
30   Steve Tipton, 1984: 29.

Literary Influences in the Counter-Culture: The Beats and Existentialists

Probably the greatest influence on the counter-culture was that of its key writers, not least of which were the Beats – described as 'dissident, countercultural, harbingers of their own kind of newness'[31] who included Gregory Corso, Allen Ginsberg, William Burroughs, and Jack Kerouac, all of whom emanated from the East Coast of the US. Kerouac's novel *On the Road*, published in 1955, was followed by a succession of other writings: Kerouac's *Dharma Bums* (1958) and *Desolation Angels* (1960), Burroughs's *Naked Lunch* (1959), and Ginsberg's poetry including the collection *Howl* (1956/7). The Beats

> simply denied the role of social critic and took an indifferent and passive posture before the problems of the world. Fallout, population, medical care, legal justice, civil rights – the beats were concerned actively with these problems when they impinged on the printing of books with certain Taboo words, or on the problem of dope addicts cut off from their source of supply [...] otherwise their approach was sardonic, apocalyptic, or impudent.[32]

In other words, the Beats led a generation into a very different form of life from traditional norms, one where values were overturned. In fact, the Beats'

> great contribution was in the expression of new motives and their creation – or recognition – of a new audience. The singular force of the beat writers is manifest in the fact that they did not merely reflect the audience of American Bohemia; they substantially altered that audience, and in doing so they liberated and clarified motives until then only imperfectly realized.[33]

Jack Kerouac himself suggests that the '"Beat Generation" has simply become the slogan or label for a revolution in manners in America'[34] although this was, as has been poignantly pointed out,

31   Robert Lee, 1996: 2.
32   Thomas Parkinson, 1971: 277.
33   Op. cit.: 285.
34   Jack Kerouac, 1971: 73.

54

primarily still a male domain, as women had little place in most of the Beat writings.[35]

Importantly, it must be added that a degree of alternative spirituality is to be found in some of the Beat writings. In this respect, it has been suggested that 'At the personal level, the ambition of the Beat writers was to recover a sense of self which married visionary tradition to a recovery of individual worth which challenged the historic, normative values of popular America [...] Yet there was another peculiarly American strain, the need for a religious metaphysic to underwrite personal authenticity.'[36]

With regards to the Beat writers themselves, while William Burroughs was seen to be 'intensely sceptical about the sacred',[37] 'Ginsberg's influence [...] extends far beyond poetry. He has been one of the first to insist that the Beat Generation is a religious phenomenon and that Beat [...] really stands for Beatitude'.[38] What is more, Alan Watts – an almost-cult figure who did much to introduce Zen Buddhism to the West – suggests that 'the "beat" mentality [...] is a younger generation's nonparticipation in "the American Way of Life", a revolt which does not seek to change the existing order but simply turns away from it to find the significance of life in subjective experience rather than objective achievement.'[39]

Other writers, too, had enormous influence on the counter-culture of the 1960s and early 1970s – especially with regard to its spiritual content. The list is long and diverse. For example, *The Third Eye* (first published in 1956) and successive books on Tibetan Buddhism by T. Lobsang Rampa (subsequently discovered to be an Irish plumber); Alan Watts published *The Way of Zen* (1957), Timothy Leary *The Psychedelic Experience* (1964), Carlos Casteneda *The Teachings of Don Juan: The Yaqui Way of Knowledge* (1968), and Ram Dass *Be*

---

35 Edward Halsey Foster, 1992: 22.
36 Clive Bush, 1996: 129.
37 Ibid.
38 Paul O'Neil, 1971: 238. Ginsberg spent more than a year in India during 1962–3 and his experiences are chronicled in his Indian journals (1996).
39 Alan Watts, 1973: 91. This view concurs with that of Theodore Roszak (1970), mentioned above.

Here Now (1971) – a book which has been called the 'Bible' of the counter-culture.

Moreover, a most important writer at this time, especially in America, was Hermann Hesse. Interest in Hesse did not begin in earnest until the late 1950s, which was almost forty years after *Demian* was first published in Germany. It is suggested that Hesse's

> American vogue [...] is based upon Hesse as the author of mind-expanding works, works in which the emphasis has shifted from the palpable straightforward narration of events to a kind of subjectivism which is related to the search for the self, mysticism, archetypal symbolism, logical paradox as psychological truth, and musical themes and forms which establish a liaison with the subconscious. These works seem not to have exerted their influence earlier simply because the audience to which they appeal [...] has only recently come into existence.[40]

To this audience, 'Hesse [seems] almost to be its prophet';[41] and he 'touched a chord which resounds in the hearts and minds – probably "soul" [...] – of thousands of young Americans'[42] who were described as the 'Hesse cult'.[43]

During the 1960s existential writers, more European than American, were widely read by counter-culturalists. Having discarded traditional norms, a feeling of alienation and disorientation was experienced by some which, in turn, created a sense of anguish *(Angst)*, yet this was also coupled with a sense that something else existed, an optimism that there was considerably more to life than had hitherto been available. The existential writers wrote about this condition in terms of a Being-ness, which some interpreted spiritually and some humanistically. This question of Being-ness centred on the notion of self-authenticity and entailed a rebellion against traditions – spiritual, social, political – where the individual has to proceed on a journey of discovery, to 'make his own decisions, find his own truths [...] that reveal the anguished journey of the spirit through the dark night of

---

40   E. F. Timpe, 1977: 141.
41   Ibid.
42   F. Pfafflin, 1977: 387f.
43   Ibid.

56

nothingness'.[44] The 1960s was perhaps the first time that large numbers of people were openly faced with such questions about the meaning of their lives. Furthermore, the journey of discovery meant 'going within' – a method that has since become a core New Age process – to find subjective, personal substance to life; and from this, it can be suggested, was created simultaneously a greater openness to the vast array of spiritual ideas which hitherto had been accessible only to the few. The existential writers were influential in raising consciousness of the problems involved in the concept of Being-ness, that the individual alone was responsible for her or his life, although these writers did not resolve the problems, as 'existentialism cannot serve as a self-sufficient philosophy. Its chief value is that of a corrective [bringing] us face to face with the urgency of ultimate questions.'[45] Moreover, many existential writers wrote about the concept of nothingness which, whether correctly or incorrectly, had the effect among some of those involved in the counter-culture of introducing them, or 'opening them up', to a new freedom, thereby encouraging their mood for experimentation in all forms of life – spiritual, social, sexual, and often all together – in fact, to whatever could be engaged with.

Instrumental at this time were such writers as Albert Camus, Franz Kafka, and Jean-Paul Sartre as well as, but to a lesser extent and from a theological viewpoint, Søren Kierkegaard. However, it is not possible in this volume to debate the different interpretations of existentialism which were – and, it is likely, in a subtle way still are – influential upon the blossoming New Age, although it is important to point out that, along with Beat Generation writers and writers such as Herman Hesse, existentialist writers also played a formative part in the genesis of the New Age.

44 Karl and Hamalian, 1973: 12.
45 David Roberts, 1968: 47.

Post Counter-Culture: The 1970s and 1980s

Even by the time of the Woodstock Festival in 1969, it has been suggested, the counter-culture was already disappearing as an identifiable social movement;[46] and this next 'phase' of the New Age commenced from around 1973 and started to conclude during the mid to late 1980s. What differentiates the counter-culture from the following period has been epitomized by in a television documentary exploring the twenty-fifth anniversary of the Woodstock Festival, entitled *The Children of Woodstock*. One interviewee in the programme (John) suggested that in the early 1970s 'what had been a very kind drug culture was turning into a very mean drug culture'[47] and, more prophetically, another interviewee (Paul) pointed out that 'the "we" or "us" generation changed into the "me" generation'.[48] Both of these interviewees pointed to the end of the sharing, cooperative state of the 1960s and the development of a more self- or ego-centred, yuppie-type materialistic way of life which occurred primarily among the middle classes in the 1970s and 1980s.

Social research also highlights the transition. Through the results of quantitative studies, it is suggested that in the sixties 'the shifts in culture barely touched the lives of the majority of Americans [...] By the seventies, however, most Americans were involved in projects to prove that life can be more than a grim economic chore.'[49] This study points out that many counter-cultural ideas of the 1960s – for example, with regard to personal relationships (albeit in a less radical form) – started to become more accepted by the American population: 'all was pluralism and freedom of choice: to marry or live together; to have children early or postpone them, perhaps forever [...] to change careers, spouses, houses, states of residence, states of mind.'[50] In the UK, an index of the change in the nature of relationships, for example,

46 William Issel, 1985: 199.
47 Leslie Woodhead, 1994.
48 Ibid.
49 Daniel Yankelovich, 1981: 5.
50 Ibid.

can be illustrated in that, between 1973 and 1983, the number of marriages declined by 14%, while the number of divorces rose by almost 40%.[51]

This period also became a time of decreasing liberalism and increasing conservatism. The trend is best illustrated by the ascending political careers of Margaret Thatcher, elected as leader of the UK Conservative Party in 1975 and whose career as a major political figure lasted until 1990, and of Ronald Reagan, who served two four-year terms of office as American President from 1980 to 1988.

In the UK, but not in US, membership of the principal Protestant churches slumped almost 40% between 1970 and 1990, according to religious research.[52] In contrast, technology boomed. An American space probe landed on Mars in 1976 and Concorde commenced scheduled supersonic services in 1977. In the following year, the first test-tube baby was born. The first heart and lung transplant was carried out in 1982. A new era in space exploration began with the first flight of the Challenger space shuttle in 1983 and, by 1987, the two-thousandth satellite was launched. In 1981, IBM launched the personal computer (PC) and, in 1983, the compact disc (CD) was brought onto the market.

During the same period there was a growth in concern for the environment, and environmental issues started to be taken up more emphatically into New Age ideology. In 1976, for example, scientists gave warnings about the condition of the Earth's ozone layer and the damaging use of chlorofluorocarbons (CFCs), especially as an aerosol propellant. Concern about nuclear safety was highlighted by near-disaster at Three Mile Island in the US in 1979 and realized by actual disaster at Chernobyl in the then USSR in 1986; and, in 1981, the Greenham Common Women's Peace Camp was established in protest at the siting of America's nuclear cruise missiles in the UK. In 1984, the disastrous Bhopal poisonous gas leak from a Union Carbide factory struck India. AIDS was identified in 1981, and by 1986 25,000 cases had been reported in the US alone.

51   Ethel Lawrence, 1985: 24, 26.
52   Peter Brierley and Val Hiscock, 1993: 253.

Popular musical influences which came to the fore included Punk, New Wave, and Heavy Metal; and two major differences between the 1960s and 1970s were said to be that, firstly, concerts became substantially larger 'grandiose spectacles' and, secondly, the development of disco technology allowed recorded music to be played instead of live performances.[53] Free festivals developed from 1973, and by the end of the 1980s, music such as Acid House, Techno Pagan, as well as raves added to the mix, bringing with them a renewed psychedelia in the form of 'designer drugs' such as Ecstasy.[54] MTV was launched in America in 1981.[55] Sid Vicious of the Sex Pistols (the first Punk band) died in 1979, John Lennon was shot dead in the following year, and Bob Marley died in 1981. In 1984 rock stars 'banded' together as Band Aid to make a record to raise funds for drought relief in Ethiopia, and in the following year Live Aid, a simultaneous concert in the UK and US, raised $60 million for African famine relief.

This, then, was the social, political, and cultural background to the second phase of the New Age, one that was markedly different to the first. On the one hand, the earlier phase represented a breaking down of many social, political, and spiritual 'taboos'; and, albeit among a comparatively small number of people, a new sense of community developed comprised of what was called the 'Aquarian Conspirators'. However, on the other hand, as I have described, with conscription and the Vietnam War ending for America, the vital focus of the protest movement disappeared. The youth generation of the 1960s became older and more settled – indeed, many participants who had 'dropped out' could be seen to be 'dropping back in' to the mores of mainstream society – and the new youth generation of the 1970s and

---

53   Jim Curtis, 1993: 243.
54   According to Steve Turner, 'in 1988, techno and acid house became the soundtrack for Britain's "Summer of Love", when empty buildings and far-flung spaces were commandeered by giant soundsystems and light shows and crowds of up to 5,000 took part in massive all-night raves' (1995: 221f).
55   According to Ann Kaplan, MTV perfectly suited current needs in that the station 'at once addresses the American adolescent's consciousness of a decentered world, while also providing a longed-for centeredness in the faces and bodies of the rock stars' (1987: 148f).

1980s had no such dynamic disestablishmentarian focus. Nevertheless, some characteristics of the 1960s did persist and, by and large, expand into a movement especially concerned with matters to do with self-authenticity. This, the development of the Human Potential Movement, together with the rise in the influence of women, the rise of channelling, and the further development of transpersonal spirituality, are now examined in greater depth.

The Human Potential Movement

A key feature of the New Age in the post-counter-culture period was the growth of the Human Potential Movement. While the genesis of this Movement occurred earlier, it was not until the late 1960s and early 1970s that the Movement became more fully developed. By this time, in the region of 150 to 200 'growth centres' had been established in the US,[56] the most notable of which was The Esalen Institute at Big Sur in California. Indeed, it has been suggested that activities practised by these growth centres had, by the early 1970s, become 'something of a fad',[57] a fad which continued at least until the early 1980s. In the UK, the Human Potential Research Project was launched at the University of Surrey in 1970 and has become the longest-established such centre in Europe.[58]

The history of the Human Potential Movement can be traced back at least to the work of psychologist William James at the turn of the nineteenth century who 'was a precursor in the three areas of human potential'[59] – the study of paranormal psychology, the existence of altered states of consciousness, and the documentation and investigation of incidences of human potentialities. Jacob Moreno and his work in psychodrama followed James in the 1920s and 1930s. How-

56   According to W. C. Schutz, cited in J. H. Mann, 1994 Vol. 2: 181.
57   Ibid.
58   Eileen Barker, 1989: 181.
59   J. H. Mann, 1994 Vol. 2: 180.

61

ever, the father of the Human Potential Movement is widely thought to be the American psychologist Abraham Maslow, who defined the 'peak' experience as being not solely religious or mystical experience but also as the 'raw material'[60] for philosophies of any kind within the realm of nature.[61] Maslow also developed Third Force humanistic psychology as an alternative to Freudian and learning theory. By the end of the 1960s, this Third Force had started to spawn a Fourth Force as a psychology of mysticism within which Maslow was again active and which became known as transpersonal psychology.[62] These two 'forces',[63] particularly the former, became the principal 'schools' of the Human Potential Movement. Although the Movement itself and humanistic psychology generally may have declined in their importance to the New Age, many of their ideas and activities remain as significant tools. These have been described as 'psychotechnologies', that is, 'systems for a deliberate change in consciousness'.[64]

Two descriptions of the Human Potential Movement provide a comprehensive picture. Firstly, a succinct four-point explanation of its principal tenets has been given as: '(1) that each of us has a great potential lying within us; (2) that this potential can be awakened through education and experimentation; (3) that the individual can change his or her situation dramatically – actual self-transformation is possible; (4) that self-realization and self-fulfilment are the proper ends of life.'[65] In more detail and at length, it is suggested that

> The human potential idea consists of an amalgamation of the existential attitude – direct experience as the touchstone – with that most basic of American ideologies, the perfectibility of man. The latter notion is what we mean by the *humanistic* orientation – a hallowed, hard-to-define tradition basic to the notion of progress in the Western world, and the fundamental principle of which is that 'man is the measure of all things' [...] God has left the world, the humanists

60   Abraham Maslow, 1964: xii.
61   See also Maslow, 1970.
62   Anthony Sutich, 1976.
63   The first two 'forces' in the history of psychology are: First Force, encompassing classical psychoanalytic theory; Second Force, relating to positivistic or behaviouristic theory.
64   Marilyn Ferguson, 1982: 91.
65   Ted Peters, 1991: 69.

claim, so that man can elevate himself to the level of God [...] Gone is the *angst* of European existential analysis. Gone too is the doubt and ambiguity, the scepticism of Freudian psychoanalysis. In other words, the demons have faded away. In their place is energy, flow, acceptance, nurture, tenderness: joy [Much] of the movement sees itself mainly as an educational adventure, primed to spread good tidings to the citizens of the New Age.[66]

It can be established from these descriptions that the Human Potential Movement is not so much concerned with treating neuroses as with assisting 'well' individuals to access and develop abilities which would otherwise remain undiscovered; and its spirituality is humanistic – that is, limited in the main to the human, rather than transcending the human.

With regard to the range of psychotechnologies incorporated in the Human Potential Movement, the difference between humanistic and transpersonal is illustrated by comparing the nature of particular courses and workshops which have been offered by the two schools. Here it is seen that some Third Force courses were more specifically technique oriented in terms of their use of psychological methods – for example, Neuro-Linguistic Programming (NLP) and Transactional Analysis, while courses to do with the Fourth Force tended to include a more holistic, compassionate, 'religious', and loving basis in their format, as we will see.

Other major players in the development of humanistic psychology include Carl Rogers (Rogerian therapy), Fritz Perls and Wilhelm Reich (Gestalt therapy – Reich also developed Bioenergetics), Arthur Janov (primal therapy); and encounter-group therapies including those subsequently developed by Werner Erhard (est) and Eric Berne (transactional analysis). On the other hand, individuals and ideas important in transpersonal psychology comprise a more complex matrix. In this regard, we find an 'increasing convergence of western physics and eastern metaphysics, of modern consciousness research and eastern spiritual systems'.[67] As a whole, transpersonal psychology incorporates concepts such as Abraham Maslow's 'peak' experience, Roberto

66   Joel Kovel, 1978: 153ff.
67   Key New Age psychotherapist Stanislav Grof, cited in Ian Gordon-Brown and Barbara Somers, 1988: 285.

Assagioli's Psychosynthesis, and Victor Frankl's Logotherapy,[68] as well as such activities as 'meditation, rebirthing, shamanic visualization, holotropic breathing and the float-tank experience'.[69] Probably the most influential theorist active in transpersonal psychology at this time was Ken Wilber.

By the mid-1980s, a branching out of the two schools became more distinct. This divergence is characterized by, on the one hand, the use of psychotechnologies to empower mainstream capitalistic enterprise through increasing the potential of its management and, on the other hand, the growth in transpersonal activities which concentrate more on the spiritual empowerment of the individual. Moreover, at the same time, there appears to have been a downswing in the direction of the Human Potential Movement, and this occurred for at least two reasons: the failed promise of what could be achieved through some of the psychotherapies; and the loss of credibility either in the therapies themselves or, more importantly, in their key proponents. A number of therapies and therapists have been listed which damaged the Movement at this time, including Feeling Therapy, problems at Esalen, scandal at the Movement of Spiritual Inner Awareness and, in the late 1980s, activities which were later to bring about the discrediting of Werner Erhard, the founder of est (Erhard Seminars Training).[70]

In the 1970s and 80s, widespread social change in terms of a new age did not happen and conservatism grew to be the dominating social influence – the 'me' generation with its inherent materialism flourished. At this time, the two forces of humanistic and transpersonal psychology were key to the development of New Age ideas and activities across America and Europe although, while the importance of humanistic psychology to the New Age appears to have waned, the ideas and practices involved in transpersonal psychology – because of

---

68   Ibid.
69   Nevill Drury, 1994: 129.
70   Carol Lynn Mithers, 1994: 405ff est was probably the most influential and widely adopted human potential training system, which had 'graduated', according to Steven Tipton, 270,000 people in the 1980s (1984: 176).

its heightened spiritual basis – continue to be a highly influential feature of the New Age.[71]

Women in the New Age

The Women's Movement as a whole was active throughout the twentieth century in a variety of directions, ranging from establishing voting rights and spiritual renewal to promoting education. Yet, even in the late 1950s, women's influence in society was not extensive (perhaps highlighted by one writer who found that 'in terms of gender, the novelty of the Beat movement for American culture was the insertion into its discourse of the "chick", the attractive, young, sexually available and above all silent ("dumb") female').[72] However, this situation was to change. Publication of Betty Friedan's *The Feminist Mystique* in the 1960s triggered the rise of the feminist spirituality movement and, by 1970, with the publication of Kate Millet's *Sexual Politics* and Germaine Greer's *The Female Eunuch* – both making powerful statements – the contemporary feminist movement became firmly established.

Women's spirituality in the 1970s and 80s is a subject which requires separate study and can only be touched upon here, although it is important to point out that spiritual concerns among women have been an influential feature in the development of the New Age. Indeed, perhaps like most spiritualities, New Age ideas have given room for the understanding that women and men have different approaches to their spirituality, differences which are perceived as harmonious, not conflicting. This difference between the genders has been assessed by saying that women's spirituality 'is more related to nature and natural processes and to the home and the domestic realm than to history-

---

71   In 1985, for example, Ken Wilber suggested that 'the humanistic psychology movement [was] running on borrowed time' (cited in Georg Feuerstein, 1992: 192).

72   Helen McNeil, 1996: 189.

making and culture [...] as more diffuse, concrete, personal, emotional, and general [whereas men's spirituality is] more focused, universal, abstract, and intellectual'.[73] Women have come to play a role in the New Age which is at least equal to, if not greater than, the role played by men – a fact that is supported numerically by head counts recorded at many New Age events, which suggest that women participants out-number men by approximately three to one. Although this is 1990s information, the same trend was in existence in the late 1970s, and it is suggested that 'wherever the Aquarian Conspiracy is at work [...] women are represented in far greater numbers than they are in the es-tablishment.'[74] It is also reported that this situation was unsurprising because, 'as the international feminist movement helped rectify an imbalance in the social and political sphere during the 1960s and 70s, it was surely only a matter of time before such expressions flowed through into different forms of feminine spirituality.'[75] And one key New Age feminist suggests that 'the feminist movement, which began as a political, economic, and social struggle, is opening to a spiritual dimension.'[76]

Women also appear to have taken the lead in the field of com-plementary health and healing. As will be shown in the following chapter, women therapists outnumber their male counterparts by four to one. One reason for this is that women historically appear to have been more in tune with or conscious of their bodies, not least through the menstruation cycle, childbirth, and the menopause. At a daylong class on Chinese medicine in California made up almost entirely of women, one delegate commented that 'Women are already into heal-ing. They are natural healers. Men have to learn how to become heal-ers.'[77] Survey findings will show that the appeal and usage of body-

---

73   Marianne Ferguson, 1995: 234.
74   Marilyn Ferguson, 1982: 249. In comparison, the ratio of difference between female and male Church of England church attenders found by sociologist Tony Walters is 55:45, and among Methodists 60:40. In the US, the ratio for Pente-costals is 2:1, and for Baptists 60:40 (1992: 75).
75   Nevill Drury, 1994: 137.
76   Cited in Katherine Zappone, 1991: 17.
77   Cited in Richard Grossinger, 1990: 325.

work therapies – acupuncture, aromatherapy, Feldenkrais, Rolfing, and the like – to women is far greater than to men.

This period also saw the upsurge of Goddess spirituality, where 'women are creating new myths, singing a new liturgy, painting our own icons, and drawing strength from the new-old symbols of the Goddess, of the "legitimacy and beneficence of female power".'[78] Women talk about the rise of a feminist religion and about becoming their own authorities, so moving away from traditional spiritualities where most of the teachers – Jesus, Buddha, Mohammad, and Moses – have been men. Historically, Goddess religion has always existed, points out one Wiccan priestess.[79] Her argument is that the influence of the Goddess has simply been suppressed primarily by male domination. She sees that the Goddess has returned through a number of avenues, not least 'via feminism to remind the world that women have value and potential, and that feminine symbols and images have power. The Goddess has returned at the head of this movement as a meaningful symbol of women's power.'[80] This priestess believes that the period we are living in is one where Goddess spirituality is growing rapidly and that women now need to work towards building (or rebuilding) 'a strong and supportive tradition'.[81]

However, it does not appear to be the case that women have sought to evoke a male-type politics or spirituality in their ideas and activities in the New Age but one which reflects their unique requirements, albeit parallel with – and not necessarily against – the male type. From academe, this argument is described more fully:

> The feminist spirituality movement includes a tremendous variety of women whose primary focus encourages the growth of woman's power to heal themselves and all creatures on the earth [...] Most agree that the main force for cultural revolution emerges when women's personal power is nurtured to effect political change. But this is not just any kind of power: these feminists are talking about potency for effecting change that only comes when one acknowledges that we are each part of a vast organism that is in trauma. A common theme

---

78 Starhawk, 1991: 34.
79 Caitlin Matthews, 1991: 6.
80 Ibid.
81 Op. cit.: 24.

consistently surfaces throughout rich diversity in [women's] writings: *We can only move beyond the ravaging of the planet and the oppression of peoples through a consciousness of interrelatedness.*[82]

The principal thesis here is that women need to play a natural (organic) part in the process of change, one where the qualities they bring are not suppressed. In this respect, many of the leading personalities in the New Age – but not the majority – have been (and continue to be) women. Much more will be said about women's activities in the New Age in later chapters, but it is clear to see that since the 1960s and in tandem with the growth of women's activities in general, women play a significant role.

Channelling

In the 1970s and 1980s the New Age saw a substantial rise in the phenomenon of channelling (a form of mediumship), a rise which has particularly occurred in the US. This activity was not new – it has, in fact, existed in various forms throughout history. Moreover, channelling is not necessarily New Age in itself, although its practice has been influential upon some of those involved with its ideas and activities. With regard to the twentieth century, a chronology of channellers has been outlined which 'would run from pioneers like Eileen Garrett, Alice Bailey, the channellers of the *Urantia Book*, Edgar Cayce, and Jane Roberts's Seth, to the more recent flood of trance technicians',[83] of which over twenty examples are given.

A sociologist points out that in this period 'it became more common for channellers to conceptualize their source in highly abstract terms as "an energy vortex" or some such, but also to give their source a personal name and even imbue it with quasi-personal charac-

---

82   Katherine Zappone, 1991: 40f, author's italics.
83   Andrew Ross, 1991: 37.

teristics.'[84] To illustrate this point, Table 1, which I have compiled from a number of sources, describes the close proximity in the dates of the emergence of the most noteworthy channelled material into the public arena either through the publication of channelled teachings or through public seminars. This unmistakably sudden increase created something of a fad among certain sections of the New Age population, again, particularly in America.

Table 1. The rise of channelled teachings in the 1970s

1970	Jane Roberts's 'Seth'
1971	David Spangler's 'Limitless Love and Truth' ('John')
1973	Kevin Ryerson's 'John'
1974	Jach Pursel's 'Lazaris'
	Phyllis Schlemmer *et al's* 'Council of Nine'
1975	Helen Schucman's *A Course in Miracles*
	Mary-Margaret Moore's 'Bartholomew'
	Pat Rodegast's 'Emmanuel'
1977	J. Z. Knight's 'Ramtha'
1978	Ken Carey's *The Starseed Transmissions*

It can be added that many of the channellers, including Ryerson and Knight, 'rose to great popularity in the 1980s with the help of publicity associated with celebrities, including the actress Shirley MacLaine'.[85]

While there is considerable triviality in much of the channelled material, one commentator believes there to be 'a number of channelled documents which address issues more immediately relevant to the human condition. The best of these writings are not only coherent and plausible, but eloquently persuasive and sometimes disarmingly moving [...] For many New Agers, this material rivals the Scriptures

84   Steve Bruce, 1995: 110.
85   Rosemary Ellen Guiley, 1991: 316.

of historical religions in its inspirational value.'[86] Probably the foremost channelled document from this period would be *A Course in Miracles*, first published in 1975. This c.1,200 page three-part channelled teaching is described as 'a mind training in the relinquishment of a thought system based on fear, and the acceptance instead of a thought system based on love',[87] which means that it is clearly at variance with how traditional Christianity is seen by some in the New Age, although it is unambiguously Christian in its style of presentation. The 'Course' 'was heard as a kind of "inner dictation" over a seven-year period by Dr Helen Schucman, a professor of medical psychology at Columbia University' (publisher's leaflet) and, since its publication, a study foundation – The Foundation of Inner Peace – has been established in California and study groups exist worldwide.

A particular difference between contemporary channelling and the historical medium or spiritualist has been pointed out: 'today's channels [...] don't contact spirits; ostensibly, they are contacted by them.'[88] This author reports that 'with tens of thousands of Americans paying $10 to $200 an hour to seek comfort and council from these higher beings (and at least one dolphin), channelling has become a very big business.'[89] This is confirmed in a specialist's study of the subject: despite scandals and notoriety of some key individuals such as J. Z. Knight, it was found that there is a 'quiet spread'[90] of techniques allowing ordinary people to experiment at home, and it is suggested that up to 30 million people might be peripherally involved.

Contact with what is known in the New Age as 'the spiritual plane' continues to be an important feature. This can be noted, for example, from William Bloom's basic New Age ideas outlined in the previous chapter. In fact, Bloom himself claims to have started to receive channelled teachings in 1987.[91] Moreover, another important New Age writer, David Spangler, frequently refers to his spirit guide

---

86   Suzanne Riordan, 1992: 107f.
87   Marianne Williamson, 1992: 18.
88   Katherine Lowry, 1987: 48.
89   Op. cit.: 50.
90   Michael Brown, 1997: 5.
91   These have been recorded in book form, see William Bloom, 1995a.

'John' from whom he receives channelled teachings.[92] Yet another commentator suggests that a positive outgrowth of spiritual guidance through channelling 'is the encouragement for individuals to develop their own connections to a source of high wisdom, especially through intuition'.[93] This action, as we will see, has broad implications to many aspects of spirituality and healing in the New Age.

The transpersonal

The notion of the transpersonal, developed in the late 1960s by Abraham Maslow as Fourth Force psychology (outlined above), became a central concept in the New Age in the late 1980s and 1990s, and three proponents in particular have been influential in its development. Christina Grof and Stanislav Grof, who developed holotropic breathwork as a 'replacement' for the use of psychedelic drugs for mind expansion, describe what is involved:

> The modern term for the direct experience of spiritual realities is *transpersonal*, meaning transcending the usual way of perceiving and interpreting the world from the position of a separate individual or body-ego [...] States involving personal encounters with the numinous dimensions of existence can be divided into two large categories. In the first are experiences of the 'immanent divine', or perceptions of divine intelligence expressing itself in the world of everyday reality. All of creation – people, animals, plants, and inanimate objects – seems to be permeated by the same cosmic essence and divine light. A person in this state suddenly sees that everything in the universe is a manifestation and expression of the same creative cosmic energy and that separation and boundaries are illusory. Experiences in the second category do not represent different perceptions of what is already known but reveal a rich spectrum of dimensions of reality that are ordinarily hidden from human awareness and are not available in the everyday state of consciousness. These can be referred to as experiences of the 'transcendent divine'. A typical example would be a vision of God as a ra-

---

92   David Spangler, 1971.
93   Rosemary Ellen Guiley, 1991: 91.

diant source of light of supernatural beauty or a sense of personal fusion and identity with God.[94]

The third proponent, and by and large the most widely-known theorist in the field of transpersonal psychology, is Ken Wilber. Wilber suggests that the concept of transpersonal is not reductive in any way; in fact, relating it to his theory for a spectrum of consciousness,[95] he believes quite the opposite is true, in that '*transpersonal* means "personal *plus*", not "personal minus".'[96] Wilber expands the meaning of 'personal plus' by indicating that in transpersonal terms people 'are no longer exclusively identified with the individual personality, and yet because they still preserve the personality, then *through that* personality flows the force and fire of the soul'.[97] Drawing significantly from Ralph Waldo Emerson,[98] Wilber describes what he believes an actual transpersonal experience can entail:

> It's not really as mysterious as it sounds [...] You yourself can, right now, be aware of your objective self, you can observe your individual ego or person, you are aware of yourself generally. But who, then, is doing the observing? What is it that is observing or witnessing your individual self? That therefore *transcends* your individual self in some way? Who or what is *that*? The observer in you, the Witness in you, transcends the isolated *person* in you and opens instead – from within or from behind, as Emerson said – onto a vast expanse of awareness no longer obsessed with the individual bodymind, no longer a respecter or abuser of persons, no longer fascinated by the passing joys and set-apart sorrows of the lonely self, but standing still in silence as an opening or clearing through which light shines, not from the world but into it – 'a light shines *through us* upon things'. That *which* observes or witnesses the self, the person, is precisely to that degree *free* of the self, the person, and *through that*

94   Christina Grof and Stanislav Grof, 1991: 40.
95   Ken Wilber's spectrum of consciousness is explored in Chapter 11 below.
96   Ken Wilber, 1995a: 280.
97   Op. cit.: 281.
98   Eileen Campbell and J. H. Brennan believe that the Transcendentalist Movement was a precursor of the New Age. They report that 'In 1836 a group of American intellectuals got together to explore the Quaker and Puritan traditions, the German and Greek philosophers and the Eastern religions. They included Ralph Waldo Emerson and Henry Thoreau [...] Transcendentalism was a philosophy which stressed an inner search for meaning' (1990: 295).

opening comes pouring the light and power of a Self, a Soul, that, as Emerson puts it, 'would make our knees bend'.[99]

It is clear here that Wilber views the transpersonal experience as a means of expanding human potential into a significantly greater form of consciousness than that of the humanistic view, one that can be interpreted as being the ultimate potential state of consciousness. Moreover, Wilber argues that this ultimate state is necessarily para- doxical – which, analogously, he describes as 'the highest rung in the ladder *and* the wood out of which the ladder is made'.[100] Wilber's views, it can be added, relate to the concept of non-duality particularly found in Zen Buddhism and Advaita Vedanta; and he suggests, in the same way as Grof, that 'If spirit is completely transcendent, it is also completely immanent. I am firmly convinced that if a new and com- prehensive paradigm is ever to emerge, that paradox will be at its heart.'[101] Wilber believes that the development of the transpersonal, that is, both the transcendent and the immanent aspects of spirituality – as well as the humanistic – are vital activities for the achievement of ultimate consciousness and a comprehensive new age. In fact, he sees them as intrinsic parts of the paradox. And it would seem that he sees that a new age is yet to come.

In practice, there are literally hundreds of different types of courses, workshops, and therapies which incorporate transpersonal aspects that are available in the New Age, and there are many guides offering directions. However, the ultimate guide in the New Age is thought to be the individual's Higher Self which, for a participant, allays suggestions of disorder. This view is emphasized by an impor- tant spiritual teacher in the New Age, Jiddu Krishnamurti, who ad- vises that 'In matters of the spirit, in matters of deep psychological investigation, one must be free from all sense of following anybody. There is no leader or guide into that realm. One has to watch, to ob- serve, see for oneself very clearly what one is, and not according to any philosopher, any psychotherapist, or psychologist.'[102]

99   Op. cit.: 280f.
100   Ken Wilber, 1990: 307.
101   Ibid.
102   Jiddu Krishnamurti, 1995: 10.

Following their own New Age direction, as Krishnamurti suggests, individuals can come into contact with a wide range of transpersonal endeavours which fall into at least six groups. These are: (1) ideas and activities which have a traditional religious basis, such as Sufi Dances of Universal Peace and the yogic teachings of the Self-Realization Fellowship; (2) teachings of some new religious movements, for example, Transcendental Meditation and Osho groups; (3) the study and practice of ancient wisdom, including the Kabbalah, Shamanism, and Gnosticism; (4) denominational or non-denominational methods of meditation, including Vipassana and Tai Chi Ch'uan; (5) psychotherapies, including rebirthing and Psychosynthesis; and, finally, (6) psychic or paranormal practices, which can include channelling, numerology, and communing with nature spirits.

New Age at the dawn of the new millennium

In social and political terms, the last decade of the twentieth century was filled with both optimism and horror. The possibility of peace came to a unified Germany, and the Cold War ended. Peace also came to Ireland and to South Africa with the ending of apartheid. The union of the USSR dissolved, the EC became larger. However, there was a spate of what became known as ethnic cleansing – in East Timor, Rwanda, Tibet, and the former Yugoslavia. Middle-of-the-road Conservatism in the UK and US weakened but the right wing – for example, the New Right in the US – became stronger.

Environmental issues were starting to be embraced as a profitable enterprise by most of the important global corporations as well as by national industries, although these activities were by no means universal; according to Greenpeace, Exxon (Esso in the UK) was a notable exception. Ethical investments were included in many of the leading pension and investment portfolios in the UK and the US. Trading in ivory was banned, as was the future production of ozone-harmful CFCs. Additionally, single-issue protest action against, for example, the building of roads and the treatment of animals no longer attracted only the radical fringes of social concern. Green commercial activities became big business.

In electronics, computer technology came of age and, in so do-ing, lost much of its Orwellian image – the PC became a household item and a means to create new (virtual) realities. The information highway opened, allowing instant communication to any individual in the world with reciprocal technology. One commentator reports that 'many of the Silicon Valley pioneers, now in their forties, were hip-pies in the 1960s'.[103] Another comments that many of the hippies of the 1960s joined the mainstream, although it is suggested that 'they are not just like their never-anything-but-straight neighbours.'[104] In fact, this description of participants of the New Age suggests that, un-derneath,

> Hippiedom is not as dead as it may appear. Their questions remain, and their in-fluence continues, many of their number living on and laboring on as mainstays of the New Age. Replace drug-induced mysticism with new forms of ecstasy. Retain the beliefs in the power and greatness concealed within each person, the positive regard for experience and understanding, the pursuit of illumination and a unified world view, and the longing for a revolution of consciousness. Add the quest for community ... and the Hippie community of yesterday re-emerges.[105]

In rock music, the technological and the New Age came together in Techno Pagan, 'a fascinating merger of the hedonism of the rave culture and the radical politics and New Age philosophies of such post-punk manifestations as travellers and "crusties"'.[106] This new style extended into clubs such as Megatripolis in the UK which con-tains a shopping mall and even a Techno-Silence room where lectures on spirituality were held.[107] However, a different New Age music also developed, which was much more serene and spiritual in character.

---

103 Steve Turner, 1995: 223. See also Theodore Roszak, 1994, and Douglas Rush-koff, 1994.
104 Lowell Streiker, 1991: 46.
105 Ibid.
106 Steve Turner, 1995: 221.
107 Op. cit.: 225.

This was music for meditation and stillness rather than for dance and featured, for example, the softer sounds of flutes and water, even the sound of dolphins and whales.

One of the principal features of the 1990s New Age was its growth, and there are many indicators which together provide substantial evidence that real growth was actually occurring. For example, one estimate is that roughly 20% of US adults have been involved in the New Age[108] – a figure which equates with Paul Ray's cultural creatives given in the previous chapter; and growth appears to be across a wide spectrum of activities. Hence, a New Age market was established which spanned therapies, workshops, holidays, and events. Retail activities grew, both in the number of shops and mail-order suppliers. In the UK, book shops now had substantial sections devoted to New Age topics.[109] In the US, New Age book shops were reported to have doubled in number.[110] Specialist magazines, too, flourished. In the UK, for example, *Kindred Spirit*, which started as a small, flimsy magazine became a 100-plus page glossy with a readership of 120,000 (publisher's estimate); and the page volume of its resource directory which advertises seminars, courses, activities, and accessories – mostly with a spiritual and healing focus – increased by 35% in just two years between 1993 and 1995. Indeed, it is the two concerns of spirituality and healing which represent what seems to have been the largest growth in the New Age of the 1990s.

The growth of interest in spiritual concerns is difficult to identify in terms of hard facts, although one way to assess this is through the levels of book sales on the subject. In 1994, the American trade magazine *Publishers Weekly* ran an editorial feature on the subject with the headline 'The New Spin is Spirituality'. The article pointed towards a significant move away from the 'recovery' genre of publishing – that is, recovery from alcohol abuse, drug addiction, divorce, sexual disorders, mourning, abortion, and the like[111] – to books which incorporated a higher spiritual content.

---

108   George Barna, cited in Jeremiah Creedon, 1998: 47.
109   Steve Bruce, 1995: 104.
110   John Naisbitt and Patricia Aburdene, 1990: 273.
111   Cited in Bob McCullough, 1994: 40ff.

Closely related to the growth in spiritual concerns was the growth in alternative and complementary healing.[112] However, the healing therapies in this instance were not so much to do with recovery as described above, but with removing 'blockages' which might bar the way to what those involved described as wholeness. Holism, in this description, is viewed in the New Age to broadly comprise the body, mind (incorporating intellect, will, emotions, and ego), spirit, and planet/cosmos not as separate parts but as a unified interconnected whole; and blockages can include physical disease, psychological disturbances, problems with relationships, and pollution. Concerning its growth, in 1994 it was reported that 'one in three Americans seek alternative health care each year to the tune of $13.7 billion.'[113]

At the start of the twenty-first century, it can fairly be claimed that interest in the healing aspects of the New Age appears to have grown substantially. However, in the same way as humanistic psychotechnologies and 'recovery' ideas and activities appear to have become less central to the New Age, so too the current interest in healing could reduce. Nevertheless, a more likely scenario would be that much of what is considered as New Age healing will be adopted in varying degrees by the mainstream as complementary to allopathic medicine. In fact, this is already happening. It can be added that this appears to be happening in the same way as many psychotechnologies of the Human Potential Movement have been adopted by mainstream business management training organizations. In fact,

> All these ideas and many others related to them have begun to enter our culture in response to a growing need not only among younger people, but among men and women of all ages and walks of life. Involvement in such teachings and practices as Buddhism, Jewish and Christian mysticism, Sufism and Hinduism, as well as Native American and African spiritual traditions, to name only a few, is no longer confined to a so-called 'new age' fringe. The search for transcendence and for inner development now calls to many of the most responsible and established members of our culture in the world of business, science, and the arts. In this sense, we are beginning to be what to some extent we were when our country was founded: a nation of seekers.[114]

112   The subject of healing in the New Age is discussed in depth in later chapters.
113   *Nexus* Vol. 2,20, 1994: 6.
114   Jacob Needleman, 1998: 14.

This view is explored from a different angle by an American journalist who suggests that towards the end of the life of any movement

> the most accessible assumptions that fuelled the movement are absorbed into the mainstream culture and the movement itself – as a cohesive entity at any rate – is largely dissolved [...] This pattern can be seen in the civil rights, women's, and peace movements, as well as the New Right, and it certainly seems true of the New Age movement as well [...] I like to think that if there is any truth to the New Age anticipation of humanity's transformation, such changes will occur irrespective of the state of the New Age movement per se. Lasting social change shouldn't be confused with the movements which help bring it about.[115]

Summary

Discussion of key historical features of the New Age appears to show that its development and expansion has been characterized particularly, but not wholly, by spiritual concerns. During the counter-culture, a great many traditional activities reduced in importance for some people, creating fertile ground for experimentation which, in turn, led to an expansion and popularization of New Age ideas and activities in general. Out of the counter-culture, either directly or indirectly, have arisen notable characteristics – described as 'Aquarian waves'[116] – which have helped to shape the New Age as it begins the third millennium. These waves include the Human Potential Movement, the rise of women's influence in particular areas, the more widespread interest in paranormal activities, particularly in the form of channelling, healing practices, and, finally, transpersonal spirituality. In fact, the rise in the range and use particularly of healing practices may well have been brought about by the increasing influence of women, and this possibility will be engaged with in later chapters. The spiritual content of the pre-1960s New Age does not appear to have

115 Jay Kinney, 1998: 16.
116 Marilyn Ferguson, 1994: 14.

78

been supplanted by subsequent events, but has been augmented both by the larger numbers of people involved and by an increase in the variety of ideas which have come to the fore, especially with regard to the transpersonal. In this respect, the situation in America seems to be changing 'from a Christian nation to a syncretistic, spiritually diverse society',[117] finding Buddhism to be the fastest-growing faith. Ken Wilber sums up the spiritual development from the 1960s to the late 1990s as a transition from what he calls 'hippie dharma' to 'new dharma'. Interviewed in 1998, Wilber saw that 'Hippie dharma is all about "Be here now", "Go with the flow" [...] New dharma is set in the political freedom of the West, which doesn't force itself on people but invites them to transcend themselves through a culture of encouragement and example'.[118]

The New Age is now becoming mature, so much so in fact that many of its ideas and activities have been adopted into the mainstream which, in turn, has further blurred the edges that some commentators seek. As we start the new millennium, it has become even more difficult to locate with any precision where boundaries to the New Age might be.

117 George Barna, cited in Jeremiah Creedon, 1998: 45.
118 Ken Wilber, 1998: 106.

3. Characteristics of Association

I love who I am and all that I do. I am the living, loving, joyous expression of life.

Louise Hay[1]

Some of the burning questions about people involved in the New Age include: who are they? What are they like? What distinguishes them from their fellow human beings? Why do they get involved? Do they take drugs? Why are so many women involved? The survey carried out for this book, together with others carried out in the US, answer these and related questions. Firstly, I explore social and demographic findings, and then we look at the more subtle issues involved in the association these people have with the New Age. On the surface, what is found demonstrates that it is not possible clearly to identify one particular type of person who is most likely to become involved, although there are certain characteristic groups within which they are more likely to be located, and it is difficult completely to dispel charges of the New Age being amorphous. But if we look more deeply into what participants say about their activities, the characteristics become much clearer.

1   Louise Hay, 1988: 100.

Gender

Perhaps one of the most radical social aspects of New Age ideology turns on a shift in emphasis from a patriarchal society to one which contains a considerably higher female content and so, in some respects, it is not surprising that many more women are active than men. In fact, women account for 70% of the UK New Age population, and for 73% in the US.[2]

Several authors, as we have seen in the previous chapter, point to the rise in women's activities in the New Age or related movements generally, and, adding to this, one academic commentator makes a direct link between the rise of both the New Age and women's spiritualities in general. This is because they 'operate out of similar worldviews [...] Both movements emerged from the late 1960s and early 1970s. They attribute various kinds of cultural malaise [...] to the same cause: the dualisms between spirit and matter, male and female, science and religion, thinking and feeling, that they see as having been fostered by Newtonian science and the established religions.'[3] She goes on to suggest that the New Age and the feminist spirituality movement are engaged in the same task of 'resacralizing the cosmos and [the] transforming of human consciousness and society's institutions'.[4]

Overall, therefore, the current size of female involvement with the New Age can be seen in part as a logical outcome of women's activities which have been developing with increasing impact over the previous three decades. Following on from this, the high proportion of women participants has important ramifications for the New Age as a whole. It means that there is likely to exist a significant number of ideas and activities which have a heightened or even specific female content and appeal, and three separate findings verify this effect.

2   Frederick Levine, 1989: 83.
3   Mary Farrel Bednarowski, 1992: 177f. Linda Woodhead, also from academe, makes similar points (1993: 174).
4   Op. cit.: 168.

In the first instance, the number of influential female teachers has increased dramatically. In fact, a sevenfold increase has been recorded between the 1970s and 1990s. In 1977 Marilyn Ferguson asked respondents to name important teachers in the survey which formed the basis of her later study *The Aquarian Conspiracy*.[5] Of the 37 names recorded, only 2 (5%) were women. Almost twenty years later, 13 (35%) women are named in the top 37 names recorded. While this increase represents a significant change, it also means that important female teachers in the New Age are still outnumbered two to one by their male counterparts. Secondly, from survey questions regarding practices, a marked female bias towards activities to do with healing and bodywork has been found, whereas there exists, albeit to a smaller degree, a male bias towards the practice of meditation and ritual activities, together with social concerns. Women also appear to be more involved in a greater number of core New Age activities than men, as well as in divinatory arts (although this is not a widely adopted New Age activity) such as astrology and Tarot reading, and in some aspects of the paranormal, such as recalling past lives. Thirdly, and specifically among the subgroup of individuals comprised entirely of those who claimed to be practising therapists (204 in number), almost four out of five (78%) were women. In comparison with the extent of non-therapist women participants (67%), this finding demonstrates that among practitioners of New Age ideas and activities the extent of women's influence is even more substantial.

More broadly, when asked to give reasons as to why New Age ideas and activities had been adopted, findings suggest that some women appear to be more active in seeking ways of improving their lives as a result of such association than men. For example, women who gave reasons for adopting New Age practices, which included 'as a response to personal trauma' and 'to improve life', outnumbered men by approximately two to one. What is more, while both women and men – almost unanimously – claimed that association with the New Age had positively changed their lives, a greater proportion of women reported that they became more self-empowered and more healed by their activities than men appear to have been. In fact, out of

5   Marilyn Ferguson, 1982.

nine categories, only one was thought by men to have more positive effects than by women – that of becoming more playful (40% to 36% respectively).

Participants themselves are aware of the increasing female content and the high numbers of women active in the New Age. For instance, some women attribute this, as a middle-aged college lecturer stated, to a 'resurgence of the female principles of caring/nurturing' or, as an older stress and bereavement counsellor and hospice nurse wrote, 'male is no longer so dominant, therefore female energies, gifts, visions, etc., [are] now more free and influential in hopefully leading to correct [the] balance between male and female.' This view is shared by some men as they, too, appear to seek a new balance. For example, in describing the New Age, a middle-aged blue-green algae distributor saw that it was 'an ending of old worn out ways of living and thinking. There is an emergence of the Ancient Feminine Ways of the Earth lore. There is a developing harmony between opposites and a movement towards non-duality.'

A final note relating to the gender of association needs to be added with regard to participant's marital status. Nearly two-thirds of the total sample reported that they were in a partnership (60%), which is very slightly less than the population average; approximately 40% were single, which is slightly higher than the national figure; and there was no noteworthy difference between the genders.[6]

Even though the above descriptions have highlighted what are the by and large most visible female characteristics, only in a few instances are the differences particularly marked; although the clear fact is that the large majority of people who are active in the New Age are women. Men appear less interested in the majority of New Age ideas and activities – or participate less in them – in relation to their appeal to women; and it must be anticipated that men who are active in the New Age hold convictions which welcome a greater balance and harmony of gender differences in society. In fact, a view commonly held by those – women and men – associated with the New Age is that

6   The UK population figures for marital status in 1991 were: married and cohabiting women 62%, men 68%; single, widowed, or divorced women 38%, men 32% (cited in M. J. Waterson, 1993: 15).

their activities essentially incorporate a harmonization of feminine and masculine elements[7] – moreover, they would argue that in time the New Age will remove most patriarchal aspects from Western (and indeed all) society.[8]

Age

Survey findings show that although participants can be found in most age groups, there is a significant concentration in one particular range. In the UK almost 60% are aged 35–54, which contrasts with the equivalent national population figure of less than 30%; and in the US the situation is similar, although there is a larger older New Age population (how much older is not possible to tell from the figures available). In both the UK and US all those surveyed over the age of 35 account for around 80% of its population, which contrasts with the equivalent national population figures for both countries at or just under 50%. The detailed findings are demonstrated separately in Tables 2 and 3.

7   Also of importance in the New Age is the awareness of, as well as the balance of, male and female aspects (the anima and animus) within each individual as described by Carl Jung (1971: 410f) whose writings, as will be shown, have been important to many of those involved.

8   An argument that the New Age is in fact as patriarchal as Western society in general is put forward by, for example, Monica Sjoo (1994).

Table 2. Age profile of UK New Age and national populations

UK Age Group	% New Age	% National[9]
under 24	3	33
25–34	16	16
35–44	30	14
45–54	27	11
55–64	14	10
over 65	10	16

Table 3. Age profile of US New Age and national populations

US Age Group	% New Age[10]	% National[11]
under 35	23	56
35–49	42	21
over 50	35	23

The finding here is that about half of all those involved appear to have been born in the decades of the 1940s and 1950s and grew up in the period of the 1960s counter-culture.

Further conclusions can be drawn from these figures. Firstly, there is a large proportion of participants who are aged 50 or over, and who were mostly born prior to the Second World War: we can also see that around a quarter or more of those involved belong to pre-

9   Resident population of Great Britain cited in M. J. Waterson, 1993: 8.
10   Frederick Levine, 1989: 83.
11   Philip's World Atlas, 1997, 7th Edition. London: George Philip (figures rounded).

counter-cultural generations, though many of whom may not have been directly involved in some of its earliest activities. Secondly, the proportion of participants in the New Age who are aged under 35 is small, yet this age group represents a large proportion of the national populations. Two reasons might account for this finding. On the one hand, a possible weakness in the survey sampling methods is that subscribers to magazines in general tend to be older or, to put it another way, more established in terms of their buying habits. On the other hand, the younger population might be more interested in other ideas, for example, to do with paganism[12] and/or 'rave' culture.[13] With regards to paganism, comparative age information has been provided for New Age participants which clearly shows a much younger age profile.[14] It can be speculated that pagan and rave activities perhaps form two platforms from which younger generations may, later in their lives, move into the New Age, although there are likely to be other more compelling routes of entry as well – for example, through healing or ecology.[15]

Thirdly, through subgroup analysis of the UK findings, and unsurprisingly, it appears that a greater number of younger participants have been associated with the New Age for a shorter period than those who are older, and that only 10% of the older population have recently become involved, as Table 4 demonstrates.

12   As Paul Heelas suggests (1996a: 126).
13   As Nicholas Saunders suggests (1995: 61). Use of the term 'rave', as Saunders suggests, is 'an outdated connotation [... to describe events] where people dance and use Ecstasy' (Op. cit.: 3). Saunders does not give actual age information of ravers in his study but cites research carried out by Harris Opinion Polls which was undertaken solely among the 16–25 age group, thereby suggesting that there might not be many 'ravers' outside of this age range. Moreover, the links between rave culture and the New Age are tenuous because, as Hillegonda Rietveld suggests, no other motivation for participation in raves can be found than that of a temporary escape from daily realities (1993: 69).
14   Michael York, 1995: 211.
15   Discussed in Chapters 7 and 8 respectively.

Table 4. Length of association with the New Age by age

Age Group	Under 35	35–54	Over 55
Sample Size	(169) %	(522) %	(217) %
up to 4 years	41	19	10
5–10 years	28	27	22
over 10 years	26	53	65
no answer	5	2	4

The figures given in Table 4 clearly demonstrate that the majority of participants – even in the younger age group – have been associated with the New Age for a considerable length of time; they also provide evidence that counter-culturalists continue to maintain interest in, and practice, 'alternative' ideas and activities. In addition, further analysis has shown that there is no marked difference between genders in each of the three age categories given in Table 4.

Returning to discussion of the largest age group, the middle-aged, these form what has been described as the baby-boom generation. In Tables 2 and 3 it was shown that this group accounts for 57% of UK participants and (most likely) around 50% of those in the US. In this regard, one commentator points out that 'the new age is a product of the baby-boom phenomenon, the '60s generation.'[16] This view is supported, for example, by my visual observation of delegates at an Alternatives conference in London, where most of the c.500 participants were aged 30–50, and by a journalist who reports that most of

16 Ken Wilber, 1987: 11. A study of 'the spiritual journeys of the baby-boom generation' by Wade Clark Roof (1993, updated in 1999), provides a comprehensive overview of the American generation's approaches to predominantly traditional religiosity; George Gallup jr and Jim Castelli also suggest that older baby-boomers are becoming more interested in religion than previously (1989: 130f); and see also Paul Heelas, 1996a: 171ff.

the 50 or so participants and staff at New Age workshops on the Greek island of Skyros were similarly aged.[17]

In summary, it has been established that the majority of participants in the New Age are in the middle-age group. However, whether or not significant numbers of younger people will become associated as they get older cannot be foretold, although, from the findings of my research, this does not appear to be happening to any large degree. Indications are, it has been shown, that the younger generations do not appear to be turning to New Age ideas and activities in such significant numbers as those who were instrumental in the New Age's occurring in the way it has. One of the prime reasons for this is likely to be the fact that many New Age ideas and activities have now become part of the cultural mainstream, and so have lost their urgency. The New Age may very well have an ageing – and therefore diminishing – population in the years to come.

Social status

Clearly, study of the surveys show that the majority of those involved in the New Age are, in the main, middle class – that is, social groups A, B, and C1;[18] and looking at the occupations of participants, the

---

17 Janet Watts, 1995: 58.
18 Each participant in my survey was assessed for social and demographic grouping by utilizing the Interviewers' Guide on Social Grading cited in Donald Monk, 1970: Appendix A. Where no occupation was given, or where classification was not straightforward – for example, if it was stated that the occupation was 'houseparent' – occupation was assessed in association with income levels. The National Readership Survey's (NRS) adults' social grade definitions are cited in M. J. Waterson, 1993: 11: A = Upper Middle Class – higher managerial, administration, or professional; B = Middle Class – intermediate managerial, administrative, or professional; C1 = Lower Middle Class – supervisory or clerical, junior managerial, administrative, or professional; C2 = Skilled Working Class – skilled manual workers; D = Working Class – semi and unskilled manual workers; E = those at the lowest level of subsistence – state pensioners or widows, casual or lowest-grade workers.

findings show that many of the professions are represented – including teaching, health, and civil service – as well as managers, administrators, and sales personnel in commerce and industry. Moreover, there are clearly defined occupations in which participants in the New Age are more likely to be found. Of significant interest, my survey results show that 20% claim to be practitioners in New Age activities, the majority to do with healing, and that one in eight participants are retired. Of the remaining classified occupations, the educational professions (12%),[19] managerial and sales (12%, and incorporating a strong male bias), and conventional health professions (7%) appear to be the most significant employment groups claimed by participants. Yet, by and large, a huge variety of occupations was given, some of which include: accountants, artists, builders, chiropractors, computer operators, dowsers, electronic testers, a grave digger, masseurs, nurses, police officers, psychotherapists, sales representatives, secretaries, shop managers, teachers (university, secondary, and primary), therapists (63 types), and yoga instructors.[20]

Turning to the matter of income levels, the income reported is across all levels, as Table 5 demonstrates.

---

19   The educational professions subgroup analysis reveals 22% earning under £5,000 per annum, although only 7% are aged under 25, thereby suggesting that few younger students are involved in the New Age.

20   The classifications of the UK and US surveys differ; but it is interesting to compare the results of the UK survey with those produced by Margot Adler in her 1985 questionnaire among American pagans. The findings are quite similar with two notable exceptions – firstly, Adler's survey reveals a bias of occupation towards the computer industry; and, secondly, Adler's survey includes no retired respondents, thus perhaps further verifying the view that pagans tend to be younger than participants in the New Age. Adler's comparable figures are: therapist 9%; unclassified (including computer personnel) 32%; retired (not listed); teacher, student, librarian 14%; managerial and sales 15%; nurse, carer, social worker 9%; houseparent 4%; writer, painter, graphic artist 11%; and secretarial, clerical 7% (1986: 446f). The findings of the American *Body, Mind & Spirit* 'Spirituality Survey' with regard to occupation were: professional/technician 25%, retired/unemployed 19%, managerial and sales combined 17%, clerical 13%, and service 12% (cited in Levine, 1989: 83).

Table 5. Income levels of New Age participants

	% New Age	% National[21]
Under £5,000	19	17
£5,000–9,999	21	33
£10,000–14,999	18	23
£15,000–19,999	16	13
£20,000–29,999	14	9
over £30,000	7	5
No Answer	5	–

As can be seen, nearly 60% of those involved earn less than £15,000 per annum, although this is a smaller percentage than the UK national average (73%). The higher income groups – that is, of over £15,000 per annum – represent 37% of participants in comparison to 27% for the UK population as a whole.

Further analysis shows that women and older participants tend to earn less, while men and participants in the middle-age group tend to earn more. This result may well be similar to the situation in the mainstream – which, if this is the case, demonstrates that there is no real marked difference between those in the New Age and society as a whole in terms of income. With regard to a person's age, the findings show that the middle-age group of participants can be found in large numbers at all income levels and that there is no predominance of, for example, younger participants at the lower income levels.

Clearly, those associated with the New Age are almost wholly middle class and a substantial majority – for instance, those working in the education and health fields, together with the large number who claim to be New Age practitioners – work in sectors of service for the benefit of the community at large. Furthermore, a similarly large number, although not the majority, claim higher than average income levels. This evidence – service to the community in a broad sense, a

21 Inland Revenue figures for the distribution of total income of individuals before tax in the UK in 1990/91 cited in M. J. Waterson, 1993: 14.

spectrum of income levels from very little to a great deal, and a range of employment types – suggests that a wide variety of individuals, albeit wholly middle class, share degrees of a common ideological focus in the New Age.

Reasons for association

Participants were asked to describe in their own words what specifically influenced them to adopt the New Age ideas and activities that they had. Of the replies, many variables were identified and these were clustered into six themes. In summary, the findings demonstrate that there exists no overarching single reason for association which, at least numerically, is particularly significant. The six identified themes include association for spiritual development, interest, or to seek wisdom, 24%; to improve lifestyle or dissatisfaction with the norm, 14%; because the ideas made sense, 10%; unconsciously led to the ideas, 9%; as a response to personal trauma, 8%; and through the influence of specific teachings or teachers, 8%. Numerous other reasons were given by a minority, of which most were mentioned by 1% or less, although two reasons were both mentioned by 3% – the experience of specific paranormal phenomena or that they had been brought up in a New Age environment. Personal recommendation as a reason for adopting New Age practices – in many other fields frequently an important contributing factor – appears to play very little overt part in the process, as only 1% mentioned this route.

The numerically widest-held theme of association relates broadly to the idea that those involved are proactive in seeking out ways and means to foster inner development or to make contact with their Higher Self. The descriptions they used included such phrases as becoming involved in the New Age for personal experience and interest, to search for truth, to answer the need for meaning and authenticity, spiritual hunger, and searching for God; and an older social services manager wrote that she selected 'tools for growth but I am not a

92

"joiner" or a follower. I try to create my own path to wholeness, seeking to integrate the eternal truths in my search for the Divine.'

Of the remaining five themes, each mentioned by between 8% and 14% of participants, the first relates to the view that adopting New Age ideas and activities is generally beneficial, and was described as to feel better, to improve lifestyle, to be more ethical, for a reason to be, for peace and happiness, and dissatisfaction – with traditional norms, or the Church, or materialism. A young TV executive wrote about 'the failure of family, school, college, or church or temple to help [her] feel empowered, whole, and serene', and a middle-aged foster carer pointed out 'how bankrupt emotionally and spiritually [her] life was' prior to becoming associated with some of the ideas.

Next, there were those who found the ideas and activities of the New Age made sense to them. This was as if, after contact with the New Age, things 'clicked' and their lives started working in a much improved way; described by a workshop leader who thought that 'they make more sense than religious bullshit and deal with reality not dogma', and a retired man wrote that 'they made sense of events in my life and explained why people act as they do. They offered ways for me to develop more of my latent qualities and understandings.'

The remaining three themes provide more specific reasons for association, and include the idea that external or other forces of various kinds exert mostly unconscious influences on participants thereby stimulating a change in direction. Participants wrote about being consciously or unconsciously led, about being activated, and having intuitive insights. Traumatic life events, coupled with a desire for self-healing, were also reasons given by some. These events included the death of a loved one, serious illness, near-death experience, or the effects of drug-related experience. A 36-year-old housewife studying nutritional medicine wrote of her experiences of 'grief, mind-expanding drugs, and personal yearning. I am searching for inner contentment, bliss with lifestyle, seeking to be more in harmony with nature and my fellow man/woman every day.' Finally, the influence of teachings or teachers was mentioned by some as being their route to association. In this theme, many names were given – firstly with regard to teachings, for example: Reiki, homoeopathy, various psychotherapies, yoga, Shamanism, and astrology; and, secondly, from teachers including: Adi Da, Sai Baba, Edgar Cayce, Carl Jung, Jiddu Krishnamurti, and José Silva.

Overall, these six themes demonstrate the spread of reasons the majority of participants gave to describe why they had become associated with the New Age. However, in the final analysis, these themes cannot be viewed as being entirely separate from one another. The conclusion must be that, as a result of many influences, the overriding reason that women and men have for becoming associated with the New Age appears to be that they discover something quite significantly wrong with their lives – mostly on a personal and individual level but also socially or both – *and* they adopt some of its ideas and activities to put things right in terms of becoming more spiritual, and more balanced, harmonious, and fulfilled. This 'something wrong' is not necessarily seen as a negative occurrence as, more often than not, it is claimed to be a challenging – even exciting – adventure leading to a spiritually transformed and, they hope, improved way of leading their lives.

Frequency of activities

In order to provide a context for the description of the frequency of activities, it is important to establish how long those involved have been active in New Age pursuits. It is clear that participants are well established in their activities, as just over half claimed association of over 10 years, and many claimed considerably longer. Moreover, a further quarter had been involved for at least five years. With regard to demographic differences, there was very little disparity in the length of association between women and men, although there is greater difference with regard to their age, as is demonstrated in Table 6. Unsurprisingly, younger people have been associated for a shorter period while, conversely, older people have been associated for much longer.

94

Table 6. Length of time associated with the New Age by age

Age Group	All	Under 35	35–54	Over 55
Sample Size	(908) %	(169) %	(522) %	(217) %
Up to six months	1	1	1	0
1 year	1	3	1	1
1–2 years	4	8	4	1
3–4 years	15	29	13	8
5–10 years	26	28	27	22
Over 10 years	51	26	53	65
No answer	3	5	2	4

What is interesting from Table 6 is the sparsity of those claiming association of two years duration or less; and that, numerically, there are more people aged 35–54 than under 35 in this group.

Several findings from the survey lead to the view that high levels of continuing activity occur in the New Age and that, in many instances, association is not usually temporary. The most important of these findings include, firstly, that 90% of participants report that they meditate at least occasionally. In fact, four out of ten claimed to meditate daily, and of these many claim to do so more frequently. As might be imagined, older participants meditate more often and the younger less so. Secondly, participants were asked to state whether they had ever and whether they currently engaged in each of a large number activities which occur in the New Age (although these activities were not necessarily New Age activities *per se*). The results are highly interesting because, while not being wholly comprehensive, they point to the most commonly used ideas and activities to be found in the New Age. Participants were further asked to name any other activities which they used, and none was mentioned to any significant degree. This means that the ideas and activities which are central to the New Age are included in the following list, where they are ordered in terms of numerical popularity and frequency of use. Table 7 reveals the most-used activity to be creative visualization.

Table 7. New Age activities 'ever' and 'currently' practised

	% Ever	% Currently
Sample Size	(899)	(783)
creative visualization	80	43
recycling	74	47
aromatherapy	73	30
massage	73	29
crystals	71	32
homoeopathy	71	28
vegetarianism	71	39
flower remedies	70	32
healing workshops	67	26
t'ai chi ch'uan/yoga	67	25
reflexology	64	17
acupuncture/shiatsu	57	15
herbalism	57	20
spiritualism	55	18
Buddhism	50	12
channelling	49	18
colour therapy	48	15
Green politics	45	13
earth mysteries	43	16
psychotherapy	42	13
hypnotherapy	39	8
past life therapy	39	8
shaman/pagan rituals	35	15
sound therapy	34	12
Alexander technique	32	6
dance therapy	30	8

transactional analysis	21	3
women's groups	20	5
ethical investing	18	10
NLP	18	4
rebirthing	18	1
veganism	14	4

Analysis of the findings given in Table 7 shows that many of the activities were currently – at the time of the research – a part of the participants' lives; and, furthermore, a number of these activities were normally practised daily or regularly. For example, almost half claimed to recycle their waste, two out of five were vegetarians, the same number practised visualization techniques, approximately 30% claimed to practice aromatherapy, the same number used crystals, flower remedies, homoeopathic remedies, and massage therapies. What is more, a quarter of participants practised t'ai chi or yoga. In total, over 80% of those involved had at some time practised more than 10 of the activities listed, the mean average being just over 15. With regards to those activities which were in use at the time of the survey, 58% were currently using at least 5 of the practices listed, some as many as 10 or more, the mean average being just under 7.[22]

Finally, frequency measures of several other activities adds further to the view that in the case of these participants New Age activity levels in general are high. For example, participants appear to be avid readers of books on New Age or related subjects – in fact, over a third of younger participants and around 60% of all others claim to have read in excess of 50 such books. Almost all claim to have read at least some books on New Age subjects. Additionally, half claim membership of – or contribute to – a variety of pressure groups, especially environmental groups such as Greenpeace and Friends of the Earth; although current membership of politically-oriented groups – such as

22   The exact mean averages are: activities ever used 15.31, activities currently in use 6.62.

Amnesty International, Tibet Support Group, or the Green Party – is considerably lower.[23]

With regard to attending a New Age event – for example, a workshop, lecture, exhibition or festival, or retreat – 86% claimed to have ever participated in at least one. Out of attendance at any of these types of events in a 12-month period, Table 8 demonstrates that workshops appear to have been most frequently attended, with approximately three-quarters of those claiming to have attended a workshop attending at least two.

Table 8. Frequency of attending New Age events
in a 12-month period

	Workshop %	Lecture %	Exhibition/ Festival %	Retreat %
none attended	46	59	52	81
Attended				
1	16	15	30	15
2–3	20	16	17	3
4–5	9	4	1	1
6–9	6	2	0	0
over 10	4	5	0	0

Clearly, the vast majority of participants attend New Age events of one sort or another, and it is likely that around half attend at least one workshop, lecture, and exhibition in a year. Demographically, there is little noticeable difference in attendance between genders, except that a slightly higher proportion of men attend workshops; and older people, in this case all those aged over 45, attend workshops and retreats more so than younger participants. In fact, visual observation I

---

23   The subject of membership of groups is further discussed in Chapter 8.

have made through attending many New Age fairs, festivals, work-shops, and retreats has demonstrated a younger attendee age profile at more lightweight events than that recorded at the more 'serious' events such as at the Alternatives conference and New Age workshops or lectures – for example, those given by the American spiritual teacher Ram Dass.

In all, participants demonstrate significant levels of activities whether privately, for example in the form of spiritual and visualiza-tion practices, the use of various therapies, and environmental activi-ties, or more publicly, for example in attendance at events. However, the large majority of activities appear to be private concerns.

Drugs

Looking at the subject of drug use, soft drugs appear to have been sampled or used by a large minority, although their continued use does not appear to be widespread. Many reported that they have used can-nabis at some point in their lives (38%), although only approximately one in eight claimed to currently use it. With regard to psychedelic drugs,[24] less than 10% reported ever having used them, and only a very small minority (2%) claimed to be current users. In all cases, drug use was rare among those over 55 years old, and strongest among the under 35s and men.

This scant use of drugs is a far cry from the 1960s blossoming of the New Age. In the processes people went through at that time to en-act change, the use of psychedelic drugs was one of the principal ve-hicles that were used – one commentator finding that it 'is impossible to overestimate the historic role of psychedelics as an entry point',[25] but she goes on to argue that 'chemical *satori* is perishable [...] For whatever glories the mushrooms and saturated sugar cubes contained, they were only a glimpse [...] Non-drug psychotechnologies offer a

24 The survey was anonymous.
25 Marilyn Ferguson, 1982: 93.

controlled, sustained movement towards that spacious reality.'[26] Another writer points out that by the 1980s New Age teachings no longer encouraged the use of psychedelics.[27] In the 1990s the use of anything other than softer, recreational drugs – probably to a similar extent as in mainstream society – does not appear to be a part of the New Age. In fact, intoxication by any substance – marijuana, tobacco, alcohol, even coffee – is seen by many as detrimental to a transformed way of being.

Paranormal influences

Many of William Bloom's six basic New Age ideas, described in Chapter 1, incorporate aspects of what can broadly be described as paranormal influence and, as reported earlier in this chapter, almost one quarter of participants have described the rise of the New Age at this time to be caused by the influx of positive external forces or energy to the planet. It is not surprising, therefore, that those involved declare there has been a considerable penetration of paranormal influences into the spectrum of New Age ideas and activities. The vast majority of participants – 82% in the UK, and 78% in the US[28] – have experienced paranormal phenomena, and of many different types including telepathy (52%), precognition (44%),[29] clairvoyance (41%), past life recall (41%), and synchronicity (41%).[30] What is more, those

---

26   Op. cit.: 94
27   Wouter Hanegraaff, 1996: 11.
28   Frederick Levine, 1989: 83.
29   As a comparison with the UK population at large, the Gallup Political and Economic Index (1989: 9), reports that, for example, the incidence in experience of precognition is 24% – just over half the incidence which is reported by participants in the New Age.
30   It will be recalled (from Table 6) that 55% of participants have also experienced spiritualism, and 49% have experienced channelling.

involved claimed multiple experiences of particular phenomenon, and 51% claimed experience of four or more types.[31]

Anyone, it is claimed, has the ability to experience paranormal phenomena,[32] and these events are reported to occur either spontaneously or be induced in a variety of ways. Methods of inducement, it can be added, include meditation and self- or assisted hypnosis. Paranormal or psychic experience was, in the same way as the use of psychedelic drugs, an important stimulus for New Age activity in the 1960s[33] although according to my survey and unlike drug use, such experience still remains a vital part of the New Age for many of those involved.

What is positive about the New Age ...

When asked whether or not associating with the New Age created positive changes to their lives, 1% (less than ten individuals) claimed it had not; practically all others reported that their engagement was beneficial. Nine variables were listed to assess more precisely which positive changes might have been most important, and the most important reasons given were 'more spiritual' (82%) and 'more meaningful' (80%). Moreover, other important reasons included being happier (72%), more fulfilled (71%), more Self-empowered (71%), and more healed (66%). The New Age appears to be least about increasing pleasures and playfulness, as these notions scored lowest out of the nine given benefits at 47% and 37% respectively. As previously mentioned, it was only with regard to playfulness that men scored more highly than women. Additionally, a quarter of participants added further positive attributes to their descriptions of the New Age. These

31   The mean average of the varieties experienced was 4.33.
32   Rosemary Ellen Guiley, 1991: 470. Rupert Sheldrake, a biologist active in the New Age, has developed the notion of morphic resonance which attempts to shed light on everyday paranormal experiences (1988, 1994).
33   Marilyn Ferguson, 1982: 93.

included becoming more wise, more sociable, more content, more positive, and having a greater sense of balance.

Overall, the findings show that those involved claim to obtain highly significant, life-enhancing benefits by adopting New Age ideas and activities. It would appear that to these people the New Age is not a meaningless or hedonistic playground, although, as has been noted, both play and pleasure do form a part of the total perceived advantages of the New Age. Increased spirituality and meaningfulness seem to be the key positive attributes for participants, and they report that their lives are much improved as a result of their activities. What is more, comparing these findings to participants' descriptions of the New Age (given above), greater spirituality continues to be seen as being one of the most – if not the most – important outcome of association with the New Age.

... and negative

Having claimed such overwhelmingly positive attributes from their association with the New Age, it is entirely logical that participants claim very little in the way of negative occurrences. Free rein was given for participants in my survey to describe any negatives they wished and just over a third stated that there had been some such instances. Yet the negative cases that were reported, paradoxically, were frequently seen to have played a positive part in an individual's spiritual growth and transformation processes.

The most mentioned negative change was not a specific 'fault', rather it was a general feeling which can be encapsulated by the expression 'there's no gain without pain'. Becoming involved in the New Age was not seen to be all plain sailing, and this view was registered by 16% of participants, that is, in the region of half of all of those describing any negative occurrence. Some examples given by participants illustrate what can happen: 'you go through hell', 'having to wade through your own shit', 'like the chrysalis and the butterfly';

and a middle-aged secretary spoke of 'not negative, but as I changed my life changed and it was difficult to get through the hurt and pain caused. All was for the best, and now the apparent negative times have led to a wonderful life.'

Two more specific negative instances were raised. The first and numerically largest of these (9%) revolves around problems to do with personal relationships caused through adopting New Age practices – although, here again, in many cases this was perceived as being ultimately positive. The adoption caused breaks with parents, with life-long friends, and even resulted in divorce. Some participants wrote about friends, relatives, or partners being negative about the New Age or of the changes which were occurring, of not being understood, and of alienation. Specifically about problems with partners, a middle-aged hypnotherapist wrote that 'I left my husband because he couldn't accept my ideas and me being stronger', and a middle-aged head teacher revealed that 'at the moment my wife thinks I'm mad and is a little frightened of the changes that she can see. Unfortunately she is not yet willing to follow me.'

Finally, 4% of participants mentioned the idea that the New Age and the 'old' age were not mutually conducive, that attempts to live in both caused problems, and this was a view held predominantly by younger people. This view is summed up by a younger woman who found it 'impossible to have a selfish, greedy outlook on [my] career – in current society, not a positive attribute for getting on.' This view was again found in the survey among mostly American Aquarian Conspirators. Here, it is reported that 'Some of the sharpest internal conflict reported in the survey was in a struggle to reconcile the old work with the new perspective'[34] and found that vocation, intuition, a clearer sense of self, wholeness, and connectedness were the qualities which came particularly to the fore in the relationship between the transformational process and a person's career.[35]

As is to be expected, the views reported here show that those involved demonstrate a highly favourable view of association with the New Age. Adoption of its ideas and activities brings about changes to

34   Op. cit.: 376f.
35   Op. cit.: 377f.

their lives which are seen to be, in the end, beneficial and rewarding on many levels – for example, spiritually, in relationships with other people, and in everyday activities. Few widely held negative views have been revealed except in terms of a discomfort which occurs for some during the process of change.

Summary

This chapter has sought to give answers to some of the more basic questions regarding the characteristics of association with the New Age. The social and demographic profile of those involved is not extraordinary, and there is no single description which can accurately be applied to clearly distinguish them from the population at large. Participants in the New Age, on the whole, are drawn from many walks of life, many ages, and many income levels. Only two facts stand out substantially – firstly, almost without exception, participants are middle class and, secondly, almost three-quarters of the New Age population is female.

Moreover, a commonly held view is that the New Age offers a way for many to improve their lives, which they see to be unfulfilled or with little deeper meaning or significance. Mainstream Western norms are viewed as shallow and without substance. Many varied 'tools' are used to carry out and maintain transformational change – their lifestyle changes and, for some, so do their relationships. They do not use mind-altering drugs, although the experience of, or openness to, paranormal phenomena is widely seen to be an intrinsic part of the influential mix of ideas. As is to be expected, those involved raise few negatives about their association but point out that it is not necessarily a wholly comfortable way of life. Furthermore, what participants have revealed so far is wholly in accord with the six basic New Age ideas outlined in Chapter 1.

A picture is now emerging which characterizes what association with the New Age can entail. It paints a portrait of those involved.

These individuals want radical (but not revolutionary) change – a transformation – and this involves creating a much stronger spiritual and meaningful content to their lives. However, they are not especially attracted to specific religious movements, either traditional or contemporary. Those involved say that they also need to move away from materialism which, in their view, has dis-eased contemporary ways of being.

4. Getting Involved

Whatever strategies I choose for learning and acting, they should, of course, reflect my individual interests, skills, and talents and the needs or characteristics of my environment; it is better for me to do what I can do best in the moment (and perhaps learn to do more later) and what is in harmony with my nature than to attempt to follow someone else's master blueprint or an idealized, abstract strategy presented in a book. For me, one of the empowering aspects about this process of emergence is that we must find our own way into it and discover for ourselves what our best contributions may be.

David Spangler[1]

The main feature of getting involved with the New Age is that it appears to occur primarily in two distinct directions which can broadly be described as inner change and external action – the former being of greater importance than the latter – and each is now studied in turn. However, with regard to actions, by no means all activities are adopted and practised by all people interested in the New Age, although many commentators – especially critics – do not attempt to separate out the varieties. Instead, they often lump all New Age individuals together as one group as if they all practised the same ideas and activities for the same reasons or to the same degree. Nothing could be further from the truth, and this is one of the reasons why the term 'New Age' is much disliked by many participants. Examination of the two directions is followed by a more theoretical discussion of the different forms of involvement individuals have with the New Age, again in two principal ways: on the one hand, according to various categories and, on the other hand, by different levels.

1   David Spangler, 1984: 90.

Going within

Any form of meaningful contact with the New Age usually involves making some type of contact with what participants term as higher levels of consciousness, and for them this is mostly a solitary process – what is known as 'going within' – through which many believe that a more significant or ultimate guidance to their lives can be found. It has been suggested that there are three general ways of encountering the New Age which, in this instance, are described as: *experience*, of the transformation going on in the world, *imagination*, in the sense of the capacity to form images, and *intuition*.[2] Of these three, knowledge gained from previous and current experiences is of course a valuable guide, although often what participants encounter by going within appears to be outside such experience; and the focus of imagination in this description revolves around bringing into focus ideas and concepts in areas where words are inadequate to comprehend or communicate what is going on. In the case of intuition, those involved stress that a form of direct wisdom exists which is not derived from sensory experience or from reason. As a consequence, intuition is seen to form a vital faculty in the New Age, one which most of all appears to facilitate the process of going within. It can be added that this process has been seen to be deeply spiritual.[3] How intuition relates to the New Age is now explored.

The psychologist Carl Jung, whose writings and ideas have made a significant impact on many involved in the New Age, has discussed intuition at length in his work *Psychological Types*.[4] Jung believes that there are 'four ways of mental functioning: thought, feeling, sensation and intuition. The first two are rational and deductive, the second two are irrational and immediate.'[5] The way in which Jung believes the power of intuition to function is described as being 'like a sensation in that it (i) perceives unconsciously, e.g. when it uses the result of an

2   David Spangler and William Irwin Thompson, 1991: 46.
3   Ibid.
4   Carl Jung, 1921.
5   K. W. Wild, 1938: 51.

unconscious perception, assumes it as a fact; (ii) perceives what is in the unconscious mind'.[6] The importance of this definition to the New Age is that by bringing intuitive perception more to the fore, those involved claim to be able to work towards, or are more receptive to, transforming their lives to a new way of being. Moreover, they would claim that an intuitively perceived fact is considerably more 'valuable' than any given fact.

Further describing what occurs with intuition, it has been described as 'our term for knowing that [which] can't be tracked';[7] and it is suggested that the term is defined as '"quick perception of truth without conscious attention or reasoning", "knowledge from within" [and] "instinctive knowledge or feeling associated with clear and concentrated vision"'.[8] Moreover, a person 'who becomes involved in the psychotechnologies realizes that those inner urgings and "hunches" do not contradict reason but represent transcendent reasoning [which] becomes a trusted partner in everyday life, available to guide even minor decisions, generating an ever more pervasive sense of flow and rightness'.[9] The importance of the right-hemisphere functions of the brain and the power of intuition in the context of the New Age is demonstrated by the same commentator in suggesting that the 'left brain can organize new information into the existing scheme of things, but *it cannot generate new ideas. The right brain sees contexts – and, therefore, meaning* [...] Every breakthrough, every leap forward in history, has depended on right-brain insights, the ability of the holistic brain to detect anomalies, process novelty, perceive relationships'

6   Op. cit.: 52. Wild has given 31 definitions of intuition (1938: 211ff), which are then condensed into two: 'A. "An intuition is an immediate awareness by a subject, of some particular entity, without such aid from the senses or from reason as would account for that awareness."   B. "Intuition is a method by which a subject becomes aware of an entity without such aid from the senses or from reason as would account for such awareness"' (Op. cit.: 226). With regard to religious intuitions, Wild asserts that 'without some such faculty it is difficult to account for the widespread if not universal "faith" in a spiritual world', (Op. cit.: 119).
7   Marilyn Ferguson, 1982: 325.
8   Ibid.
9   Op. cit.: 114f.

(author's italics).[10] In fact, she argues that without intuition the human race would still be in the cave.[11]

In the New Age, therefore, it can be seen that intuition is a human faculty which is not confined by rational thought and which can access higher realms of the human psyche – the conscious, the personal unconscious, and the collective unconscious, if all these states are believed to exist. Many other individuals who are influential to the New Age have written about the role and importance of intuition, and these include Roberto Assagioli,[12] the originator of Psychosynthesis, and Fritjof Capra,[13] a philosopher and physicist. Particularly regarding spirituality, what seems to happen is that 'through deep levels of spiritual intuition, insight, and attunement [...] we encounter the movement and activity of metaphysical forces at work in the world'.[14] Intuition, in this case, must be seen as the most important means through which ideas and activities in the New Age are approached. Moreover, intuition has just the same importance in relation to paranormal phenomena.[15]

10   Op. cit.: 326. It is widely accepted that the two halves of the human brain – the left and right hemispheres – are responsible for different human functions. Language is one of the most obvious functions of the left hemisphere, while the right hemisphere incorporates creativity including, for example, visual recognition and musical ability. See, for instance, T. S. Bennett, 1994: Vol. 1, 183.
11   Marilyn Ferguson, 1982: 326.
12   Roberto Assagioli, 1980: 217ff.
13   Fritjof Capra, 1984: 21ff, 1988: 32, 324. A more detailed study of the psychological view of intuition is given by Tony Bastick, 1982; and the transpersonal view is given by Charles Tart, who suggests that 'intuition is seen as something that can be cultivated, and as something that can give a more profound understanding of many things than reason' (1975: 94). For discussion of transpersonal religious views of intuition see other essays in this volume discussing the Buddhist, yogic, and Christian views. In addition, a comprehensive list of sources with regard to intuition is given in Rosemary Ellen Guiley, 1991: 287f.
14   David Spangler and William Irwin Thompson, 1991: 46.
15   Rosemary Ellen Guiley points out that intuition 'is integral to all forms of divination and psychic consultation' (1991: 286), which includes astrology, channelling, dowsing, I Ching, palmistry, tarot reading, and many other similar such arts which, as we have seen, are used by some of those involved in the New Age.

There is more to be said to get wholly to the crux of what intuition means to those involved in the New Age. First of all, going within is reported to be about listening to what inner voices might be saying. This entails creating the space – time, environment, and receptivity – to be able to 'hear' or intuit clearly, and is one of the reasons why creative visualization and meditation are so important in the New Age. It will be recalled from the previous chapter that almost all of those involved in the New Age claimed to have carried out these practices. This 'listening' includes the attempt, consciously or otherwise, to separate out what the right half of the brain is saying from the left half – that is, putting reason and rationality to one side and becoming intuitively open to that which transcends them. Participants talk about listening to the heart, which is love, not the mind, which is thought and praxis; and many of the meditative processes which are used – including Buddhistic meditation techniques – have this end in mind. David Spangler is right when he talks about the process of going within as being deeply spiritual to those in the New Age, although where what is 'heard' comes from is open to debate. Some participants believe they can intuit God within, in that quietening the mind reveals the existence of a transpersonal and mystical presence – Absolute Reality, or Light, or whatever term is used; others believe that external energies from higher beings can be received, and these beings are described for instance as guiding spirits, guardian angels, or input of various kinds from the Akashic Records. There are many ideas although, in the main, they can be reduced to either a non-dual or dualistic spiritual basis.[16] Which ever might be the case, most of those involved are certain that the human (as mind and body) is not all that exists.

These issues raised with regard to intuition are central to the New Age, and will be referred to time and again as our exploration unfolds. A picture has been provided of how intuition affects the activities of people who could be described as New Age networkers which suggests that:

16   Discussion of non-dual or dualistic spirituality in the New Age will be found in later chapters, particularly the last.

Perhaps the most significant characteristic of people who network is their finely developed sense of intuition, the ability to *feel* what is going on around them. Intuition enables people to know where to go to get information, whom to trust, and in what way to share [...] Sometimes networkers know precisely where to go to find the information they need; more often, they operate on hunches.[17]

Intuition is the fundamental means by which individuals in the New Age claim to obtain what they see as authentic guidance, and hence it can be argued that through such guidance, the possibility of an inner change – that is, what they see as amounting to a transformation of consciousness – could occur. Frequently the intuitive choice appears to be irrational although in reality, to the individual concerned, within intuitive wisdom is found the loci of what they see to be truly authentic.

Physical access

The New Age, as we have seen, is comprised of individuals who each follow many different paths of activities, selecting what they wish to proceed with at any one time. For example, a person who has experienced reflexology may wish to also see how acupuncture might benefit them, or a student of the Self-Realization Fellowship may wish to add an ecological dimension to their spiritual path. This section seeks to identify the *means* by which an individual accesses particular features of the New Age, although it does not attempt to identify the *reasons* why these choices are made.

In the first instance, academics have suggested that the New Age is anti-institutional and decentralized in character and that 'New Agers embrace a loose form of organization called "networking", in which informal contacts among New Age groups are maintained by newsletters, shared phone lists, and word of mouth.'[18] Also from academe,

17   Jessica Lipnack and Jeffrey Stamps, 1982: 257.
18   Philip Lucas: 1992: 205f. Networking is a term used to describe the means by which individuals access ideas and activities in the New Age and how they

another commentator discussing New Age spirituality believes that networks are 'leaderless'[19] and that they 'are cooperative, not competitive'.[20] Consequently, as opposed to the traditional hierarchical and vertical structure of organizations in mainstream society, it can be said that networking in the New Age is much more horizontal and democratic in structure.

In the second instance, and turning to a theoretical analysis of networking as a social and cultural phenomenon in their study of movements as a whole, two observers have found that within reticulated structures of movements

> Cells, or segments of movements [...] are linked into a network in a variety of ways. One type of linkage is the overlapping membership of individual participants. Another kind of linkage is formed by personal ties between leaders of different cells or segments. A third type of reticulation is the activities of traveling evangelists or spokesmen who move across the network contributing to its cohesion and ideological unity. This network also provides a very effective grapevine communication system and logistical financial support system [...] A fourth and very important type of reticulation is what, in a religious movement, would be called a revival meeting. In social or political movements they are termed conferences, mass rallies, or demonstrations. But the function is very similar. It is a mechanism through which various segments of the movement [...] come together temporarily for a specific purpose.[21]

As will be seen, many of the means of access to the New Age appear to involve – in differing degrees – most of the ideas incorporated within these findings. However, because those people who are active in the New Age appear to be following individuated spiritual and healing 'paths', the need for the individual's network to be part of a more structured movement seems to be diminished.[22]

> make contact with other like-minded individuals. The term itself is widely used in many areas – for example, in computer terminology – yet it can be seen that the principles behind the concept of networking as a whole aptly describe some of the processes involved in the New Age.

19   Lisa Woodside, 1993: 160.
20   Ibid.
21   Luther Gerlach and Virginia Hine, 1973: 165f.
22   See Chapter 1 above.

With regards to the practical application of networking, the basic form – or first step – in the process of becoming involved in, or increasing activity in, the New Age appears to be most frequently enacted by means of self-education through reading about the particular subject of interest. The basic sources of this form of information are bookshops and specialist magazines and, increasingly, the Internet. Following this, if the interest in a particular topic is sufficiently strong, further information and instruction can be sought, most likely by attending a workshop or having a consultation.

Naturally, there are other ways of becoming involved in the New Age, but access through literary sources, at least in the first instance, appears to have become increasingly significant. Retail sales statistics show that, during the 1980s, the distribution of books, videos, and audio cassettes on New Age topics increased substantially in volume. Specialist New Age book shops – of which Mysteries in Covent Garden, London, claims in its advertisements to be 'Europe's leading psychic shop and New Age centre', and the Boddhi Tree Bookstore in Los Angeles, California, which is described as 'possibly the largest New Age bookstore in the world'[23] – have increased dramatically in number, and many New Age general shops now have book and networking sections. Additionally, multiple retail chains of booksellers now dedicate large sections of shelf space to New Age, health and healing, and environmental issues.[24]

Specialist magazines, too, have proliferated over the last fifteen years, although they have yet to break into the larger general magazine market. This suggests that there is no significant mass-market attraction to New Age ideas and activities although, it must be pointed out, mass-market magazines – especially womens' magazines – frequently include articles on New Age and related subjects. An example of this has been Leslie Kenton's health and beauty column from 1974 to 1988 in the magazine *Vanity Fair* where 'she rapidly achieved guru status [persuading] her readers to indulge in an array of what were

23 J. Gordon Melton, 1991: 371.
24 See *Publishers Weekly*, 25 September 1987; Steve Bruce, 1995: 104ff; Paul Heelas, 1996a: 113f.

then seen to be outlandish practices'[25] but which have since become common practice.

Low penetration of New Age specialist magazines into the UK mass market can be further illustrated by the fact that, in 1995 alone, two such magazines (*Body Mind Soul*, and *i-to-i*) ceased publication although, in the US, there is much greater variety. In fact, there is a group of nationally or internationally circulated specialist New Age magazines which have established a reputation for their editorial and, in some instances, their networking resource contents. In this regard, it is interesting to see how the principal specialist magazines on New Age subjects have proliferated.

Table 9. Proliferation of specialist New Age magazines

Title	Country	Year of first Publication[26]
Resurgence	UK	1966
The New Journal	US	1974
Yoga Journal	US	1974
One Earth	UK	1976
Human Potential	UK	1978
Body Mind Spirit	US	1981
Magical Blend	US	1983
New Age Journal[27]	US	1983
Caduceus	UK	1987
Kindred Spirit	UK	1987

As can be seen from Table 9, the majority of these specialist magazines were launched between the mid-1970s and mid-1980s, and it would appear that few other major specialist New Age magazines have been launched and remained in circulation since 1987.

25   *Independent on Sunday* magazine, 10 September 1995: 15.
26   Some dates are approximate.
27   The *New Journal* was renamed as *New Age Journal* at this time.

In addition to the more general New Age magazines, there exist a significant number of single-focus specialist magazines which can be included in the range of New Age magazines as a whole and which are in national or international circulation. Examples of these include *Stella Polaris* (UK), first published in 1951 by White Eagle Lodge; *Green Egg* (now relaunched) in 1968 (US); *Whole Earth* in 1975 (US); *Gnosis* in 1986 (US); and two magazines on shamanism – *Shaman's Drum* (US), and *Sacred Hoop* (UK). More-single focus magazines have been launched mainly in the 1990s and these include: *Sage Woman, Personal Transformation, Shambhala Sun, Tricycle, Pan Gaia,* and New Age spiritual guru Andrew Cohen's *What is Enlightenment?*

Not surprisingly, there is a huge number of regional (and even more local) specialist magazines of this type – for example, published in the UK are *Cahoots* in the north of England, *South West Connection* in Wales and the west, and *South East Connection* in the London and the south east; additionally, as an example of those published in the US, *Inner Self* for the Florida area. It is interesting to note, however, that the more general entertainment-listing publications – such as *Time Out* in London and *Village Voice* in New York – contain very little in the way of New Age topics and hardly any networking information at all.[28]

It must also be pointed out that the wider-circulating American specialist magazines listed in Table 9 do not contain much in the way of networking resource information; the focus of these magazines is primarily based on editorial features together with product advertising, while information relating to networking resources is to be found primarily in regional and local magazines. However, in the (smaller) UK, specialist magazines do provide substantial networking-resource sections. As an example, Table 10 provides an analysis of activities by type which were networked in the magazine *Kindred Spirit*, Issue 28.

---

28   The *Village Voice* is much more than simply an entertainment-listing publication.

Table 10. New Age networking in *Kindred Spirit* Issue 28

Type of Activity	No.
Exhibitions	
National exhibition (London)	1
Regional exhibition (Manchester)	1
Provincial exhibitions	6
Conferences	1
Workshops, Courses, and Seminars	
Over one week long[29]	33
One week long	5
Large weekend workshops	11
Small weekend workshops	142
One day workshops	21
Classes/courses (mostly evenings)	13
Lectures	11

From the information given in Table 10, in total 245 entries had been listed for actual dated New Age activities. In addition, there were 102 separate entries offering ongoing and undated courses, seminars, and workshops where readers were requested to apply for further details and/or course prospectuses. In this single issue of *Kindred Spirit* magazine, therefore, while it is not possible accurately to quantify the precise number of events which were available, an estimate would suggest there to be well in excess of 500 events networked in this one issue of one specialist quarterly magazine. Therefore, it is fair to say that opportunities for getting involved with the New Age at the basic level of networking through books and specialist magazines are comprehensively available.

---

29   With regard to the duration of these courses, a course length of one to two years is not uncommon.

Other forms of access to New Age ideas and activities also exist. Education plays an important role in an individual's approach, and an indication of acceptance by the mainstream is illustrated by the number of courses which now have local and national government support. For instance, in Lancaster, UK, the Adult College runs courses on yoga, shiatsu, reflexology, t'ai chi, meditation and self development, and the art of healing.[30] The Department of Continuing Education's Open Studies programme run by Lancaster University offers courses which include Tibetan Buddhist painting, Alexander technique, herbal medicine, NLP (neuro-linguistic programming), and self and human potential.[31] Courses leading to academic qualifications are offered by several universities. For example, the University of Exeter offers postgraduate degrees in complementary health studies, and the University of Surrey – through its Institute for the Development of Human Potential – offers a variety of degrees and diplomas. The Maharishi (Transcendental Meditation) College of Management and Technology at Mentmore Towers, Buckinghamshire, opened its doors in 1996 and planned to become a fully fledged university within five years. In the US, the situation is more developed. For example, the John F. Kennedy University in California has a graduate school for holistic studies, which their prospectus describes is dedicated to the study and exploration of consciousness. The school comprises four departments – Interdisciplinary Consciousness Studies, Transpersonal Psychology, Arts and Consciousness, and Holistic Health. Many more such examples exist. In fact, one source[32] lists 49 US and Canadian institutions offering undergraduate degree programmes incorporating New Age topics, together with 26 offering graduate programmes, and a further 27 offering unaccredited degree programmes. Moreover, also listed are 143 institutions offering other kinds of New Age education, and examples of such institutions include the Academy of Chinese Culture and Health Sciences to the University of the Trees and the Whole Life College.

---

30   City of Lancaster *Adult College Course Guide*, Spring 1996.
31   Lancaster University *Open Studies Courses Guide*, January–April 1996.
32   J. Gordon Melton *et al.*, 1990: 517ff.

However, given the criticism by some that the New Age is amorphous, the question needs to be asked: Does there exist an integrated form of structure through which access to its ideas and activities is available? To answer this question it is necessary to survey the possible existence of a closer-knit type of network where, for example, attendance at seminars, workshops, and lectures might lead like-minded individuals to cooperate more closely in specific fields of interest.

One of the most notable forms of closer-knit New Age network in the UK is likely to be that of Alternatives, founded by William Bloom and others in the early 1980s, and based at St James's Church in Piccadilly, London – an Anglican church where the former rector was the Reverend Donald Reeves. Alternatives describes itself as being

> dedicated to creative spiritual alternatives to currently accepted Western thought. Our purpose is to provide a friendly atmosphere in which to taste the best of these ideas. We are dedicated to the freedom of each individual to choose their own path of personal and spiritual growth. We are dedicated to exploring new consciousness.[33]

Alternatives provides a forum whereby many New Age (or, as Alternatives seems to prefer to call it, 'new consciousness') ideas and activities can be experienced. For instance, on Monday evenings throughout most of the year, talks are held on a wide range of topics whose titles include (from the above-cited programme) Journeys through Time (past-life therapy), Rebuilding Communities, The Eco-Spiritual Revolution, Work as an Expression of Who We Are, and Feng Shui Made Easy. Additionally, occasional workshops of various durations are held on such subjects as attitudes to money, psychic protection, Holotropic breathwork, and the contents of James Redfield's book *The Celestine Prophecy*.[34] In May 1994, a two-day conference and networking event 'A New Consciousness' attracted approximately 500 delegates, many of whom were regular attendees at Alternatives' events. The Alternatives circle of influence is further extended by a

---

33   Alternatives' *Summer/Autumn Programme*, 1995.
34   James Redfield, 1994.

network of subscribing 'friends' who numbered perhaps as many as 1,000 in 1991.[35]

Apart from occasional social events, the above-described activities encompass in total what the Alternatives network sets out to accomplish. Alternatives is dedicated, as it has stated, wholly to help individuals discover their own pathways to personal or spiritual growth. Consequently, it seems that Alternatives would argue that there is no requirement or benefit in creating a more formal or hierarchical structure to their network or, necessarily, of their being part of a larger association.

Other such networks exist within the New Age as a whole in the UK and many more exist in the US and elsewhere; some are more closer knit than others. These networks include the Centre for Creation Spirituality[36] (also housed at St James's), The Isle of Avalon Foundation (formerly the University of Avalon) in Glastonbury, The Schumacher Circle (a network of seven networks including the Schumacher College, The New Economics Foundation, and Intermediate Technology) based in South Devon, and Neal's Yard Agency for Personal Development which is described as 'The Travel Agent for Inner Journeys' in London. International networks also exist – for example, Earth Stewards, The Lucis Trust, and Brahma Kumaris. There are, naturally, many other networks which incorporate New Age ideas and activities but where the New Age may not be central to their particular focus. These networks include, for example, LETS (Local Exchange Trading Systems), the Gaia Foundation, and the Natural Medicines Society. Moreover, many specifically New Age destinations offer workshop holidays throughout the US, in Peru, Hawaii, and Europe, including Cortijo Romero in Spain and Atsitsa on the Greek island of Skyros. With regard to the latter, the Skyros Club meets monthly in London and attempts to bring together people who have visited the island; and Œkos is a network of these people who seek a way to bridge the gap between Skyros and everyday life. And, as technology becomes increasingly more sophisticated, the possibility of new networking arenas are beginning to open up. Most notably, this

35   Michael York, 1995: 43.
36   The UK branch of Matthew Fox's church in California.

has happened with the advent of the information Superhighway, the World Wide Web. The prime difference between Internet and traditional communication technologies is that the Internet is fully democratic, practically instant, and removes geographic limitations.[37] In this case, it would appear that computer technology incorporates a great many ideas which particularly suit its use in the New Age; and an example of such use can be seen in the way by which Timothy Leary used the Internet up to (and including) his death in 1996, thereby giving a new meaning to his (in)famous counter-cultural advice to 'turn on, tune in, and drop out'. However, one influential commentator on the New Age does not believe the Internet will have much value,[38] and, in the end, it may be found that computerized communication will not add significantly to the practice of networking in the New Age.

The answer to the question regarding whether there exists a more integral structure through which access to the New Age is available appears to be that while there are many networks, there is little evidence of the development of any integrated structure. This is wholly in accord with the fourth central idea of the New Age given by William Bloom in Chapter 1, that those involved are free to choose their own path – each of which is different (subtly or wholly) from the next; each being particularly influenced by the inner guidance received by going within. As a consequence, the possibility – even desirability – of creating structures among participants does not appear to exist.

A New Age individual's network is likely to be comprised of many varied ideas and activities, and association with each could demand different levels of involvement and commitment – for example, commitment to Alternatives' Monday evening meetings may be low in comparison with commitment to a new religious movement such as a Gurdjieffian or Osho group. However, as has been demonstrated, networks form a resource for individuals to gain access to ideas and activities either as a means for passive information gathering or for entry into some form of participation, although there seems to be no overarching or structured mode to these entry methods.

37   Tracy Laquey, 1994: 6ff.
38   Theodore Roszak, 1994: 171f.

The physical means by which access to New Age ideas and activities can be achieved is readily available at relatively low cost to every person in practically every High Street throughout the world via a wide variety of books, magazines, or the Internet. New Age networking remains highly individuated. However, the existence of overriding organizational infrastructures which could move towards influencing change to particular aspects of society may occur in instances where networks combine to form larger networks. This can be seen to be happening with the environmental Real World Coalition[39] of over 30 such networks, including not only environmental organizations such as Friends of the Earth, but also humanitarian aid organizations such as Christian Aid and Action Aid.

Forms of involvement

It has become fairly obvious that individuals are likely to participate in New Age ideas and activities in different ways, and it is to a more theoretical assessment of this variety to which attention is now drawn. Some critics agree that an element of genuine 'seekers' in the New Age does in fact exist although, even in the early 1970s, a Tibetan Buddhist teacher foresaw what he described as the possibility of a 'spiritual materialism'.[40] Highlighting the dangers of setting the practice of one spiritual path against another, he argued that they become 'dangerous [...] purely external entertainment, rather than an organic personal experience'.[41]

More recently and as we will see in more detail below and in the final chapter, other commentators – notably Paul Heelas, David Spangler, and Ken Wilber – have reported that involvement individuals have with the New Age can be seen to differ and the whole genre is being called, according to a journalist, 'pastiche spirituality' or 're-

39   See Michael Jacobs, 1996: 135ff.
40   Chogyam Trungpa, 1987: 14.
41   Ibid: 19.

ligion à la carte'.[42] Wilber, drawing on an earlier survey,[43] argues that only about one in five New Age individuals are seriously involved in its ideas and activities. Wilber relates this argument to his ideas for a spectrum of consciousness and suggests that 'about 20% of the New Age Movement is transpersonal (transcendental and genuinely mystical); about 80% prepersonal (magical and narcissistic)'.[44] Whether Wilber's estimate is right or wrong, what is clear is that there are different types of involvement people can have with the New Age.

Categories of involvement

One means of assessing categories of involvement individuals can have with the New Age is put forward by Paul Heelas, who suggests a spectrum that describes participants specifically in relation to the values of the capitalistic mainstream to which, he believes, the New Age is strongly linked. At one end of this spectrum is 'world rejection' where 'emphasis is very much on avoiding the contaminating effects of life in the mainstream'[45] and at the other 'world affirmation', where 'importance is attached to becoming prosperous'.[46] Heelas's use of the term 'world' needs clarification. Its use refers the world of mainstream capitalism and its rejection or affirmation in the light of New Age ideas and activities and not to any broader sense as might be found, for example, in New Age ecological views where individuals can be world- (nature-) affirming, because of the planet's perceived

---

42 Jeremiah Creedon, 1998: 42.
43 Ken Wilber reports that his survey estimate is based on research among students protesting against the Vietnam War at Berkeley, California, who were given the Kohlberg test of moral development. The findings showed that 20% based their objections to the war on moral grounds whereas the remainder were protesting because they did not want to fight and not because the war was seen to be either right or wrong (1993: 267).
44 Op. cit.: 268.
45 Paul Heelas, 1996a: 30.
46 Ibid.

abundance, but reject outright the idea of prosperity as found in capitalism, or in those spiritual individuals who also reject the materialist world but welcome the world that they believe God (or whatever name is used) created. As we have seen in the previous chapter, a large proportion of New Age individuals appear not to fall comfortably into Heelas's spectrum. Moreover, this academic also believes that the spirituality of those involved is humanistic;[47] yet the majority of participants to my survey talked about a spirituality which was transcendent, that is, not confined to the purely humanistic. Nevertheless, the spectrum is interesting and, for his analysis, Heelas[48] draws from such social theorists as Max Weber, Sydney Ahlstrom, Roy Wallis, and Dick Anthony and Bruce Ecker,[49] and develops their ideas into a New Age context.

Heelas's spectrum is divided into five categories, the first of which, at the world-rejecting end, is the *spiritual purist*. People in this category reject materialism, he suggests, and, citing others, he believes that here, '"authentic spiritual transcendence or realization" is all that matters'.[50] Heelas's description of this category appears confusing. If, as he states, the New Age is humanistic, then those in this world-rejecting category fall mainly outside the New Age because these people describe their spirituality as transcendent, that is, beyond the purely humanistic. Yet, in contrast, this category appears to fit with Ken Wilber's level of 'transcendental and genuinely mystical' individuals, noted above, a level which he sees to contain all those who are serious about the New Age. If this is the case, the top category of the spectrum (together with, as we will see, the bottom category) both fall outside of what Heelas considers to be New Age.

47 Op. cit.: 28.
48 Op. cit.: 29ff.
49 Dick Anthony and Bruce Ecker developed the Anthony Typology as a framework for assessing spiritual and consciousness groups in terms of spiritual validity and potential harmfulness 'along three descriptive dimensions: its metaphysics, its central mode of practice, and its interpretative sensibility' (1987: 36). The Typology incorporates four main groupings (multilevel charismatic and technical, and unilevel charismatic and technical) divided into either monistic or dualistic dimensions (Op. cit.: 37ff; see also Ken Wilber, 1990: 274ff.
50 Ibid.

Next in this spectrum comes the *counter-cultural*, which are described as being 'less radical [than world-rejecting and] can be taken to include all those activities which emphasize *Self-actualization* [where] the emphasis is on becoming a whole person: and in ways which are not catered for by conventional institutions'.[51] The middle portion of Heelas's spectrum, the *mainstream-transformer*, describes individuals attempting to make the best of both worlds where 'participants learn to detach themselves from – while living within – the capitalistic mainstream.'[52] Even greater acceptance of the capitalistic mainstream can be found in the *self-enhancer* who tends 'to emphasize the intrinsic value of, say, making money'.[53] It would appear that these three categories, taken as a whole, are thought by Heelas to describe most of those who participate in the New Age.

Finally, at the other end of the total spectrum can be found the *self- or mainstream-empower* who, according to Heelas, are at the 'very fringe of – or beyond – the New Age as envisaged by the purist or counter-culturalist [where] inner spirituality is accorded little intrinsic value'.[54]

One way to interpret the contrast between Heelas's two extremes of categories, the spiritual purist and the self- or mainstream-empowerer, can be illustrated in the notion that, for the purist, the world appears naturally abundant and sufficient for all as long as there is cooperation, while for the empowerer individualistic growth and material prosperity need to be competitively sought. Summarizing the division between the two, Heelas suggests that while purists see capitalistic modernity 'as irredeemably flawed, the empowerers suppose that it can be made to work properly'[55] – that is, in the main, for personal prosperity.

The five categories of involvement Heelas believes individuals can have with the New Age is not the end of the matter, as there can be seen to be at least one further development which needs to be borne

51   Op. cit.: 31.
52   Ibid.
53   Op. cit.: 32.
54   Ibid.
55   Ibid.

in mind. In this regard, it can be assumed that individuals within each of the five categories determine their activities from the whole range of what the New Age has to offer, which means that, at each level of Heelas's spectrum, the considerable diversity of an individual's involvement needs to be taken into account. No such analysis can provide a wholly accurate categorization, not least because there are many areas of overlaps, as the social theorists that Heelas remodels themselves point out, where particular aspects of one group activity can also be represented in one or more of the other categories of involvement.[56] Heelas's spectrum seems to assume that individuals approach their New Age participation from a single activity, whereas there exists the probability that individuals actually approach the New Age from a number of categories at the same time, as will be demonstrated below. In fact, the characteristics of overlap and a multifaceted approach appear to feature throughout the New Age which, as has been shown, is comprised of an extremely wide variety of ideas and activities – and many types of people, not least those of different ages and genders.

Levels of involvement

Ken Wilber, it will be remembered, suggests a two-tier 20:80 split with regard to the way in which individuals become involved with the New Age. David Spangler, too, suggests that there are levels of involvement people may have, and in his case four are proposed: superficial, attraction to its glamour, change in terms of a paradigm shift, and transformatory in terms of an 'incarnation of the spirit'.[57] By simplifying the difference between Wilber and Spangler, three principal levels of involvement can be seen.

The first level I describe as *unwitting* or, as Spangler suggests, superficial involvement – that is, involvement in its weakest sense.

56   Dick Anthony and Bruce Ecker, 1987: 58.
57   David Spangler, 1984: 78ff.

This is where the individual practises an idea or activity which can be classified as New Age but which is not necessarily thought to be New Age by the participant. For example, it is not necessarily the case that a person who has a tarot reading is interested in anything other than the personal advice and future predictions such a reading might give, or that aromatherapists and their clients necessarily need to experience anything other than the pleasurable and healing properties of the art, or that attendees at management training seminars involving psycho-technologies want anything other that to increase their material prosperity. Spangler describes this involvement aptly as being where 'one can acquire new age shoes, wear new age clothes, use new age toothpaste, shop at new age businesses, and eat at new age restaurants where new age music is played softly in the background'[58] but not have any greater interest. This level of involvement appears to be marked by the person being occupied with one – or at most a very few – ideas and activities which can be considered New Age, but these have made virtually no impact in the form of a change on their life. It can be remembered from the previous chapter that the mean average number of activities being undertaken by participants at the time of the survey was nearly seven, and the mean average number for ever using any New Age activity was more than double this figure.

The second level I describe as *partial* involvement. This is where an individual knows that the ideas and activities which they practise are New Age, although contact with them has created little in the way of spiritual transformation to their lives. One commentator uses the term 'simple waking awareness'[59] to describe this pretransformational level of consciousness. These individuals carry on living in mainstream society in much the same way as they had prior to their contact with the New Age. Moreover, it can be argued that there is a scale of involvement with the New Age which encompass Spangler's second and third levels of glamour and change respectively. At one end of the scale, individuals start to try out New Age ideas and activities, whereas at the other end involvement starts to become more meaningful.

58   Op. cit.: 78.
59   Marilyn Ferguson, 1982: 71.

At this partial level of involvement an individual can be active in terms of attending workshops, lectures, courses, and exhibitions. However, at the lower level of partial involvement, Spangler suggests that 'the new age has become populated with strange and exotic beings, masters, adepts, extraterrestrials [...] with dynamic, magnetic leaders and followers who have subtly surrendered their individuality to the image of the cause, the teacher, or the group.'[60] Moreover, this lower level can be compared to Wilber's second level in his spectrum of consciousness, which he describes as being epitomized by mythic and narcissistic, prepersonal levels of consciousness. At the higher level of partial involvement, Spangler argues that the New Age is seen in relation to 'social, economic, and technological terms rather than spiritual ones'.[61] By this description we can understand Spangler to mean that these individuals would be assessing their social and economic position with a view to 'downsizing' or otherwise reducing the way their lives impact on society: for example, by implementing an ecological way of life or the use of alternative technology. Here, Wilber's fifth and sixth levels of consciousness – which he describes as the egoic – might fit with Spangler's description.

The third and final level can be described as *full* involvement. Individuals at this level are differentiated by their claims that contact with the New Age has brought about what they take to be a life-changing spiritual transformation. Spangler, for example, describes this level as 'the emergence of a new, holistic culture [...] concerned with identifying, naming, and exploring the nature of the sacred experience that lies at the heart of that culture. This is not just a religious search, for the experience of the sacred is not only religious. It is also intellectual, artistic, emotional, and physical.'[62]

It is not possible to quantify in terms of percentages the number of participants involved at each of these three levels of involvement, although Ken Wilber has estimated that perhaps 20% of all those active are fully involved. What is clear is that there exist distinguishable

60   David Spangler, 1984: 79.
61   Op. cit.: 80.
62   Op. cit.: 81.

levels at which, or through which, individuals make contact with New Age ideas and activities.

In comparing the different levels of involvement with the characteristics of association discussed in the previous chapter it would appear that respondents to my survey were primarily drawn from those who were more fully involved, and whose lives have been transformed through their contact. They display, most of all, a depth of spirituality – as it were, religious, but without necessarily membership of a specific religion – a non-aligned religiosity – which is practically impossible to pin down into anything other than the broadest of categories; what William Bloom has described as 'not being boxed in'.[63]

As can be imagined, the task of attempting to classify levels of involvement in greater detail than the suggested three-tier categorization is extremely difficult. Nevertheless, what it means to be fully involved with the New Age is likely to be that an individual needs to have experienced a spiritual transformation that has led to an uncompromising practice of New Age ideas and activities which, in turn, results in a new direction being taken in her or his life as a whole.

Summary

Access to the New Age can clearly be made in two principal directions, which are not mutually exclusive. By 'going within' and following intuitively derived guidance, an individual seems able to discover what she or he might categorize as their authentic Higher Self – a process which in itself could be transformative. And, through external contact via a very wide variety of means from books to networks, the vast panoply of the more public New Age territory is accessed with ease and often without great cost.

Furthermore, clearly a particular feature of the New Age is that there exist different forms of involvement individuals can have with its ideas and activities, and analysis of these can be used to help make

63   William Bloom, 1990: 12.

sense of the many disparate aspects entailed in their participation. As has been shown, this includes analyses of both categories and levels of involvement although, while there is some similarity between the two means, in the end, both methods are not fully successful in pinning down a wholly accurate portrayal of what involvement in the New Age is like – this is simply because participation is primarily individualistic and frequently multifaceted. Nevertheless, use of such assessments demonstrates that in the New Age as a whole there appear to be broad measurements against which involvement can be gauged; and a clearer, less amorphous picture of the New Age comes into focus as a result.

5. Essential Concepts

Clear your mind of dogmatic theological debris; let in the fresh, healing waters of direct perception. Attune yourself to the active inner Guidance; the Divine Voice has the answer to every dilemma of life.

Paramahansa Yogananda[1]

There are many terms which go to make up the complete New Age lexicon, although within its ideas and activities certain terms have a special significance. In fact, within William Bloom's basic New Age ideas a number of these terms have been revealed, and the most used are now reviewed in detail. Bearing in mind the differences in meaning between the same terms which might be possible,[2] this chapter

---

1   Paramahansa Yogananda, 1994: 377.
2   Ludwig Wittgenstein (1967) established that throughout societies and cultures multitudes of different 'forms of life' exist within which the use and meaning of language is dependent upon the 'game' or context in which they are used. Related to the New Age and because of its segmented nature and wide range of ideas and activities, it would not be surprising to find that the New Age itself contains innumerable forms of life. As a consequence, there is little likelihood of complete uniformity existing in the understanding of the terms which are used other than at a basic level. Ferdinand de Saussure (1964) too, in his seminal work *Course in General Linguistics* (first published in 1915), pointed to problems associated with the meanings given to words particularly regarding distinctions between *langue*, the communal language system, and *parole*, individual manifestations of the same system. Saussure's argument is especially relevant to the New Age where participants follow individuated paths and, hence, build their own meaning systems. Again, it can be argued that in the New Age no two participant's meaning systems are likely to be precisely the same, although within each person's vocabulary many similarities may be found, especially in the basic underlying significance of the concepts which are used. In this respect, Paul Heelas suggests that in the New Age 'beneath much of the heterogeneity [...] one encounters the same (or very similar) lingua franca

131

describes six terms which are met with frequently in the New Age. Selection of these terms has been made from what participants have said in my survey and from a detailed analysis of key New Age commentators' writings. The terms considered are: spirituality, transformation, connectedness, love and compassion, Higher Self, and God.

Spirituality

Attempts have been made to produce a form of words which might be definitive for the term 'spirituality', yet not one has been universally adopted; moreover, scholars from specific fields have endeavoured to produce various forms of words which attempt to suit their particular disciplines.[3] For each person, New Age or not, spirituality is one of the most difficult words to define; it can be used in place of and meaning something similar to religiousness (without the institutional connotations). In this regard, perhaps the term can only signify an extremely broad area of meaning to do with all that is contained within the realms of higher human sensibilities.[4] However, the term is widely used in the New Age and, as we have seen, the vast majority of those involved believe that it is primarily about spiritual affairs, so some description of what its meaning might entail is needed.

to do with the human (and planetary) condition' (1996a: 2). (A discussion of Wittgenstein's and Saussure's work can be found in R. Harris, 1988).

3   Some examples, although by no means a comprehensive selection, can be found in – ecological: Jonathan Porritt and David Winner, 1988, Charlene Spretnak, 1986; feminist: Katherine Zappone, 1991; humanistic: David Cave, 1993, Erik Craig, 1992, David N. Elkins *et al.*, 1988, Joel Kovel, 1990; psychological: David G. Benner, 1989, Cynthia K. Chandler *et al.*, 1992, Joel Kovel, 1991, J. Melvin Witmer and Thomas J. Sweeney, 1992; and transpersonal: Ken Wilber, 1995a.

4   Further study has found that spirituality is not dependent upon being religious (that is, belonging to a particular religion); what is prerequisite is some form of continued reverential experience, maintained practice, and a life imbued with love. See Stuart Rose, 2001b.

To start with, in the process an individual in general may go through to approach their spirituality it is suggested that

> Throughout history, religious traditions have noted that those people who long for a transformative or complete understanding of themselves and of their place in the world must somehow find a teacher or set of teachings to help them along. That guide may be a person, an idea, or a set of values; whatever it is, it establishes the orientation and outlines the procedures the seekers should follow in order to make real the transformation for which they hope. Many traditions further maintain that, having found (or having hoped eventually to find) that guide, the seeker then must practise various regimens that will help him continue along the way to ultimate transformation. Such endeavours constitute spiritual discipline, the means by which people find their fullest potential in the context of any particular religious ideology.[5]

Furthermore, the same writer suggests that there are three ideal types of spiritual discipline which each variety of spirituality shares to some extent. These he believes are *heteronomous* discipline, which is governed by external authority, *autonomous* discipline, which is where authority exists at the very depths of one's personal being, and *interactive* discipline, which is marked by a combination of both external and internal sources of authority.[6] Within the New Age, the obvious conclusion to be drawn is that spiritual activity is principally governed by autonomous authority – very little seems to be determined as heteronomous. He then finds that there are six different ways in which spiritual practice can be conducted and which, again, are not mutually exclusive. These categories are ecstatic and constructive disciplines, restraints of the body and of the mind, the cultivation of love and, finally, the promotion of enduring personal relationships.[7] In varying degrees, all six are found in the New Age, although the most important is likely to be the cultivation of love.

In further determining the characteristics of New Age spirituality, there appears to be two principal strands – transcendent (or transpersonal, mystical) and humanistic. Put simply, the two terms are used to denote other-worldly or this-worldly types of spirituality respec-

5   William K. Mahony, 1987 Vol. 14: 19.
6   Op. cit.: 20ff.
7   Op. cit.: 23ff.

tively, but greater explanation than this is required. In the first regard, the term 'transcendent', as noted in Chapter 2, relates to something which is not subject to the limitations of the material universe, and its use in conjunction with the term 'spirituality' is applicable to much in the New Age including God and the other key words (discussed below), the doctrines of *Karma* and reincarnation, together with channelling, past-life regression, and contact with the supernatural. In the second regard, the term 'humanism' relates to all that is secular and is described philosophically as being 'very definitely non-religious [and] not a specific system of beliefs [...] Humanism is so called because, in the words of the Ancient Greek thinker Protagoras, it regards "human beings as the measure of all things" [It] is the acceptance that human reason is all we have, all we can rely upon.'[8] This description does not exclude the combination of the two terms 'spirituality' and 'humanism' into 'spiritual humanism', but where the latter is used it refers to that which is primarily non-transcendent and, within the New Age, some ideas and activities can be so classified including a number of psychotechnologies such as encounter groups, gestalt therapy, hypnotherapy, neuro-linguistic programming, and transactional analysis.

What is more, as we have seen Paul Heelas summarizes the New Age as 'a highly optimistic, celebratory, utopian and spiritual form of humanism'.[9] Heelas's understanding of the New Age leans more towards Emile Durkheim's concept described as the religion of humanity or cult of man[10] than towards any more transcendent meaning.

8   Eric Matthews, 1991: 3f.
9   Paul Heelas, 1996a: 35.
10   Defining the precise nature of Durkheim's religion of humanity is difficult because of the lack of a specific treatise. However, in essence, Durkheim's concept was based on a 'glorification' (his word) of the human being and human potential. Durkheim replaced concepts of transcendental religiosity with the humanistic view that people were ultimate. His 'proof' was empirically grounded, as people positively existed. The strength of a society not bound by traditional religiosity was seen to be in its 'collective conscience', the sum of humanity being greater than its parts, which Durkheim saw as being equally able to provide the kind of social morality which traditional religions had provided to societies – but in his view better, because of its celebration of unrestricted human possibilities. Durkheim's ideas regarding the concept of a religion of humanity can be drawn from several works which include: *The Division*

However, from what we have seen so far, I can state that those I have surveyed are most likely to view their spirituality as transcendent and not humanistic. Of course, this does not exclude an additional practice by the same individuals of ideas and activities which have a spiritually humanistic nature.

To add to this somewhat tangled situation, use of the term 'spirituality' in the New Age can be found applied generally to a variety of ideas connected with higher human sensibilities. In this respect, one American academic, in his wider study of the spiritual journeying of America's baby-boom generation, suggests that they 'speak of creation spirituality, Eucharistic spirituality, Native American spirituality, Eastern spiritualities, Twelve-Step spiritualities, feminist spirituality, earth-based spirituality, eco-feminist spirituality, Goddess spirituality, and men's spirituality, as well as what would be considered traditional Judeo-Christian spiritualities'.[11] There are many more such variations although, in the New Age, they would be seen to be interconnected and harmonious.

A typical New Age view of spirituality is given by Marilyn Ferguson, who describes it broadly as a mystical experience[12] containing two key principles – those of 'flow' and 'wholeness'.[13] God, she suggests, 'is experienced as flow, wholeness, the infinite kaleidoscope of life and death, Ultimate Cause, the ground of being [...] mystical experience nearly always leads one to a belief that some aspect of consciousness is imperishable'.[14] Similarly, David Spangler, who has been called the shaman of the New Age,[15] suggests that there are four levels[16] at which the New Age can be met and explored,[17] the highest of which is where

---

of *Labour in Society* (1947), *Suicide* (1951), and *Sociology and Philosophy* (1953). See Heelas's discussion of this aspect of Durkheim's thought (1996b).

11 Wade Clark Roof, 1993: 243.
12 Marilyn Ferguson, 1982: 398.
13 Op. cit.: 417.
14 Op. cit.: 420ff.
15 As noted on the book jacket of David Spangler, 1984.
16 Discussed in Chapter 4 above.
17 David Spangler, 1984: 78ff.

the new age is fundamentally a spiritual event, the birth of a new consciousness, a new awareness and experience of life. It is humanity becoming more fully integrated with the being of Gaia, more fully at one with the presence of God. It is a deepening into the sacramental nature of everyday life, an awakening of the consciousness that can celebrate divinity within the ordinary and, in this celebration, bring to life a sacred civilization. It is the new age as a state of being, a mode of relationship with others that is mutually empowering and enriching.[18]

Moreover, those responding to my survey were asked to write a brief description of what the term meant to them (we will see more of this in the following chapter). Overall, the majority of the hundreds of descriptions were steeped with a transcendent content. They wrote of energy emanating from a divine source, the love and light of the divine eternal spirit within us, awareness of transcendent being, discovery of soul, connection with the ground of being, of being a co-creator with God. A younger care assistant wrote that spirituality to her was 'something beyond the realms of the material part of the world. To do with God, universal love, love of mankind, healing, helping positive emotions and actions. In touch with the inner self and God' and, lastly, a social worker wrote that she used the term 'to describe my personal connection to the Universal energy, my link with ALL that is. I see it as separate from religion or groups of people – it is direct and personal.'

The notion of a spirituality which is transcendent, therefore, is fundamental to the New Age. In fact, I see this to be its *raison d'être*. Both New Age writers and participants describe encountering dimensions beyond the purely human, beyond reason and the rational. What they claim to experience is unique to each person, and its description cannot be reduced to the limitation of words; which is why the term 'spirituality' cannot, in the end, be fully defined.

18   Op. cit.: 81.

Transformation

The term 'transformation' in the New Age represents change. However, the particular type of change described by commentators is not subtle or partial but a metamorphosis, a complete change or, as it has been described, self-transcendence.[19]

It is helpful to provide an illustration of what is meant by the term 'transformation', and an example can be found in one of the most widely read books in New Age literature, first published in the early 1970s. This is the allegorical story written by Richard Bach about the transformation of Jonathan Livingston Seagull and is the tale of a seagull who, unlike other seagulls in his flock, delights in flying and pushing back the physical, emotional, and spiritual barriers which he sees retarding the development of his – and, ultimately, all seagulls' – potential for flying. His transformation is brought about through continued self-development, and the notion of transformation as a whole is summed up in Jonathan's final conversation with his pupil, Fletcher Lynd Seagull.

> 'You need to keep finding yourself, a little more each day, that real, unlimited Fletcher Seagull. He's your instructor. You need to understand him and to practise him.'
>
> A moment later Jonathan's body wavered in the air, shimmering, and began to go transparent. 'Don't let them spread silly rumours about me, or make me a god. O.K., Fletch? I'm a seagull. I like to fly, maybe...'
>
> 'JONATHAN!'
>
> 'Poor Fletch. Don't believe what your eyes are telling you. All they show is limitation. Look with your understanding, find out what you already know, and you'll see the way to fly.'
>
> The shimmering stopped. Jonathan Seagull had vanished into empty air.
>
> After a time, Fletcher Gull dragged himself into the sky and faced a brand-new group of students, eager for their first lesson.
>
> 'To begin with,' he said heavily, 'you've got to understand that a seagull is an unlimited idea of freedom, an image of the Great Gull, and your whole body, from wingtip to wingtip, is nothing more than your thought itself.'[20]

19   Ken Wilber, 1995a: 42ff.
20   Richard Bach, 1994: 92f.

Bach's account can be interpreted from both a humanistic or transcendent standpoint although, in either case, he describes complete transformation as a result of a determined effort to reach one's ultimate potential.[21]

With regard to what is thought to occur in a person's transformation in the New Age, commentators describe the event as a 'personal spiritual-psychological transformation that is identical to what is generally termed as a "religious experience"'.[22] Here, these authors point to the idea that a transformation needs to include a combination of *both* spiritual and psychological aspects and not exclusively one or the other – a notion, it can be remembered, that Ken Wilber also suggests.[23] Moreover, many New Age healing techniques are described as transformational processes – for instance, two New Age therapists describe the transpersonal psychotechnology of rebirthing as 'a significant emotional transformation brought about by insights, new thoughts, and understanding of life and oneself'.[24] Apparently going one step further, from academe the suggestion is made that transformation can include not just the individual but society as well, creating, it is argued, 'a new healing religion'.[25]

It is fair to say that the term 'transformation' is one of the most widely used words to describe the paradigmatic shift in consciousness that is reported to occur among many of those involved in the New Age. Noting its importance, a New Age author depicts the transformation process as being 'the key process of the New Age. It implies not only a sense of change but also a sense of healing, self-realization and self-becoming. The process is seen as a natural one, an opening out to new possibilities, further growth and increased awareness.'[26] This view, suggesting that transformation is the key process in New Age ideas and activities, appears to be shared by many commentators. In fact, the word is often used in the titles of books on New Age subjects

---

21   Whether Bach himself is writing in terms of human potential or a potential which transcends the human is not clear.
22   J. Gordon Melton *et al.*, 1991: 301.
23   Ken Wilber, 1990: 307.
24   Leonard Orr and Sondra Ray, 1983: xvi.
25   Catherine Albanese, 1992: 75.
26   Stuart Wilson, 1989: 83.

– for example, in Marilyn Ferguson's[27] *The Aquarian Conspiracy: Personal and Social Transformation in the 1980s*, in Shakti Gawain's[28] *The Path of Transformation: How Healing Ourselves Can Change the World*, and Shirley MacLaine's[29] *Going Within: A Guide for Inner Transformation*. Such is the apparent importance of the term that it is also used it in the title of this study.

With regards to the nature of transformation, Marilyn Ferguson describes the experience as 'specifically the transformation of consciousness [...] of being *conscious of one's consciousness*',[30] which cannot be quantified.[31] Ferguson uses an analogy of an aircraft passenger and its pilot to describe the change that she believes occurs as a result of a transformational experience:

> A mind not aware of itself – *ordinary* consciousness – is like a passenger strapped into an aeroplane seat, wearing blinkers, ignorant of the nature of transportation, the dimension of the craft, its range, the flight plan, and the proximity of other passengers. The mind aware of itself is a pilot. True, it is sensitive to flight rules, affected by weather and dependent on navigational aids, but still vastly freer than the 'passenger' mind.[32]

Ferguson suggests that 'transformation is a journey without a final destination',[33] and goes on to express the idea that there are four major stages to this journey.[34] The first stage, she reports, can only be seen in retrospect: it is the entry point or trigger which starts the process, perhaps by means of one of a number of psychotechnologies, creative visualization, wearing a crystal, or attending a workshop. As reported earlier, Ferguson also suggests that in addition 'it is impossible to overestimate the historical role of psychedelics as an entry point [...] especially in the 1960s.'[35] The second stage is seen as one of ex-

---

27   Marilyn Ferguson, 1982.
28   Shakti Gawain, 1993.
29   Shirley MacLaine, 1991.
30   Marilyn Ferguson, 1982: 71.
31   Op. cit.: 192.
32   Op. cit.: 72.
33   Op. cit.: 93.
34   Op. cit.: 93ff.
35   Op. cit.: 93f.

ploration; while the third stage is one of integration, of catching up where 'intuition has leaped ahead of understanding'.[36] Finally, the fourth stage is what is described as a conspiracy, a joining together of like-minded individuals who work towards extending the transformation of consciousness out into the world at large – to transform society. Here, it can be noted how important Ferguson sees community activity to be to the New Age, a sentiment which is echoed by two American academics,[37] one reporting that 'New Age theorists have in common a perception of this particular time in history as one of drastic change – paradigmatic change – that will effect all the institutions of the culture, not just organized religion.'[38]

Jiddu Krishnamurti, one of the most radical spiritual teachers of the twentieth century and influential to the New Age, too, taught about the importance of transformation as both an inner change and a change of society, although he advises that inner change is more important. This is because, he suggests, 'the transformation of the world is brought about by the transformation of oneself, because the self is the product and a part of the total process of human existence.'[39]

Furthermore, Krishnamurti indicates that transformation can only come about in relation to a thorough and deep self-realization, and he argues that

> to transform oneself, self-knowledge is essential; without knowing what you are, there is no basis for right thought, and without knowing yourself there can be no transformation. One must know oneself as one is, not as one wishes to be which is merely an ideal and therefore fictitious, unreal; it is only that which *is* that can be transformed, not that which you wish to be.[40]

Other commentators on the New Age appear to agree with Ferguson and Krishnamurti. One sees that it is important for individuals to transform their selves first and then join with others in the hope that

---

36   Op. cit.: 98.
37   Catherine Albanese (1992: 75) and Mary Farrel Bednarowski (1995: 16).
38   Mary Farrel Bednarowski (Ibid.). The concept of community' in the New Age is discussed in Chapter 8 below.
39   Jiddu Krishnamurti, 1974: 23.
40   Ibid.

140

'if we all were to transform ourselves and raise our culture to "the next phase of human evolution" then the world would surely be a much better place in which to live.'[41] What is more, another suggests that if such a social transformation were to take place it 'would amount to one of the most thoroughgoing transformations in the history of mankind'[42] which he uses the Greek word *metanoia* to describe.

Clearly, the notion of transformation is vital to the New Age, as it forms the 'bridge' between a participant's existing worldview and the new. As has been shown in these descriptions, what is reported to occur in an individual is an awakening of consciousness so life-changing that the previous 'sleep-like' state may not easily be regained. In the New Age, it must be said, those involved would argue that to revert is not desirable at all.

However, a question has been raised by Ken Wilber with regard to the possibility of misinterpretation among some New Age individuals of whether or not a transformation has occurred.[43] He argues that there might exist two levels, what might be called partial and full. On the one hand is what he calls 'translation', which he describes as rearranging the furniture on the same level, and on the other 'transformation', which he sees as changing levels. Wilber suggests that many people mistakenly believe they have experienced a transformation whereas, in reality, they have merely rearranged their lives without bringing about actual change. Wilber also points out that individuals can experience a series of transformations, each one producing greater significance to the individual.[44]

---

41   Nevill Drury, 1994: 126.
42   Willis Harman, 1991: 19.
43   Ken Wilber, 1995a: 60f.
44   In relation to Wilber's allied concept of a multilevelled spectrum of consciousness – whereby he points to the possible existence of different degrees of spiritual awareness – it can be argued that the less extensive forms of transformation he suggests may equate with his description of mythical and egocentric levels of consciousness, whereas the more extensive forms may entail the transpersonal stages – that is, incorporating an increasingly greater spiritual content.

Connectedness

Several words commonly used in the New Age relate to the concept of connectedness – or, as is sometimes expressed, interconnectedness or interrelatedness. These include 'harmony', 'holism', 'unity', and 'wholeness'. Linked to this concept, therefore, are ideas about health, society, and ecology.

Outlining the importance of connectedness in areas of influence to the New Age, scientist, philosopher, and ecologist Fritjof Capra suggests that the essence of the Eastern worldview

> is the awareness of the unity and mutual interrelation of all things and events, the experience of all phenomena in the world as manifestations of a basic one-ness. In ordinary life, we are not aware of this unity of all things, but divide the world into separate objects and events. This division is, of course, useful and necessary to cope with our everyday environment, but it is not a fundamental feature of reality.[45]

Capra argues that this unity can not only be seen in mysticism but in the quantum theory of physics (in this case, New Science) where, he argues, unity 'becomes apparent at the atomic level and manifests it-self more and more as one penetrates deeper into matter, down into the realm of subatomic particles'.[46]

Capra's ideas appear to be mirrored in the shamanic world view, perhaps the most ancient of belief systems, many of the ideas of which can be found at the heart of the New Age. A Shamanic teacher, for example, describes one of the principal shamanic world views as be-ing that 'all parts of the world are interconnected, on all levels of real-ity, so whatever happens to one individual affects all others and what-ever happens to the others affects the individual, at every level from the physical to the spiritual.'[47] He goes on to suggest that shamanic concepts are 'remarkably similar'[48] to a wide spectrum of scientific

45   Fritjoff Capra, 1988: 141f.
46   Ibid.
47   Lewis Mehl, 1988: 129.
48   Ibid.

thought, thereby building on Capra's views. A further and related development on the theme of connectedness is seen in the concept of the Gaia hypothesis, developed by scientist James Lovelock, whereby it is argued that 'the entire range of living matter on Earth [...] could be regarded as constituting a single living entity.'[49]

Turning to a more general understanding of the importance to the New Age of the concept of the connectedness of all life, there is the suggestion that 'from Oneness arises Wholeness, and from Wholeness arises Harmony. Ultimately these are not three separate elements but one continuous process [...] Oneness, Wholeness, Harmony – this is the central theme of the New Age.'[50] In the same way as spiritual writers of influence to the New Age such as the theologian Pierre Teilhard de Chardin,[51] here this commentator also intimates that the natural extension of the concept of connectedness leads to a direct union with an ultimate reality,[52] and this idea will now be examined further.

According to Ken Wilber,[53] in the full sense of the term 'connectedness' there can be no duality. By this Wilber suggests that all aspects of life – however 'good' or 'bad' – are without exception part of an interconnected whole; or, in other words, he believes there cannot exist a separation between aspects of life which are thought to be holistic and those which are not. In this way, Wilber highlights the difference between the concept of monism – which is dualistic in that he considers it to exclude such elements as an individual's outer personality – and non-dualism which is fully inclusive. The difference appears to be, in Wilber's view, a further example of a mistaken notion (reported above) held by some New Age individuals.

---

49   James Lovelock cited in William Bloom, 1991: 166.
50   Stuart Wilson, 1989: 31.
51   Pierre Teilhard de Chardin, 1959.
52   The idea of an uninterrupted connection to an ultimate reality is not exclusively New Age. As has already been established, monistic religious traditions include forms of direct connectedness with the divine. Moreover, some theistic traditions also embrace this view, as can be seen in the Quaker Testimony which is 'based on the realization that there is that of God in everybody, that all human beings are equal, that all life is interconnected' (Harvey Gillman cited in Quakers, 1995: 23.12).
53   Ken Wilber, 1981, 1995a: 518ff.

In addition to all these views, a large number of those active in the New Age are reported to claim that there exists substantial evidence which confirms the existence of a connectedness with other realities. This evidence relates to the field of paranormal phenomena (psi) which occurs in many New Age ideas and activities including channelling, clairvoyance, psychokinesis, telepathy, and – for the purpose of the following illustration – synchronicity. Synchronicity is the notion that meaningful coincidences exist in the world, and is a concept which was much developed by Carl Jung. In his essay 'On Synchronicity', Jung suggests that

> Synchronistic phenomena prove the simultaneous occurrence of meaningful equivalencies in heterogeneous, causally unrelated processes; in other words, they prove that a content perceived by an observer can, at the same time, be represented by an outside event, without any causal connection. From this it follows either that the psyche cannot be localized in space, or that space is relative to the psyche. The same applies to the temporal determination of the psyche and the psychic relativity of time. I do not need to emphasize that the verification of these findings must have far-reaching consequences.[54]

Jung's 'far reaching consequences' are illustrated in his view that, for example, 'A synchronicity exists between the life of Christ and the objective astronomical event [the beginning of a new aeon], the entrance of the spring equinox into the sign of Pisces.'[55] Following on from Jung's theories regarding synchronicity, other possible far-reaching consequences have been pointed to, in that

> Modern interest in synchronicity is appropriate, since even rudimentary awareness of the phenomenon sensitizes a person to the realities and possibilities of universal harmonies and complementariness, even where none was thought possible. The resulting openness to alternative worldviews could lay a philoso-

---

54 Carl Jung, 1976: 518. An idea much related to Jung's views on synchronicity is developed by the biologist Rupert Sheldrake with regards to his concept of 'morphic resonance', 1988.

55 Carl Jung, 1976: 248. From an astrological view, the Piscean age is believed to be coming to an end and a new age, an Aquarian age, is beginning (see, for example, Fred Gettings, 1990: 9; John Anthony West, 1991: 139).

phical foundation, if not also a theological framework, for new political, cultural, and even ecumenical unities.[56]

Overall, the concept of connectedness appears to be an essential element in New Age ideas and activities. Moreover, this connectedness is claimed to be manifest in what is termed as the 'universal life force' called variously *Prana, Ch'i, Qi, Ki, Mana, Od, Orgone,* or bioenergy. This energy 'transcends time and space, permeates all things in the universe, and [is the energy] upon which all things depend for health and life',[57] and which many healing therapies attempt to harness, such as acupuncture, shiatsu, and kinesiology. It can be remembered that William Bloom takes the idea of a universal life force one step further in his basic New Age ideas by suggesting that 'All life, in all its different forms and states, is interconnected energy – and this includes our deeds, feelings and thoughts.'[58]

Love and compassion

At the start of this book it was suggested that the most overt of the two principal connections which linked all elements of the New Age together is the 'energy' of love. Study of the many New Age writings further demonstrates that love and compassion are seen to be core values in many of the ideas and activities; and, moreover, the two concepts appear to be inextricably connected. It is not the intention here to attempt to describe the concept of love in the New Age in depth but to illustrate how several authors who are influential have portrayed its significance.

With regards to the concept of love, from the spiritual point of view, Jiddu Krishnamurti suggests that

56   Rosemary Ellen Guiley, 1991: 597.
57   Op. cit.: 626ff.
58   William Bloom, 1990: 13.

When the things of the mind don't fill your heart, then there is love; and love alone can transform the present madness and insanity in the world – not systems, not theories, either of the left or the right. You really love only when you don't possess, when you are not envious, not greedy, when you are respectful, when you have mercy and compassion, when you have consideration for your wife, your children, your neighbour [...]

Love cannot be thought about, love cannot be cultivated, love cannot be practised. The practice of love, the practice of brotherhood, is still within the field of the mind, therefore it is not love. When all this has stopped, then love comes into being, then you will know what it is to love. Then love is not quantitative but qualitative. You do not say, 'I love the whole world', but when you know how to love one, you know how to love the whole world. Because we do not know how to love one, our love of humanity is fictitious. When you love there is neither one nor many: there is only love. It is only when there is love that all our problems can be solved and then we shall know its bliss and happiness.[59]

A further view regarding love, this time from a shamanic healing perspective, says that 'love is the source that moves and guides the effective healer – a love that springs from a deeper Source than the individual ego and which has been called by many names in different spiritual traditions [...] We need only to live its energies to make its presence known through our work.'[60]

From these two examples, it appears that the love described does not to relate to romantic love but to something much greater. In this regard, Bhagwan Shree Rajneesh (Osho) makes a distinction between the types of love by differentiating between exclusive love, which he suggests can be experienced towards one person or ideal to the exclusion of other people or ideals, and inclusive love, which can be felt for all people and all ideals.[61] It can be added that Rajneesh's view of inclusive love applies to the love which, it is claimed, is experienced in higher forms of spirituality.

We can look at this universality of love a little further. In an academic study of religious love it is suggested that three types of love as a whole exist. The first two types are identified as being carnal and friendly love, but the third type is described as 'divine love manifested

59   Jiddu Krishnamurti, 1974: 173f.
60   Lewis Mehl, 1988: 133.
61   Bhagwan Shree Rajneesh, 1970.

as self-giving grace and represented as *agape* (Greek), *caritas* (Latin), *karuna* (Sanskrit, Buddhism), *prema* (Sanskrit, Hinduism), *rahman* (Arabic), and *hesed* (Hebrew)'.[62] Moreover and in much the same way, one of the most influential writings from the earlier part of the contemporary New Age, Ram Dass's *Be Here Now*, gives examples of the similarity in the concepts of love as they have been expressed in twelve of the world's religions, as well as by many of their spiritual teachers from Rabindranath Tagore and Ramakrishna Paramahansa to C. S. Lewis and Thomas Merton.[63]

The love that New Age participants claim can be experienced is also described as being unconditional. In this regard, Pierre Teilhard de Chardin (also influential to the New Age), describes unconditional love as 'a unifying energy, in fact it is "the supreme spiritual energy" linking all elements and persons in their "irreplaceable and incommunicable essence" in a universal process of unification'.[64] Regarded in this way, the concept of unconditional love in the New Age can be seen to be interchangeable with its equivalent as found in all religions. There is no difference. In fact, this is further shown to be the case in a study I have undertaken among priests, rabbis, and other religious 'professionals' from five major traditions, as well as certain key New Age figures, the findings of which show that while there is no absolute agreement, their description of spiritual love demonstrate a remarkable cogency.[65]

Turning to the relationship between the concept of compassion and that of unconditional love in the New Age,[66] New Age Christian teacher Matthew Fox makes the point that he believes compassion is

---

62   Bruce Long, 1987, Vol. 9: 31.
63   Ram Dass, 1971: 75f.
64   Cited in Ursula King, 1980: 205.
65   Stuart Rose, 2004.
66   Thomas Merton describes compassion as 'the keen awareness of the interdependence of all living things which are all part of one another and involved in one another' (cited in Matthew Fox, 1988: 50); and Ken Wilber suggests that the only true compassion is where 'all beings are treated as one's Self' (1995a: 291) – other, less true forms are seen by Wilber as being egocentric, sociocentric, anthropocentric, or worldcentric.

not altruistic because it does not exclude the love of the self. Fox suggests that

> the entire insight upon which compassion is based is that the other is *not* other; and that I am *not* I. In other words, in loving others I am loving myself and indeed involved in my own best and biggest and fullest self-interest. It is my pleasure to be involved in the relief of the pain of others, a pain which is also my pain and is also God's pain. Altruism as it is commonly understood presumes dualisms, separateness and ego differences that the compassionate person is aware are not fundamental energies at all.[67]

Similarly, in the definition of love given by M. Scott Peck, the Christian psychiatrist influential to the New Age, he suggests that love is 'the will to extend one's self for the purpose of nurturing one's own or another's spiritual growth [...] Thus the act of loving is an act of self-evolution even when the purpose of the act is someone else's growth.'[68] Moreover, the combined experience of unconditional love and compassion for the self is said to lead towards building stronger communities, in that

> compassion begins with ourselves. When we are kind and caring toward ourselves, we are nurturing our spiritual growth and cultivating compassion for others [...] Compassion is the tender opening of our hearts to pain and suffering [...] Compassion is the basis of all truthful relationship: it means being present with love – for ourselves and for all life, including animals, fish, birds, and trees. Compassion is bringing our deepest truth into our actions, no matter how much the world seems to resist, because that is ultimately what we have to give to this world and one another.[69]

Finally, with regard to the essential nature of love and compassion in everyday life, the Dalai Lama suggests that 'love and compassion are necessities, not luxuries. Without them, humanity cannot survive. With them, we can make a joint effort to solve the problems of the whole of humankind.'[70]

---

67   Matthew Fox, 1979: 33.
68   M. Scott Peck, 1993: 81ff.
69   Ram Dass and Mirabai Bush, 1992: 4ff.
70   Cited in op. cit.: 4.

In the order which the foregoing three terms of transformation, connectedness, and love and compassion have been described, it can be seen that to some extent there exists a logical sequence. For participants in the New Age, transformation constitutes the start of a process – the opening up of individual awareness to a new, some would say higher than human, reality. This reality is not seen as being comprised of separate facets because all that can be experienced is believed to be part of an interconnected whole. The most important unifying feature of this whole appears to be unconditional love combined with compassion. Moreover, the New Age view of experiencing love and compassion towards oneself is thought to be a vital means of being able to fully (wholly) give love and compassion to others and to extend it into community activity. However, it can be added that the notion of loving oneself in this way has resulted in some critics arguing the New Age is narcissistic.[71]

Higher Self

Some argue that those active in the New Age believe there are two basic levels of being at which individuals can live their lives. These two levels cannot be compared directly with ideas in psychology relating to the different levels of consciousness – that is, including the unconscious and the conscious – because the suggestion is that both levels of being can be experienced within consciousness.

The two levels are described here as 'self' and 'Higher Self'. In the first instance, self is seen to be inferior because it is centred on itself – that is, egocentric – and is experienced as existing separately from all other beings. However, in the second instance, the Higher Self is believed to be superior because it is seen to be integral in a much wider and more comprehensive level of being.[72]

71 Claims of narcissism in the New Age will be explored in Chapter 11 below.
72 As mentioned above, Ken Wilber (1995a) and others are critical of this notion; see also Georg Feuerstein, who draws a distinction between self-transcendence

William Bloom describes two aspects of human consciousness in the following manner:

> All life, as we perceive it with the five human senses or with scientific instruments, is only the outer veil of an invisible, inner and causal reality. Similarly, human beings are twofold creatures – with: i. an outer temporary personality and ii. a multi-dimensional inner being (soul or higher self). The outer personality is limited and tends towards materialism. The inner being is infinite and tends towards love.[73]

With regard to lifting this outer veil, Marilyn Ferguson describes what she believes can happen when the Higher Self is approached through what she notes has historically been described as a transformatory awakening:[74]

> A new understanding of *self* is discovered, one that has little resemblance to ego, self-ishness, self-lessness. There are multiple dimensions of self; a newly integrated sense of oneself as an individual [...] a linkage with others as if they are oneself [...] and the merger with a Self yet more universal and primary.[75]

Ferguson's notion of a more universal Self is described by another as 'our personalized reflection of the Divine Spark [...] our centralized God space'[76] – and both point to what has been called the Higher Self as having a highly sacred content.

Ted Peters provides a review of how writers and teachers – such as Sri Aurobindo Ghose, Ralph Waldo Emerson, Werner Erhard, Marilyn Ferguson, Willis Harman, and Marion Woodman – have described the Higher Self.[77] Peters argues that most of these individuals agree on the nature of the Higher Self with the exception of Erhard

---

and the spiritual seeker, where seeking is described as being a 'mode of the ego-personality' (1992: 103).

73 William Bloom, 1990: 13.
74 Marilyn Ferguson, 1982: 103.
75 Op. cit.: 104.
76 Shirley MacLaine, 1991: 82.
77 Ted Peters, 1991: 64ff.

who, he believes, provides a more limited description.[78] In his critical analysis of the New Age,[79] Peters describes the two levels of selfhood as where

> the doctrine of the higher self usually begins by acknowledging that life here on Earth is darkness, a sleepy haze. We bumble through life in a sort of hypnotic sleep, not clear on what forces are governing the course of personal events. We feel that our life is a lonely combination of inconsistent decisions, random events, accidental happenings. At times things may appear to be meaningful, but overall life has no visible purpose or unity. If we could penetrate the haze to apprehend the light of truth, we would realize that a hidden higher and eternal self is directing us. Our life happenings are not simply a series of accidents or random events. There is purpose, direction, and influence from a source of which we are at best only dimly aware. Occasionally the higher self breaks through to the mundane level. When it does, we experience a moment of inspiration.[80]

In the New Age, access to higher levels of consciousness is not thought to be accomplished easily and, as Peters intimates, considerable effort needs to be maintained by individuals to rise above the 'sleepy haze' in order that they may remain connected to the higher reality.

God

Finally, what the Higher Self is seen to connect with in the New Age can be broadly described as God. It must be noted, however, that in ideas and activities which have a humanistic or egocentric basis, the

---

78 Ted Peters's interpretation of Werner Erhard's view of the Higher Self is that Erhard teaches 'us to rise out of our "State of Mind" and into our "State of Self" [...] where such things as ego activity and personal identity take place' (1991: 66); whereas Peters's interpretation of the other authors listed is that they suggest ways to transcend the ego.
79 Examined in Chapter 10 below.
80 Ted Peters, 1991: 66.

notion of God is replaced with that of highest human possibility or potentiality or 'the perfectibility of man'.[81]

No duality is seen by many of those involved in the New Age between God and what they call the Higher Self – the two are claimed to be interconnected and inseparable. In this case, when God is spoken of here it is likely to be in a reverential sense, although this is not necessarily the same way that members of traditional theistic religions might speak of God. Paradoxically, however, many New Age commentators (for example, William Bloom[82]) acknowledge that both the New Age and theistic religions speak of the same God – that is, in their view there appears to be no ultimate or meaningful difference between the two concepts. The difference occurs in the particular way each group speaks of God or, in Wittgensteinian terms, in the particular language of their different forms of life.

In the New Age, participants seem not to be particularly concerned with using a single or mutually acceptable term to denote what they mean by God, although in theistic religions the opposite is mainly the case. Hence, in the New Age there exists a variety of terms which are used in reference to God. This variety has been expressed thus, that 'all life – all existence – is the manifestation of Spirit, of the Unknowable, of that supreme consciousness known by many different names in many different cultures.'[83]

To illustrate this variety further, the following list of examples of variations of the term God has been compiled from a number of sources influential to the New Age:[84] Absolute Truth, the Divine, the Divine Force, the Divine Mother, the Divine Spark, God, Goddess, Great Spirit, Infinite Light, Paramatman, Shakti, the Silence Out Of Which All Sound Comes, the Source, Spirit, the Supreme Being, Supreme Consciousness, Transcendental Reality, Ultimate Cause, Ultimate Unifying Principle, Unity Consciousness, Universal Energy, and

81   Joel Kovel, 1978: 153.
82   William Bloom, 1990: 13.
83   Op. cit.: 12f.
84   The list has been compiled from such writers as William Bloom (1991), Marilyn Ferguson (1982), Georg Feuerstein (1992), Stanley Krippner (1988), Jiddu Krishnamurti (1987), Mother Meera (1994), Gordon Melton *et al.*, 1991, and Ken Wilber (1995a).

the Unknowable; there are many more. Additionally, with regard to the use of the terms Energy and Light a further range of words can be added including Vibration, as well as 'prana, mana, odic force, orgone energy, holy spirit, the chi, mind, and the healing force'.[85]

Most of all, across world religions and New Age spiritualities, and in which ever way God is thought about, God is seen to represent the highest love. And it is perhaps true to say that the scriptures which talk of love are those that are most adopted into New Age thinking and beliefs.

What is more, even within traditional Western religions there are theistic notions – primarily based on mysticism – which appear to have also been adopted at least in part into New Age ideas and activities. Most notably, these include aspects of Sufism from Islam, and Cosmic Wisdom (a concept which includes the notion of a Cosmic Christ and cosmic consciousness) from Christianity, as expressed by Pierre Teilhard de Chardin[86] and Matthew Fox.[87] In some respects, therefore, aspects of contemporary interpretations of theistic religions appear to fall within the broad definition of New Age spirituality and, in consequence, bring with them their own particular names and words for God.

With regard to how God is viewed in the New Age, David Spangler warns participants about the problems of only seeing God in an immanent sense. He says that

> The idea of God within, improperly understood, can also make us lose sight of the other image of God as an external presence and force in the world. Instead of seeing ourselves as cocreators we imagine ourselves as creators. But what, then, can we create except forms in our own image? Where is the possibility of transformation in that? If the God within is not complemented by a living experience of God as that which transcends us, it becomes an idol, wrought in the image of our own personalities. We are then more limited than before, since we have lost a sense of that which can help us transcend ourselves.[88]

85   Gordon Melton *et al.*, 1991: 304.
86   Pierre Teilhard de Chardin, 1978: 55ff.
87   Matthew Fox, 1988.
88   David Spangler, 1984: 156.

Spangler, in a similar way to Stanislav Grof and Ken Wilber, believes that the qualities of God in the New Age are both immanent and transcendent, and not just one or the other.

A final point needs to be made with regard to the gender of God as described in the New Age. Here, there appears to be considerable agreement. God is seen as having both male and female attributes, as one single entity or energy without division. This situation is described by the suggestion that 'all the gods are one god; and all the goddesses are one goddess, and there is one initiator.'[89] In this instance, the word 'God' is seen to be masculine because of the way it has been used in the historical monotheistic traditions, and what is described as 'the initiator' appears to be over and above any genderization. However, it needs to be noted that there exist groups, particularly pagan, which might be considered to be New Age, and which concentrate more or wholly on the Goddess or feminist aspects of spirituality; for example, the Fellowship of Isis and the House of the Goddess Network.

Summary

This description of key terminology has demonstrated the most significant features which are reported to be involved in the paradigmatic shift which New Age individuals suggest is required in order to break free of 'ordinary' life and which, they believe, leads to a more natural, higher level of being. The New Age is seen to be, at heart, deeply spiritual. Transformation is seen as the important entry point, although the nature of this transformation, as understood by those involved, can vary substantially. Moreover, there appears to be little dispute that the primary focus of the transformation – through the core qualities of interconnectedness and unconditional love combined with compassion – is to make contact with higher levels of consciousness. Finally, an ultimate, inclusive reality is seen to exist which, in a variety of forms,

89   Dion Fortune cited in Caitlin Matthews, 1991: 9.

appears to provide a sacred focus to the New Age, although there seems to be no overarching agreement as to what the precise nature of this might be. Among the many writers who are influential to the New Age, a significant level of common ground exists with regard to the key concepts which, as has been shown, comprise an essential basis to the core New Age ideas described by William Bloom.

PART TWO

ENCOUNTERING NEW AGE DOMAINS OF INTEREST

Introduction

Great innovations never come from above; they come invariably from below, just as trees never grow from the sky downward, but upward from the earth.

Carl Jung[1]

Through observation of the New Age it becomes apparent that its ideas and activities can be separated into core domains or fields of interest; and this further assists in clarifying both the scope of New Age practices and the structure of ideological frameworks which individuals develop. Three principal domains have been identified, and each will be discussed in the following chapters. The domains involve matters concerning a change or empowerment of an individual's spirituality, their healing practices, and their community activity, which includes environmental concerns.[2] The most influential domain is that of spiritual empowerment, not least because it frequently seems to play a key directional role in the other two.

It is arguable whether there are just these three domains or whether there are more. In fact, other attempts have been made to divide New Age ideas and activities in similar ways – although I place greater emphasis on healing – plus New Science/new cosmology, whose description is mostly beyond the remit of this book.[3]

By and large, the three core New Age domains are suggested because they broadly encompass the majority of its principal ideas and

1   Carl Jung, 1976: 471.
2   The term 'community' is not used in the narrow sense of a face-to-face physical community of people – for example, the Findhorn Community – but in its broader sense of fellowship and mutual social cooperation.
3   William Bloom suggests: new paradigm/new science, spiritual dynamics, new psychology, and ecology (1991: xvi); while Mary Farrell Bednarowski proposes new cosmology, immanence of the divine, individual and social transformation, and ecology (1991: 209).

activities. However, not one of these three groupings is mutually exclusive, as each frequently incorporates influences from all domains. In this regard, a significant overlap can be seen to exist between the domains of spiritual empowerment and healing practices. A reason for this overlap is that while healing may be enacted without affecting an individual's spirituality, it frequently acts as a form of spiritual empowerment. The converse is also true, in that spiritual influences often have beneficial healing results. Additionally, one area in particular incorporates considerable overlap of all three domains – that of service – and this will be described briefly below.

It needs to be pointed out, however, that the spread of New Age interests is simply too big for any one person to be involved to any great degree in all of its ideas and activities, although it is common for participants to become involved in some or many of those selected – or intuited – from across each of the domains. This is the principal reason why study of the New Age is particularly difficult: no two individuals are likely to have precisely the same interests or reflect precisely the same philosophy. Nevertheless, the categorization of ideas and activities into three core domains illustrates that there are observably distinct features to the New Age, analysis of which goes towards demonstrating that within what appears at first sight to be amorphous in complexion can, in fact, be shown to have (using William Bloom's term) some scaffolding. Thus, the domains explored here focus on variations of possible approaches which participants can adopt.

Service

A particular area in the New Age where spiritual empowerment, healing practices, and community activity overlap to a large degree is in the concept of service. In fact, it is suggested that the '"service" aspect of the New Age – service to individuals, to communities, to the universe – is one that does not receive much publicity in the popular understanding of the movement, but it is a prominent theme.'[4] What is not made plain here is that some New Age writers – for example, Ram Dass and William Bloom – see that such service also incorporates a great deal of spiritual merit for the individual.

The notion of service as a form of spiritual practice for Ram Dass originates from his teacher, the Indian mystic Neem Keroli Baba, whose principal teachings Dass reports include the idea that the only way to an individual's salvation is through service to fellow human beings.[5] Dass suggests that through service the sense of individual separateness is diminished while the sense of unity is increased. Dass also believes that acts of service go towards Self-healing[6] and, using examples from the life of Mahatma Gandhi, he demonstrates how spiritually-imbued service has also healed community problems.[7]

Similarly, William Bloom points out that 'there is a powerful thrust in the movement to better the conditions and quality of life for all people and beings on the planet'[8] which he suggests is bound up with the ethics of the New Age, and these he states are 'compassion, caring, and unconditional love'.[9]

Finally, the way in which the concept of service appears to manifests itself clearly among those active in the New Age is through their sense of vocation. On this point, two commentators have found that, firstly, 'a large proportion of New Agers work in the caring professions'[10] and, secondly, that 'participants in the Aquarian Conspiracy questionnaire represented nearly every vocational field.'[11] It can also be recalled that among participants to my survey a large number

4   Mary Farrel Bednarowski, 1991: 214.
5   Ram Dass, 1979: 248.
6   Ram Dass and Paul Gorman, 1994: 224.
7   Op. cit.: 174. In Gandhi's earlier days in South Africa, he first developed a need to do service for the community and this, he found, brought him peace (1993: 202f), the rest is history. And service is also of prime importance in the teachings of Sathya Sai Baba, who is influential to some of those involved in the movement (see, for example, Sai Baba: 1991).
8   William Bloom, 1991: 183.
9   Ibid.
10   Ibid.
11   Marilyn Ferguson, 1982: 376.

claimed vocational occupations. However, it needs to be noted that not all of those who participate in New Age ideas and activities necessarily also carry out acts of service. In fact, it is impossible to quantify the extent of service activities by those involved as some of their activities are not 'visible', including, for example, the many instances and types of distance healing.

Bearing in mind the interconnected nature of the domains and the notion of service, each of the domains is now studied separately.

6. Spiritual Empowerment

What exists in truth is the Self alone. The world, the individual soul, and God are appearances in it, like silver in mother-of-pearl; these three appear at the same time, and disappear at the same time.
The Self is that where there is absolutely no 'I' thought. That is called 'Silence'. The Self itself is the world; the Self itself is 'I'; the Self itself is God; all is Siva, the Self.

Sri Ramana Maharshi[1]

Ideas and activities which go to make up the domain of spiritual empowerment are primarily to do with effecting and maintaining a transformation of an individual's life. This change is reported to occur as a total transformation of an individual not only in terms of her or his way of thinking but in a complete change with regard to the way they lead their lives – a change which is described as 'not just a matter of seeing things differently but of seeing different things'.[2]

Spiritual empowerment has already been shown to be of great significance to the New Age, yet its importance raises several issues relating to how participants approach their individual spiritual quests which include, for example, what characteristics their spirituality might entail, whether 'God' is important, how they identify and evaluate their spirituality, and which teachers are most influential. To address these issues, this chapter examines the nature of spirituality as those involved themselves report it. Of course, spirituality cannot be quantified by any technical measure because spirituality is itself an indeterminate concept which denotes a certain type of experience or understanding. However, in order to proceed, the less than perfect 'tools' which are generally available for such an analysis – that is, in-

---

1   Ramana Maharshi, 1969: 8.
2   Marilyn Ferguson, 1982: 397.

dividual descriptions taken at face value without the possibility of further verification – are those which will be generally used.

Spirituality and participation in the New Age

Measures of the spirituality of participants and the extent to which it is taken to occur in their lives are gauged by comparison with a benchmark for the overall importance of spirituality *per se*. In this respect, Gallup polls provide a reasonably reliable indication. In one of their standard monthly surveys[3] among a sample of one thousand adults – the social and demographic profile of which is designed to reflect the population at large – respondents were asked to gauge the level of importance that spiritual well-being played in their lives. The results show few people reporting spirituality to be more important than anything else, although a quarter reported it to be very important, and the remainder believed it was either not very important or quite important. These findings demonstrate that spiritual well-being is not a central feature in most people's lives. In fact, out of eight subjects, the importance of spirituality came seventh. More important were health, love, sleep and rest, pleasure and fun, and material security.[4]

This situation, as might be expected, is not reflected in the survey I carried out for this study. Here, participants were asked whether and to what degree they believed that spiritual affairs were involved with their ideas and activities. While the two surveys are not technically comparable, the juxtaposition of the results is interesting in that it

3   Gallup Political and Economic Index (1993).
4   The Gallup findings in response to the question 'How important is spiritual well-being in your life?' were: more important than anything else 3%, very important 24%, quite important 39%, and not very important 32%. The total findings for the eight-part question for those claiming 'more important that anything else' and 'very important' were: health 85%, love 65%, rest and sleep 60%, pleasure and fun 48%, material security 40%, achievement and success 29%, spiritual well-being 27%, and the approval of your employer and colleagues 23% (Ibid.).

164

shows a significant reversal in the importance of the spiritual content of participants' lives. In fact, 56% saw that spiritual affairs were always involved in their activities and, in total, more than 90% claimed that it was always or often the case.

The conclusion which can be reached with regard to these two sets of information is that participants in the New Age lead lives with a significantly higher spiritual content than the population at large. Moreover, it is possible to contend – given these facts together with evidence from previous chapters regarding participant's description of the New Age – that heightened spirituality is a fundamental quality among those engaging with its ideas and activities. Further views from my survey findings also confirm this. For example, virtually all participants considered themselves to be spiritual people, and more than 90% reported that they were actively pursuing a spiritual path. What is more, 90% of participants also claimed that they meditate, although some differences occurred. While there was little difference between the genders with regard to meditation practice, there was in relation to the frequency of such practice in their age groups. In fact, 25% of younger, 40% of the middle, and almost 60% of the older age group claimed to meditate each day – that is, there were more than twice as many older participants who meditated frequently than younger.

A final note on the measure of the spiritual nature of participants concerns the principal attribute which they claimed was present in their spirituality. Asked whether they believed spirituality could be experienced without love or whether they believed love was always present in spirituality, it was no surprise to find that almost 90% gave an answer reporting that love was always present.

Perhaps one of the most interesting findings of my survey regards the use of the term 'spirituality'. As briefly reported in the previous chapter, those involved were asked to write in their own words a description of what they meant when they used the term. Overall, the findings show that spirituality is seen to be a particularly meaningful and essential part of most participants' lives.

The number of times particular words had been used was evaluated in a large sample of these descriptions and it was found that six were mentioned more than any others.[5] These were 'Universal Force', 'God', 'love', 'Higher Self', 'more than physical', and 'connectedness'. In the case of the most often used description, spirituality was seen either as awareness of, or connection to, a *Universal Force* (35% used this notion). This was also expressed as: 'Universal or Cosmic Energy', 'Vibration', 'Essence', 'Light', and 'that which flows through each individual's incarnations'. It is of note that within this description there is no reference to a theistic God or any form of central being; in its place was the concept of a sacred energy which these individuals believed permeated everything everywhere.

Four words were each used by just under 20% of participants. Briefly these were, firstly, where the word *God* was mentioned, its use was very much in the traditional sense of Creator, as a higher being, and spirituality was seen as a connectedness to this being. Secondly, *Love* was seen as being closely linked with the notion of compassion,[6] and in its relationship with spirituality it was frequently expressed as being unconditional. Thirdly, *Higher Self* appeared to be used more to describe a process of going within to make contact with, as one participant put it, 'inner superstuff'. However, whether participants using this description were referring to a universal force, or God, or the perfectibility of man was not clear from this manner of enquiry.

A different phrase was used in approximately the same number of descriptions, that of *more than physical*. Sometimes this was phrased as 'more than our senses', 'more than material', 'lessening of the ego', 'loss of self', 'or beyond earthly existence'. This definition, it is believed, was used either by those who found describing their spirituality problematic or who had no fixed view of what spirituality might mean – although, again, it was not clear which. The expression 'more than physical' was not used in the same way as the previous description, that of going within to make contact with the Higher Self, nor did it appear to be used to describe particular levels of consciousness: it simply appeared to represent an individual's general perception of matters of higher or ultimate concern. A final word, used by

5   Some participants may have used more than one of these words in their descriptions.
6   This confirms the description given in Chapter 5 above.

12% of participants, was *connectedness*, and this could well link with all of the above descriptions in a variety of ways, although it was also used in a separate context, that of oneness, common brotherhood, wholeness, and harmony.

The conclusion which can be drawn from this analysis is that there appears to be little, if any, dispute among participants with the commentaries made in regard to the language of spirituality in the New Age that were given in Chapter 5. Most often, spirituality was seen as some form of connection with an all-pervading force or energy which was not believed to be separate from each individual; but it appeared to be referred to as distinct from the ego, although there were variations to this view. Furthermore, there appeared to be an element of theistic dualism in some descriptions; yet, overall, the representations were not dualistic in the theistic sense – in fact, there seems to be substantial evidence that monistic or non-dualistic views are held by many or most participants.

In summary, the majority of participants – having been engaged with its ideas and activities for some considerable time, who overwhelmingly claim to be actively spiritual, and who believe the New Age to be mostly involved with spiritual affairs – predominantly gave a transpersonal and mystico-transcendent description of their spirituality which frequently incorporated sacred elements. Moreover, the conclusion can be drawn that, if these participants are typical, the New Age itself, at its centre, appears to be primarily comprised of individuals who hold beliefs in an immanent *and* transcendent view of ultimate reality – as Stanislav Grof, David Spangler, and Ken Wilber have suggested – where the New Age is not only seen as a matter of finding spirituality within but where it is also a matter of connecting with a spirituality which transcends what is claimed to lie within.

God and the New Age

Following on from these findings, several questions were asked in an attempt to establish what participant's ideas about God might involve. It can be remembered that there are many descriptions given to the concept of God, the majority of which are not theistic in character.

In the first instance, participants were asked whether or not they considered that all New Age ideas and activities always included at least some notion of God or an eternal/divine spirit.[7] The findings show that 40% believed that at least some notion of God or divine spirit was 'always' present, and a further 43% believed this 'often' to be the case. In total, therefore, more than four out of five believed that God was mostly present in the New Age, with most of the remainder reporting that this was only sometimes the case. Practically no individual suggested that this was never the case. These participants, therefore, in the main see that their activities are frequently imbued with a sense of the sacred.[8] It can be added that women appeared to be a little more certain of the sacred content of their activities and men less so, and the same finding occurred between older and younger participants respectively.

Ensuing from this question, two additional questions were asked along the same theme to assist in further clarifying beliefs in God contained in the New Age; and here the second result might be seen as surprising. First of all, an attempt was made to gauge the extent to which those involved believed in the concept of spiritual perenniality by asking whether they believed there existed varying types of spirituality – for instance, New Age, Buddhist, or Christian – or whether spirituality was universally the same. The finding clearly shows that almost three-quarters saw spirituality to be universally the same wher-

---

7   The survey phraseology was intentional in order that the findings could be clearly separated into groups of those who believed there to be a spiritual element in all aspects of the New Age and those who did not.

8   The American survey found that 95% of those involved believed in God, although the majority reported that their idea of God was different to that of the Bible (Frederick Levine, 1989: 111).

ever it occurred, while the remainder believed there to be types. Secondly, this view was probed further by asking wh not participants believed there could exist the concept of a separate theistic God – as seen in Christianity, Judaism, and Islam – in New Age ideas and activities. The results here show a surprisingly mixed outcome. The majority view, shared by just under 40%, indicated that the theistic concept of a separation between God and humanity was not in accord with New Age ideas, yet 30% were undecided, and a little over 20% believed 'definitely' it was the case that theistic concepts can exist in the New Age. This mixed finding, and especially that one in five believed in a theistic view of God, is highly interesting because practically all participants claimed to be involved in the New Age,[9] yet it goes against views held by some authors[10] who claim that the New Age incorporates a wholly monistic spiritual basis.

In combination, these two findings demonstrate that the New Age is not viewed by some participants as being exclusively monistic and that it does not exclude any 'variety' of spirituality. The logical conclusion of this view must be, therefore, that an element of participants believe theistic religions – or at least theistic concepts – and New Age ideas and activities are compatible and, as a consequence, that Christians, Jews, and Muslims can hold New Age beliefs. While this conclusion might appear to be paradoxical if the New Age is seen to be wholly monistic, there are numerous examples of New Age teachings which go to confirm the ambiguity (for example, *A Course In Miracles*); and perhaps the most important notion to arise here is that many spiritual teachings appear to be practised ambivalently – that is, either independently of other teachings or as complimentary to them. The New Age has no dogma or institutions and, in this regard, does not attempt to – and could not – prohibit participants from following any idea or activity which they intuitively see as beneficial to the development of their spiritual life.

Two examples will assist to clarify this all-embracing concept of New Age spirituality. Firstly, at a two-day conference staged by Al-

---

9   In answer to a question on their involvement, 97% of participants claimed to have adopted New Age practices.
10   For, example, Paul Heelas (1996a: 37) and Ted Peters (1991: 59ff).

ternatives in London with the theme 'A New Consciousness', an Anglican service of Holy Communion was held at the conference venue, St James's Church in Piccadilly. In this service, the Reverend Donald Reeves, the then Deacon of St James's, announced that the Eucharist was open to everybody present (the congregation being predominantly comprised of New Age individuals) and invited the entire gathering – regardless of beliefs – to participate. The Eucharist commenced with a *Tripudium* (an ancient non-Christian meditative dance) by all around the altar. When Donald Reeves broke the bread he announced that he was doing so to the four corners of the world, that it was for Buddhists, Hindus, Jews, Muslims, and Christians alike – in fact, Donald Reeves made a plea to 'let them soon be one'. Following this, the congregation – whether they had been confirmed or not, and whether they were Christian or not – were invited to take the sacrament.

Spiritual teachers who are important to some participants give the second example. Mother Meera was asked by a devotee whether they should stop believing in Jesus and believe in her. The Mother replied, 'Whomever you believe in, believe with all your heart. All divine incarnations are equal. Be sincere, open, and my help will be given to you always';[11] and Sathya Sai Baba teaches his disciples that 'All religions, all faiths, are but phases or facets of the same universal faith or discipline'.[12]

Overall, we can conclude that belief in the concept of God or a divine spirit in the New Age is strong, although it is not restricted to any one description. In many respects, the particular 'variety' a participant might adopt appears to be of less relevance in comparison to their reported overarching need to lead a spiritually empowered life.

11   Mother Meera, 1994: 52.
12   Douglas G. Davie, 2000: 111.

Identifying varieties of spiritual empowerment

To identify the varieties of spiritual empowerment, the first – and basic – point to clarify was whether those involved demonstrated a fidelity to any one type of spirituality. With this in mind, participants were asked whether a particular teacher or teaching was followed, and they clearly – over 75% – answered that this was not the case. This finding is important because it confirms the idea that the New Age has no uniform structure and that there is no formalized ideology common to most participants. It also goes to substantiate the previously stated view that New Age practice is very much a path or quest which individuals follow primarily on their own. The minority (21%) who reported that they did follow a particular teacher or teaching were further requested to state who or what that was. In response, although over eighty teachers or teachings were mentioned by name, none were given by more than a handful of participants each – the most mentioned name being Sathya Sai Baba (given by 15 individuals). This finding clearly shows that membership of new religious movements is not a feature of these participants' spiritual activities. Furthermore, those involved were also asked whether more than one teaching was followed at the same time and, here again, the results show that two-thirds did in fact follow multiple teachings.

These findings confirm the commonly accepted view that while belief in the overarching ideas of the New Age appear to be widely held by those involved, there are few rigidly adhered-to modes of practice which are followed in any particularly structured way. New Age spirituality is comprised of mixtures of activities and, what is more, represents the diametrically opposite position to religions, cults, and new religious movements which, on the whole, frequently incorporate more formal methods of practice and exclusivity from one another. In fact, this New Age mix can, in principle, incorporate both esoteric and exoteric teachings at the same time.

Looking more closely at a detailed analysis of the means of spiritual empowerment, participants were asked to state or list what spiritual discipline or teaching had created the greatest influence on their

171

lives. In response to this request, the majority gave more than one name, although it can be deduced that these influences were not necessarily concurrent. In fact, a large list of names has been compiled yet, in all, no clear teaching or even type of teaching appears (numerically) to have been more influential than any other. The influences given by a total of just under 30% of those involved, the largest group of names, were described as the influence of many teachers, none specific, or a combination of Eastern and Western. This latter category, for example, included various combinations of Christianity and Buddhism and, more specifically, a retired academic working as an autogenics therapist lists Quakerism, Buddhism, Jiddu Krishnamurti, Meister Eckhart, Matthew Fox, the Essenes, and Gnosis.[13] Approximately 20% gave answers which more specifically comprised of Eastern (or Eastern-influenced) spiritualities and new religious movements. In total, these two groups account for half of all replies. However, other groups include Christianity (7%), healing (7%, which included elements of spiritual healing as well as healing therapies), channelled teachings such as *A Course in Miracles* (6%), and pagan and ancient wisdom teachings (4%).

From these findings it can be concluded that the means of spiritual empowerment employed by participants stems from contact with, or synthesis of, a number of teachings or influences. The resulting spirituality is not rigid but seems fluid and malleable and is developed according to the progression of each person's spiritual quest. In this respect, for example, a participant might believe it to be perfectly acceptable to carry out their spiritual practice in many different locations – a Christian church, a Buddhist temple, a circle of standing stones, and in any other space which they consider (or make to be) sacred including, of course, their homes.

---

13   A personal account of spiritual progression in the New Age, which typifies the kind of path taken, is given graphically by Ihla Nation (1998: 19ff), who describes her life as travelling over many years from childhood Lutheran Christianity, through Seth (books), U. S. Anderson (books), the Mile High Church of Religious Science in Colorado, serious study of Hinduism and Buddhism, and finally to classes on A Course In Miracles where, she writes, 'a genuine transformation of consciousness took place' (Op. cit.: 22).

Appraisal of the multiplicity

An underlying notion in New Age ideas and activities which has become apparent is that it would be rare indeed to find one teacher or teaching that could completely encompass an individual's spiritual quest. In this regard, trial and error and spiritual growth in steps and stages appear commonplace.[14] Teachers who are important in the New Age themselves advise participants to utilize many sources of inspiration in order to achieve spiritual empowerment. Jiddu Krishnamurti, for example, suggests that

> If you look to one person as your teacher, then you are lost and that person becomes your nightmare. That is why it is very important not to follow anybody, not to have one particular teacher, but to learn from the river, the flower, the trees, from the woman who carries a burden, from the members of your own family and from your own thoughts.[15]

From another perspective Ram Dass identifies that

> Some people fear becoming involved with a teacher. They fear the possible impurities in the teacher, fear of being exploited, used, or entrapped. In truth we are only ever entrapped by our own desires and clingings. If you want only liberation, then all teachers will be useful vehicles for you. They cannot hurt you at all.[16]

Put in a different way, Marilyn Ferguson believes that 'The radical Centre of spiritual experience seems to be knowing without doctrine.'[17] Here, Ferguson suggests that the role of the spiritual teacher is important only as a facilitator who can assist in enabling an individual in their quest for Self-understanding. Ferguson maintains that

14 Georg Feuerstein, for example, illustrates some of the parameters found in the range of spiritual teachers (1992: 131).
15 Jiddu Krishnamurti, 1974: 240.
16 Georg Feuerstein, 1992: 143.
17 Marilyn Ferguson, 1982: 414.

Teachers and techniques in the spiritual disciplines must be considered together, for the teacher does not impart knowledge but technique. This is the
'transmission' of knowledge by direct experience [...] Doctrine, on the other
hand, is second-hand knowledge, a danger. 'Stand above, pass on, and be free'
is the advice of Rinzai, the same sage who advises the seeker to kill the patri-
archs or the Buddha if he should encounter them. 'Do not get entangled in any
teaching.'[18]

Likewise, an academic suggests: 'If New Agers themselves have
got it right, we are in the realm of the koan, not the Ten Command-
ments. That is to say, religion, as normally understood in the west, has
been replaced by teachers whose primary job is to set up the "contexts" to enable participants to experience their spirituality and authority.'[19] All these authors suggest that teachings have a reduced importance in providing definitive paths to reach higher levels of spiritual
practice, and, moreover, that the provision of 'techniques' and 'contexts' now appears to replace spiritual direction. What is more, these
views seem to be fully upheld by participants who, in the main, believe that satisfying spiritual needs is their responsibility and not the
teacher's.

This view, however, does not paint an entirely comprehensive
picture, as it has been shown above that some of those involved include specific religious traditions and movements in their notion of
what they believe the New Age can entail. This being the case, more
formalized paths of spiritual empowerment cannot be excluded from
New Age practice.

How participants decide which paths to follow obviously entails
subjective appraisal of each teacher or teaching – and one of the principal 'tools' used in this capacity is intuition. This process, outlined in
Chapter 4, is succinctly described by a co-director of a New Age resource centre who reported that 'if something resonates with me I use
it, if not I don't. I take bits from different teachings/cultures that speak
to me and put them together with my life,' and a massage therapist
declared that she 'looked into many [teachings], but I have experienced the greatest "influence" from my own Higher Self or God-Self.'

18   Op. cit.: 415.
19   Paul Heelas, 1996a: 23.

Through qualitative interpretation of the survey findings, it is apparent that participants appraise the potential worth that teachers or teachings may provide, and this incorporates different levels of 'usefulness' although, from the nature of the research method, it is not possible to determine with any certainty what the characteristics of these levels might entail. However, what is clear is that participants, especially those who are more fully associated with the New Age, adopt a variable plurality of spiritual teachings, some of which may be continued with over the course of time, while others may be discontinued according to either or both their perceived value and the unique direction of each person's spiritual path. Finally, as must be anticipated, each teaching can result in very different levels of consequences among participants who appear, in the end, to trust intuitional guidance for spiritual direction.

intuition takes over from custom or tradition

Spiritual teachers

Turning to the matter of identifying the relative importance of teachers, those involved were asked to name individuals whose ideas had an important influence on their lives, firstly by contact[20] and, secondly, through their writings. In each case, the total number of names recorded was substantial yet, interestingly, if we compare the two sets of the ten most influential names given with regard to their importance by contact or by their writings, no name is found to be common to both categories.

With regard to individuals who have been important by *contact*, the finding shows that no one specific individual was of overriding

---

20 The term 'contact' can be applied either as contact with influential individuals through workshops – that is, attending a workshop led by the individual concerned – or through more personal contact. On the whole, the former use of the term is what appears to have been understood by the majority of participants, although no prompts were given in the question as to the type of contact which was to be described.

importance among 60% of those involved; yet among 40% the reverse was the case. The person who was most important was, in one-third of cases, well known by, or related to, the participant. This finding further confirms the view previously given that there is no overridingly important teacher or teaching in the New Age.

An additional analysis was carried out with regard to the names which were mentioned. The 10 names which received the highest number of mentions were, in descending order, Denise Linn, Sir George Trevelyan, Matthew Manning, the Dalai Lama, Mother Meera, Sri Sathya Sai Baba, Gill Edwards, Ram Dass, Stuart Wilde, and the Cosmic or Jesus Christ. No one name was mentioned by more than 3% of those involved. In all, 595 names were given, of which the vast majority were mentioned only once. Furthermore, it can be pointed out that the teachings or activities of the majority of those listed are predominantly to do with spiritual and healing concerns.

With regard to individuals who had been important through their *writings* the situation is quite different, as the vast majority claimed that the influence of many writings had been important.[21] This result appears to suggest, logically, that actual contact with an individual is likely to have greater influence than that achieved through reading what they say.

In 1977 Marilyn Ferguson distributed over 200 questionnaires to named people who were engaged in many areas of New Age ideas and activities, and the findings subsequently formed the basis of her study *The Aquarian Conspiracy*. Respondents were requested to name individuals 'whose ideas had most influenced them, either through personal contact or through their writings'.[22] Ferguson reported a list of the top seven most frequently mentioned names in order of frequency of mention, plus a further list of 30 names which were often mentioned by respondents, although these were not ranked in her volume. I repeated the question nearly 20 years later, albeit split into two separate parts, and generated a total of 771 names of individuals whom those involved claimed had had an important influence on their lives

---

21   This category includes thinkers, gurus, channelled or other spirit beings, saints, key practitioners, and artists, as well as all manner of teachers.
22   Marilyn Ferguson, 1982: 462f.

through their writings. While the basis of the two surveys cannot be compared exactly because of the differences in the sampling methods and questions used in each, it is interesting to review the names that each survey generated, and these are reported in Table 11.

Table 11. Most influential New Age teachers in
1977 and 1994

1977 List	1994 List[23]

1. Top seven names in order of priority:

Pierre Teilhard de Chardin	Louise Hay
C. G. Jung	C. G. Jung
Abraham Maslow	Shakti Gawain
Carl Rogers	White Eagle
Aldous Huxley	Richard Bach
Roberto Assagioli	David Icke
Jiddu Krishnamurti	Rudolf Steiner

2. 30 other names most frequently mentioned
(in alphabetical order):

Sri Aurobindo	Alice Bailey
Gregory Bateson	Helena Blavatsky
Ruth Benedict	Barbara Brennan
Elise Boulding	Paul Brunton
Kenneth Boulding	Fritjof Capra
Martin Buber	Ken Carey
Albert Einstein	Carlos Castenada
Werner Erhard	Edgar Cayce

23 The 1994 list has been edited to exclude mention of traditional religious teachings – for example, the Bible, Buddhist scriptures, and Taoist writings.

Heinz von Foerster	Deepak Chopra
Erich Fromm	Ram Dass
Buckminster Fuller	The Dalai Lama
Willis Harman	Gill Edwards
Hermann Hesse	Dion Fortune
Oscar Ichazo	Kahil Gibran
Alfred Korzybski	Jiddu Krishnamurti
John Lilly	Denise Linn
Marshall McLuhan	Shirley MacLaine
Margaret Mead	Matthew Manning
Thomas Merton	Mother Meera
Swami Muktananda	M. Scott Peck
Gardner Murphy	Bhagwan Shree Rajneesh
Joseph Chilton Pearce	Sathya Sai Baba
Karl Pribram	Sanaya Roman
Frederic Spiegelberg	Betty Shine
D. T. Suzuki	Sogyal Rinpoche
Tarthang Tulku	Julie Soskin
Paul Tillich	Sir George Trevelyan
Alan Watts	Lyle Watson
Alfred North Whitehead	Stuart Wilde
Maharishi Mahesh Yogi	Paramahansa Yogananda

As can be seen from the top part of the lists, only one name is common to both – that of Carl Jung – and, not without coincidence, Jung holds second place in both lists. In the lower part there are no names common to both lists, although Jiddu Krishnamurti at seventh position in 1977 is also mentioned in 1994 as being important.[24]

The difference between the two sets of lists can, to a large extent, be accounted for by the New Age ideas and activities prevalent in the two periods. As has been shown in the historical account of the New

24   In the 1994 survey as a whole – that is, from over 700 names – a further eight names from the 1977 list were mentioned, although the actual number of mentions for each was low. The eight names were Roberto Assagioli, Herman Hesse, Aldous Huxley, Abraham Maslow, Carl Rogers, Pierre Teilhard de Chardin, Alan Watts, and Maharishi Mahesh Yogi.

Age given in Chapter 2, in 1970s America – especially in California where Marilyn Ferguson was based – ideas surrounding the Human Potential Movement had become widespread and, therefore, it is not surprising to see names such as Assagioli, Maslow, and Rogers appearing as important at this time. Equally, the same premise can be applied to the list from 1994, when healing practices had become more widespread and, therefore, the names of Gawain and Hay are to be expected. Additionally, in comparing both lists with regards to the inclusion of spiritual teachers, it would appear that each contains 12 such names.

Turning to the matter of identifying the names in each list, it is not relevant to describe each one individually. However, with regard to the types of teachings involved, as well as 12 spiritual teachers the 1994 lists include 12 healers, 6 astrologers and other psychically-oriented writers, and 7 miscellaneous writers. It must be pointed out, however, that there exists a degree of overlap in categories among some of the individuals involved. Interestingly, the more recent top seven names of those important through their *writings* include few specifically spiritual teachers, yet the list of individuals who have been important by *contact* during the same period contains the names of many spiritual teachers. The most mentioned teacher in 1994, Louise Hay, a 'metaphysical counsellor',[25] has published a number of self-help guides aimed at improving the health of the body, mind, and spirit. However, by contrast, the most-mentioned teacher in 1977, Pierre Teilhard de Chardin, was a Jesuit priest who, posthumously, expounded the concept of a Cosmic Christ together with the notion that humans were co-creators in the evolutionary scheme of (Christian) life.[26]

25 Louise Hay, 1988.
26 Two survey variables should be noted. Firstly, the 1977 survey was carried out in the USA while the 1994 survey was carried out in the UK. Secondly, the 1994 list appears to have been influenced by the dates of publication of various writings. The prime example of this is David Icke, who is listed in fifth place. The survey was carried out shortly after the publication of Icke's book The Robot's Rebellion, which had attracted some notoriety from its reviews. It is anticipated that had the 1994 survey been carried out six months later, Icke's name might have been replaced with that of James Redfield, whose best-selling

The overall conclusion which can be drawn from the above lists of key individuals is that the New Age has been – and, most likely, will remain – in a state of evolution in that teachers who are seen to be important at one moment in time may not be so important in the next moment. It has to be suggested that the importance of some teachers listed above frequently depends on the marketing 'hype' surrounding publishing events; and publishing in general, as noted in Chapter 4, is of prime importance as a method of access to the New Age. However, the extent of interest in spiritual concerns – as suggested by the numbers of spiritual teachers listed in each period – appears to have remained constant, whereas the ranking of others listed has changed considerably, particularly in the movement from psychotechnologies to healing.

Summary

This chapter has provided evidence which describes, at least in part, what spiritual empowerment means for participants in the New Age. In summarizing these findings, it is valuable to compare them with the six basic ideas that William Bloom[27] proposes described in Chapter 1.

Firstly, Bloom suggests that, in New Age ideas, all life is thought to be comprised of aspects of spirit and, clearly, those involved have demonstrated that spirituality is an extremely important element in their lives. Secondly, Bloom believes that a single energy pervades all life forms, and the manifestation of this energy is love. Plainly, in the descriptions of spirituality which have been given, there is no dissent

The Celestine Prophecy had only just been published. So, too, it must be expected that inclusion of some of the names contained in the 1977 lists might be the result of contemporaneous publications – for example, John Lilly had at least four books published or in print between 1973 and 1976. The four books were: The Centre of the Cyclone (1973), The Human Biocomputer (1974), Simulations of God (1975), and The Dyadic Cyclone (1976). For bibliographical details see Nevill Drury, 1994: 183.

27   William Bloom, 1990.

from this view. In fact, the vast majority believed that love was always present in their spirituality. The same is true of Bloom's third basic idea, whereby it is thought that there exists a Higher Self which tends towards love.

Bloom's fourth point is that each person appears to be following a succession of incarnations and is free to choose a spiritual path. Overwhelmingly, participants reported that they are actively following a spiritual path, and large numbers also claimed to have participated in recalling their past lives. Moreover, many of the individuals who have been important by contact or through their writings base much of their work on the idea that being human is but one of a succession of incarnations, and it must be expected that a large number of participants would therefore concur with their views. It can be added that Marilyn Ferguson's survey found that at least 75% were sure or moderately sure that consciousness did not end with bodily death.[28] Similarly, in Bloom's fifth and sixth ideas, the participants appear to strongly confirm the existence of spiritual guides and the appearance of seemingly many more such guides at this particular time.

In this case, therefore, there can be no doubt that participants would wholly support Bloom's contentions. This evidence adds significant weight to my supposition that the survey sample is representative of individuals who are more fully associated with the New Age and that the majority of these individuals exhibit what they take to be a profound, mystical and transcendent spirituality.

---

28   Marilyn Ferguson, 1982: 422.

7. Healing Practices

All healing is essentially the release from fear. To understand this you cannot be fearful of yourself [...] All sickness comes from separation. When separation is denied, it goes [...] Thus is your healing everything the world requires, that it may be healed.

A Course in Miracles[1]

The healing domain of the New Age incorporates a very wide variety of practices which participants claim to use to rid themselves of problems which block the way to optimum and holistic health of the body, mind, and spirit. In many respects, these healing practices can be regarded as both the most visible 'face' of the New Age and the most adopted out of all of its ideas and activities – in fact, certain of these therapies have been embraced by the medical mainstream both as complementary to its normal practices and, in a few cases, as alternative to them.

While many of the individual practices which comprise New Age healing are widely known, not very much is known about the users of the therapies and activities or the practitioners themselves. Following an introduction to the subject of healing in the New Age as a whole and some of the therapies involved, a way in which it is possible to quantify a more precise scope to this otherwise wide-ranging domain of ideas and activities is given.

---

1   *A Course in Miracles*, 1985: 19, 514, 536.

The domain of healing practices

The domain of healing practices in the New Age appears to be closely allied to the domain of spiritual empowerment, differing primarily in that it is predominantly to do with the health and well-being of the whole person, whereas the nature of spiritual empowerment is more to do with individuals seeking to transform or develop themselves through an educative or experiential process. To describe how close the two domains are, it has been reported that the

> holistic healing movement that gathered momentum throughout the late 1970s is rife with symbols evoking an explicitly religious interpretation of the healing process [...] It entails commitment to a belief in the interpenetration of physical and nonphysical spheres of causality to a degree that is inherently incompatible with the naturalistic framework of our modern scientific heritage.[2]

Moreover, another commentator sees that, 'With the linking of health and spiritual concerns, health becomes an idealization of a kind of self, healing is then part of the ongoing process by which that self is accomplished, and well-being is the individual's resulting subjective experience'.[3]

Healing practices are, therefore, where individuals seek to rid themselves of problems which bar the way to an optimum state of health of the body, mind, and spirit. Health, according to the World Health Organization (WHO), is 'not the mere absence of symptoms or infirmities but a state of physical, psychological, spiritual and social well-being'.[4] The alliance between the two domains of spiritual empowerment and healing practices lies in the main in the benefit optimum health brings to the spirituality of the individual in the form of firm foundations on which transformation or development can be enacted and maintained.

---

2   Robert Fuller, 1989: 91f.
3   Meredith McGuire, 1993: 153.
4   Cited in *One Earth* Issue 20, 1995: 24.

Additional to healing the body, mind, and spirit is the notion of healing the planet. While for some in the New Age this is a critical issue, it is too large a subject to discuss here, although aspects of it are touched upon in the following chapter. Nevertheless, one aspect must be introduced at this point. In New Age ideas and activities, an individual cannot consider themselves wholly in balance, wholly well, if they live in a sick environment. As the deep ecologists argue, "'no one" ... all humans, whales, grizzly bears, whole rain forest eco systems, mountains and rivers, the tiniest microbes in the soil, and so on ... "is saved until we are all saved".'[5] This is why holistic healing, if it is to be fully comprehensive, necessarily needs to incorporate planetary healing.

Returning to the discussion of healing the body, mind, and spirit, there appears to be no general agreement as to what might be the precise scope of healing practices in the New Age: this appears to be for two reasons. Firstly, many such practices are not necessarily specific to the New Age and are used simply as alternatives or complementaries to allopathic forms of medicine. Secondly, the sheer number of types of practices and their varying uses prohibits much determining classification.

What is more, there exists a number of tensions between allopathic medicine and the introduction of many of the new or renewed healing practices, and, relatedly, between the two concepts of alternative and complementary practice. In respect of the latter, the term 'complementary' – which, according to the British Centre for Complementary Health Studies, was only brought into use in 1981[6] – has become the more established, and less confrontational, term to describe the whole genre. Moreover, with regard to tensions between the medical mainstream and complementary medicine, the point is made that 'it is not the *technology* of modern medicine that is at odds with alternative medicine; it is the philosophy behind the development and exploitation of that technology.'[7] Here, it is suggested that these tensions are caused by the clash of the more mechanistic aspects of medi-

5   Bill Devall and George Sessions, 1985: 67.
6   Simon Mills, 1993: 25.
7   Richard Grossinger, 1995: 471.

cal science with the more holistic approaches to the treatment of health in general. Yet, as more and more evidence becomes available concerning the pros and cons of complementary medicine, these tensions appear to be reducing and the development of a more comprehensive approach to healthcare is beginning to emerge.[8]

Turning to the question of what might be considered as 'disease',[9] there appear to be significant differences between allopathic and complementary notions. From the allopathic point of view, illness is seen to be a biological or psychological malfunction and, correspondingly, health is simply considered as the absence of illness. In contrast, from the complementary and New Age perspective, illness is considered much more as an effect – and not necessarily the cause – of physical, psychological, social, spiritual, and environmental imbalance: dis-harmony, or dis-ease. In this case, New Age types of healing are seen to restore what can be described as a natural balance to the whole being.[10]

There are differences, too, in the means by which healing is brought about. In allopathic health care, the patient is mostly passive

---

8   Studies into the type, quality, benefits, and use of complementary medicines can be found in numerous academic journals such as the *British Medical Journal* and *The Lancet*, together with more specifically focussed journals such as *Complementary Therapies in Medicine, Complementary Digest*, and *Holistic Health*. See also publications by the British Medical Association (1993), and the Health Education Authority (Anne Woodham, 1994). Further evidence for the growth of complementary medicine is illustrated by the considerable number of professional associations and accreditation bodies which now exist – some of which have been in existence for over 50 years. The Institute for Complementary Medicine in London, for example, claims the affiliation of nearly 300 professional organizations, together with 400 linked bodies, and maintains a register of practitioners incorporating 17 divisions of complementary therapies which include aromatherapy, Chinese medicine, nutrition, colour therapy, counselling, and hypnotherapy. See also British Medical Association, 1993, chapter 6, a survey of non-conventional therapies which lists in detail 27 such professional organizations.

9   This word is frequently hyphenated in New Age writings as 'dis-ease', thus pointing to the difference in interpretation of the word between allopathic and complementary philosophies.

10   These ideas are expressed by Fritjof Capra, 1984, in his chapter addressing 'Wholeness and Health'.

in the process of treatment, although in complementary medicine the patient (or client) is wholly involved in the process of care – here, the patient represents the primary focus in the means of bringing about her or his own cure. This approach

> will be multidimensional, involving treatments at several levels of the mind/body system, which will often require a multidisciplinary team effort [...] Health care of this kind will require many new skills and disciplines not previously associated with medicine and is likely to be intellectually richer, more stimulating, and more challenging than a medical practice that adheres exclusively to the biomedical model.[11]

One vital element needs to be discussed with regard to the scope of this domain, and this relates to what healing can be used for. It can be said that there are two different 'needs' which can be satisfied – those of repair and of nurture. In the case of repair, healing denotes activity surrounding damage or disease to the physical, psychological, or spiritual aspects of the person – often experienced as combinations of these aspects – which takes the form of a *distress* healing requirement. On the other hand, there is not necessarily any damage or disease involved directly in the notion of nurture; in this instance, nurture relates to tuning, nourishing, and balancing all aspects of the person, and is more of a *considered* healing requirement. The overall objective of healing in the New Age is, by and large, to create and then maintain a harmony and holistic balance – that is, nurturing rather than repair – without which growth in other domains can be impaired.

The practices: not new and not necessarily New Age

There are very many different forms of healing which can be found being used in the New Age; and these forms of healing, as a genre, are

---

11   Op. cit.: 369.

not new and not necessarily specific to the New Age. In fact, whether or not a particular healing activity can be considered New Age or not is contestable, as will become clear. To give an indication of the types of practices involved, in the first instance some of the principal non-Western and more ancient practices are introduced and then Western and more recent developments are traced.[12]

There is evidence to suggest that Shamanism is the oldest form of healing, having its roots in mysticism and magic.[13] Shamanism is said to be 20,000 years old, stemming from Siberia, Asia, and North America. The Shaman's primary function is 'to heal and restore the individual's connectedness to the universe'.[14] Today contemporary Shamanism (or neo-Shamanism), according to the Eagle's Wing centre in London, is the adoption of the ancient shamanic teachings 'to help urban, suburban and all people of today [...] to heal the inner wounds and to create a way of life that is sustainable'.[15]

In company with the growth of shamanistic techniques, the West is also experiencing a growth in Neo-Pagan activities including Wicca and the women's and men's movements. At the heart of all of these activities is a heightened contact with the Higher Self and with nature through many ritualized forms of group activity celebrating, for instance, the seasons or rites of passage.[16]

Since the 1960s in the West, there has been a substantial rise in the use of traditional, ancient, and Eastern systems of medicine including Ayurveda (the Science of Life) from India and Chinese medicine, of which acupuncture, shiatsu (finger pressure), and herbology are the main branches. The principles of Chinese medicine 'are embedded in Confucianism and Taoism'[17] originating over 2,500 years ago. Here, treatment is very much to do with the concept of harmony – the bal-

---

12 General descriptions of the various types of bodywork therapies or psychotech-nologies can be found in Kate Brady and Mike Considine, 1990; Rosemary Ellen Guiley, 1991; Joel Kovel, 1978; and Anne Woodham, 1994.
13 Helen Graham, 1991: 165.
14 Rosemary Ellen Guiley, 1991: 540ff. See also Nevill Drury 1989 and Michael Harner 1990.
15 Eagle's Wing pamphlet.
16 For further examples of these see Vivianne Crowley, 1994.
17 Effie Poy Yew Chow, 1985: 115.

ance of yin and yang – which is disrupted in illness.[18] In 1986 it was estimated that there were 500 registered acupuncturists and 600 doctors who use acupuncture in the UK;[19] and many New Age magazines list scores of clinics and practitioners.

One further, but quite different, example of ancient healing practice is aromatherapy. This is the art of using oils extracted from aromatic plants to enhance health and beauty. The use of plant essences dates back to beyond Egyptian times, as has been shown by the discovery of scent bottles in Tutenkhamun's tomb.[20]

A thousand years ago in the Middle East, the philosopher Avicenna – influenced by the Ancient Greeks – wrote a work entitled *The Canon of Medicine* which 'the *Encyclopaedia Britannica* calls "the single most famous book in the history of medicine, in East or West"'.[21] In this work Avicenna developed a system of healing called Unani Tibb. Tibb literally means 'medicine and healing of the physical, mental, and spiritual realms',[22] which demonstrates that the concept of holism actually existed hundreds, if not thousands, of years ago. Even today there are reported to be 28,000 practitioners of Unani Tibb in India alone. Tibb is described as 'a truly unified, holistic medicine',[23] where a person's temperament – that is, their mental state – 'provides an altered biotic environment in which (disease) can thrive',[24] thus explaining in the eleventh century why, for example, some people contracted diseases while others did not.

From a different viewpoint, there are many forms of meditative practice which have become widely used since the 1960s – most notably Yoga, of which there are nine principal systems.[25] The term 'Yoga' is a derivation of the Sanskrit word meaning 'union' or 'one-

18   Ibid.
19   *Which?*, October 1986: 447.
20   A. Stanway, 1982: 84ff.
21   Hakim Chistie, 1988: 16.
22   Op. cit.: 2.
23   Op. cit.: 6.
24   Op. cit.: 19.
25   The nine systems are union by knowledge (Jnana), love and wisdom (Bhakti), action and service (Karma), voice and sound (Mantra), vision and form (Yantra), Kundalini, Tantra, Hatha, and Raja (mental mastery).

ness'; and this is yet another example of an ancient holistic approach to healthiness. In the West, the Yoga most widely practised is the Hatha Yoga, which includes postures and breath control;[26] and an Indologist suggests that it 'does not seek mere transcendental experiences. Its objective is to transform the human body to make it a worthy vehicle for Self-realization.'[27]

This practice of meditative techniques in the West such as Yoga has expanded since the 1960s and now includes t'ai chi ch'uan. Tai chi is a form of 'moving meditation, exercise, and stress reducer',[28] and is a type of martial art which dates back over 5,000 years. Tai chi can be described as a healing practice which dissolves blockages of *ch'i* – a life-force energy comprised of yin (female) and yang (male) energies – in the body, thus creating the harmony and balance which are required for health and happiness.[29]

Perhaps the best known new religious movement which practises meditation is Transcendental Meditation (TM). TM became popular in the West following the Beatles' visits to the Maharishi Mahesh Yogi in India during the late 1960s. This meditation technique has been found to be beneficial in the treatment of stress and, some believe, 'may confer long-term benefits on health'.[30] In the organization's own literature the benefits of practising TM are given as 'increased intelligence and creativity; improved memory and perception; better physical coordination; slowing of the ageing process; and more fulfilling personal relationships' (pamphlet). Advanced forms of practice, especially siddhi (paranormal powers including yogic flying), claim to have far-reaching – and healing – social effects and this is one of the reasons why TM has launched a worldwide political party, the Natural Law Party. TM, as an organization, now spreads information and products of the ancient Ayurvedic medicine system across the West; and Ayurveda itself is strongly linked with yoga.[31]

26   James Hewitt, 1983: 8.
27   Georg Feuerstein, 1990: 133.
28   Rosemary Ellen Guiley, 1991: 598.
29   Op. cit.: 599.
30   H. Graham, 1990: 118.
31   Georg Feuerstein, 1990: 218.

Apart from ancient, often Eastern, healing and meditative practices frequently used in New Age ideas and activities, the West has developed its own holistic healing practices. These fall into two broad types – those concerned more with physical healing, and psychotherapeutics.

One of the most widely used alternative holistic therapies in the West, developed by the German physician Samuel Hahnemann in the eighteenth century, is homoeopathy. This therapy is based on the concept of similars – that is, that which makes us sick can also make us well.[32] Although in decline in the first half of the twentieth century, since the 1960s homoeopathy has shown considerable growth. While not especially New Age, homoeopathy's recent widening appeal has played an important part in the transformation of healing practices generally from their previous allopathic base. This transformation is specifically characterized by individuals' taking greater responsibility and activity in healing themselves by looking beyond traditional norms for treatment. In this case, homoeopathy (like acupuncture) has become widely available and accepted in the mainstream and has been available on the National Health Service (NHS) in the UK since 1948. A 1993 Gallup Poll suggests that 6% of the UK population have at some time consulted a homoeopath.[33] However, as already mentioned in the examples of healing therapies given above, it is increasingly difficult to create a clear distinction between what is incorporated in New Age healing and what are simply alternative or complementary forms of healing to the traditional allopathic norm.

There are many other healing techniques which have been developed more recently in the Western World – for example, from Australia the Alexander technique, which relates physical posture to emotional well-being, kinesiology, and Rolfing. This development of healing practices – whether considered New Age or not – appears likely to continue and to penetrate further into the therapeutic and allopathic mainstream.

The second broad type of Western healing practices is psychotherapeutics. As briefly described in Chapter 2 with regards to the

32   Harris Coulter, 1985: 57ff.
33   Gallup Political and Economic Index, 1993.

ential Movement, this comprises a huge range of therapies adly stem from the development earlier in this century of ilysis. In one healing guidebook alone, *Holistic London*, the page for psychotherapy lists the availability of 56 different therapies ranging from art therapy and biosynthesis to rebirthing and transactional analysis. The editors report that 'What they all have in common is they all try to help the client in changing [...] to better understand his or her self, feelings and relationships.'[34]

The healing process

As mentioned above, New Age individuals tend not to delegate full responsibility for their own healing to third parties – for example, to medical practitioners – but start to take over at least some of this responsibility for themselves; and the concept of self-responsibility is a recurring theme in the ideas and activities of the New Age as a whole, as has been seen. The fact that a healer is not necessarily required in the process of healing is an important point. Indeed, an American study of healing suggests that

> If we are to understand alternative healing among middle-class Americans, it is misleading to emphasize healing that comes from *outside* the person needing healing – typically an expert 'healer'. Very little of the healing described by respondents to this study was performed by specialized, 'expert' healers. Rather, most groups believed that healing was mainly endogenous – a transformation process within the person.[35]

The majority of healers in a great many disciplines in the New Age would argue that their work is, in the main, to assist in facilitating the energies within the individual to heal themselves. New Age healing is not a passive activity – it requires active contact with or toward the Higher Self to help clear the blockages which hold back the possi-

34   Kate Brady and Mike Considine, 1990: 1.
35   Meredith McGuire, 1988: 165.

bility of full holistic health. Teachers play a part, but more as guides than prescribers. In essence, *the self heals itself.*

What is more, sources of help are widely available – these can take the form of varieties of both healers (including teachers, therapists, practitioners, channellers, and others) and their methods – but there are very few guides. This leads to the view that, perhaps to a greater extent than in the domain of spiritual empowerment, the individual appears to self-select whatever healing type might suit her or his requirement at any given time without necessarily following any preformed framework, 'path', or guidance.

With regard to those involved, it has already been pointed out that numerically there are a great deal more women than men; and this is particularly so in the case of those healing activities which incorporate bodywork therapies. It is perhaps fair to suggest that, especially among women, spirituality can be approached not just cerebrally but also through the body. Women are generally more in touch with their bodies, and the New Age offers a new (some would argue renewed) means of exploring their spirituality through the body. As I have suggested elsewhere, there is also strength in numbers and, as the number of women involved increased from the 1960s, so confidence grew and more and more became involved.[36]

As described above, healing is not just concerned with repairing damage: to a large extent it also involves nurturing and maintaining health. In this respect, even pampering the body, mind, and spirit in a playful, loving, and pleasurable way is seen by many of those involved to be therapeutically beneficial and natural, not sinful in the theistic sense or unacceptably hedonistic as some critics suggest.[37]

As we have seen, New Age healing is comprised of a wide range of practices which can be grouped under at least five main categories. These are: (1) non-Western and often ancient practices including acupuncture, qigong, and herbalism; (2) meditative practices including t'ai chi ch'uan, Transcendental Meditation, and many forms of visualization; (3) newer and often Western originated holistic practices

36   Stuart Rose, 2001a.
37   This subject is returned to in Chapter 11 below with regard to critics of the New Age who see its activities as being narcissistic.

including the Alexander Technique, colour therapy, homoeopathy, and Rolfing; (4) psychic practices including channelled healing and past-life therapy; and, finally, (5) psychotherapeutic practices including hypnotherapy and psychodrama. It will be noticed that this description of the range of ideas and activities bears a close resemblance to the description of spiritually empowering practices given in the previous chapter. The principal – and important – reason for this is that many of the same activities can be used for different purposes. For instance, visualization processes can be used to enhance spiritual development or to help with the relief from disease (e.g. cancer), and acupuncture is claimed to be just as beneficial when used to revitalize the life-force energy (*ch'i*) as an aid to psychological well-being or as a relief from physical pain.

In summary, it is not possible to separate out different types of healing processes and label some New Age and others differently, but it is possible to create a differentiation between the two by addressing the reasons why individuals choose the healing processes they do. The difference clearly rests in the motivations each individual has in adopting their healing path. If there is an effort to reach what is claimed to be the Higher Self, and if this is accompanied by feelings of unconditional love and compassion combined with a sense of Self-responsibility, then it can be argued that the motivation is indeed New Age and, hence, the healing processes are being used for a New Age purpose. However, if the same healing processes are used simply to repair, for non-directional nurture, or to entertain, they should not be seen as being used for New Age purposes. Put another way, just because a person might 'treat' themselves with acupuncture and aromatherapy does not automatically make either the treatments or the user New Age. The word 'treat' is used deliberately as its double meaning is particularly apt. Are they, in fact, following a spiritual and transformational path or do they simply want to feel better, to follow the view that, as Freud suggested, 'what decides the purpose of life is simply the programme of the pleasure principle'?[38] If this argument is accepted, then it means that a distinction can be drawn between alternative health *per se* and healing in the New Age.

38   Sigmund Freud, 1970: 13.

The importance of healing practices

In the previous chapter, a benchmark was given for the importance of spiritual well-being as a whole, and a similar benchmark is provided here; and the picture with regards to health is quite different to that of spirituality. Whereas the importance of spiritual well-being was reported to be the seventh lowest of the eight categories in the Gallup survey, the importance of health is by far the highest. Of the total respondents, 85% name health as being very important or more important than anything else in their lives.[39]

Also as reported above, my survey asked participants to give their views on the extent of involvement that healing and, relatedly, holism[40] have in the New Age. The findings showed overwhelmingly that both were seen as being always or often involved (90% and 88% respectively). The differences among social and demographic groups were not particularly marked; in fact, there were no discernible differences between the views among the three age groups while, in both instances, women showed a small bias towards being more certain about the involvement of healing and holism in the New Age than men.

The level of these results echoes the extent of agreement found in the Gallup findings with regards to the importance of health.[41] Moreover, they demonstrate that – bearing in mind considerable differences between the samples and between what the terms 'health', 'holism', and 'healing' can be thought to entail – there is significantly less difference in the comparative interest in health and spiritual issues between the general and New Age populations. However, while health can be seen to be very important to New Age participants, it does not

---

39 Gallup Political and Economic Index, 1993. The Gallup findings in response to the question 'How important is health in your life?' were: more important than anything else 14%, very important 71%, quite important 13%, and not very important 1%.

40 The concept of holism is more expansive than healing, as it also includes matters to do with, for example, the environment and spiritual empowerment.

41 These questions are, as stated in the previous chapter, not strictly comparable to the Gallup results.

appear to have the overriding importance that has been found to exist in the general population as a whole. This finding is the outcome of a multi-choice question in my survey where participants were requested to select influences which had created important positive changes to their lives.[42] The results show that the ranking given to healing was significantly lower at sixth position (66%) than that given to either the concept of spirituality, ranked first (82%), or meaningfulness, ranked second (80%).

Overall, therefore, with regard to the priorities which participants demonstrate, it can be concluded that while healing activities have a central importance in the New Age, they appear to be subordinate to the claimed importance that other qualities – including spirituality, meaningfulness, and happiness – seem to have.

Measure of practices

As reported in Chapter 3 (Table 7), participants were asked to state whether they had 'ever' and whether they 'currently' used any of 32 pursuits representative of the many ideas and activities involved in the New Age. The findings clearly prioritized the overall use of the principal types of healing practices and, in the main, showed that the use of bodywork therapies – such as aromatherapy, massage, flower remedies, and reflexology – were substantially higher than those of psychotechnologies – such as psychotherapy, hypnotherapy, past-life therapy, transactional analysis, and NLP (neuro-linguistic programming).

There are two material reasons which go towards accounting for this difference. Firstly, in contrast to psychotechnologies, many bodywork therapies can be conveniently self-administered. In fact, study of the most-used therapies or activities reveals that the top eight can all be self-administered or self-managed. Secondly, it is obvious that there is a significant cost differential between self-administered or

42   Reported in full in Chapter 3 above.

self-managed activities and therapist-assisted activities. Many of the most popular therapies can either be purchased as over-the-counter (OTC) remedies or be used without requiring long-term use of a therapist – although, in the first instance, a therapist might advise such use. Indeed, self-help books, instruction manuals, and cassette and video tapes are widely available to advise on how a person might treat themselves using visualization techniques, essential oils, flower remedies, crystals, and the like. One journalist suggests that there is a 'quiet revolution going on'[43] within complementary healthcare and reports that over one-third of the British population tried out alternative therapies between 1984 and 1987; and it has been reported elsewhere that in the United States 'one in three Americans seek alternative health care each year, to the tune of $13.7 billion.'[44]

A conclusion which can be drawn from this situation is that, viewed in isolation from the nature of participants, these findings illustrate how easy it can be to become unwittingly or partially involved in the New Age, as an individual can purchase therapies without ever subscribing to the more expansive New Age ideologies which might incorporate them. Visits to any pharmacy or drug store demonstrates the breadth of therapies available, including ranges of homoeopathic and herbal remedies as well as many other related items, for instance, do-it-yourself acupuncture kits. It is suggested that many alternative health therapies are 'far from alternative and fringe [they now] dominate popular conceptions of the relationship between body and mind'[45] and often form part of 'a journey of personal transformation'.[46]

Also as reported in Chapter 3, multiple use of therapies was found to be substantial. This finding was not unexpected because, in holistic healing practices, nurture and/or repair to the whole person is frequently carried out on different levels at the same time. In this regard, we have above described the multidimensional nature of holistic health care,[47] and the situation is further illustrated in the description

43   Rosalind Coward, 1989: 4.
44   *Nexus*, 1994 Vol. 2, 20: 6.
45   Rosalind Coward, 1989: 13.
46   Op. cit.: 197.
47   Fritjof Capra, 1984: 369.

of a five-day healing workshop given in Chapter 9, where, at one event, eleven of the healing practices listed in the same earlier chapter were used. That the same practices appear to have been used regularly leads us back to the conclusion that such New Age practices are more to do with the *considered* healing requirement for the maintenance and nurture of good health rather than for a *distress* or shorter term requirement for repair.

The social and demographic profile of many New Age participants, given in Chapter 3, shows several marked characteristics including biases towards female, middle-aged, and middle-class individuals. What is interesting is that, by study of the subgroups with reference to their reported use of healing practices, differentiating characteristics are brought into focus.

Firstly, with regards to the gender of those involved, an important question to examine relates to whether the same healing practices were followed by both women and men equally or were there particular differences? Analysis demonstrates that there are substantial differences. On the one hand, women claimed to incorporate a wide mix of bodywork therapies in their activities while, on the other hand, men claimed to concentrate much more on psychotechnologies and dietary concerns.[48] To describe the difference in another way, women's healing activities involve high levels of physical touching and movement while men's healing activities appear to be more cerebral.

Secondly, it has also been possible to examine whether the use of healing practices was concentrated in any particular age group, and the findings show clearly that, again, there were substantial differences. The younger age group was characterized primarily by dietary and bodywork practices;[49] whereas the middle age group demonstrated a higher propensity for psychotechnologies. The older age group, however, showed a distinct difference to the other two groups in that there was less propensity for psychotechnologies or for the type of body-

48   Additionally, it can be remembered that it was found that men have a higher propensity for interest in Buddhism, earth mysteries, Shaman or Pagan rituals, and green politics.
49   In this instance, the prime influences on dietary practices among the younger age group are most likely to be based on ecological principles.

work and dietary practice prevalent in the younger age group; their practices were characterized by therapies which were more gentle or passive in their nature.

In quantifying the use of healing practices by gender and age, it has been possible to demonstrate which healing activities were most used by the participants as a whole and which by particular demographic groups.[50] Clearly, and logically, cheaper and self-administered activities are used more widely than those which require the assistance of a therapist. The most widely used healing activity of all, creative visualization, is used in a variety of ways, and these are now explored.

Visualization

There is one healing practice which deserves particular mention because it appears to be the most used of all healing practices and because, although not limited to the New Age, the nature of its use spans practically all aspects of the New Age itself – that is, the practice of visualization. Visualization techniques are sometimes described as 'creative visualizations', 'positive affirmations' (which do not always include a visual content), or 'guided goal-oriented imagery' and are used in both spiritual empowerment and healing practices.

In my survey it was found that 80% of those involved had used visualization techniques, and over 40% were using them at that particular time. Visualization techniques can be practised with or without the help of a therapist (in this instance, sometimes called a teacher, facilitator, or guide). Moreover, it is reported that they are 'widely employed in the arts, sports, business, alternative medicine, religious practices, psychotherapy, the mystical and the occult arts, psychical

---

50   Fulder and Munro's survey into complementary medicine pinpoints the middle-aged as being mostly concerned with complementary healthcare (1985: 545). They also find that two-thirds of patients are female, (542), and middle class (544), which are the prime social and demographic characteristics of New Age participants.

research, and in personal self-improvement'.[51] It is also suggested that guided imagery is starting to play an important part in healing processes, and its benefits are still being developed. What happens appears to be that 'Sick organs and parts of the body are manipulated by vivid images on the part of the patient and the healer [...] Since the 1970s imagery has been used increasingly as an alternative or supplemental treatment for a variety of illnesses and disorders, in particular cancer.'[52]

Visualization techniques are not new in the twentieth century. In fact, their use can be traced back through history to the Ancient Greeks, to Eastern religions, and to Shamanism. In the contemporary West, two well-known teachers and authors on the subject are Norman Vincent Peale and Shakti Gawain. Although Peale himself was a Christian writing in the decade before the counter-culture, his ideas can be seen to have been influential to New Age teachers, in particular Louise Hay. What Peale suggests is that 'You can make yourself ill with your thoughts and by the same token you can make yourself well by the use of a different and healing type of thought'[53] and he suggests that 'one of the greatest laws of the universe'[54] is encapsulated in the following procedure which he believes 'channels God's power into personality':[55]

> To change your circumstances, first start thinking differently. Do not passively accept unsatisfactory circumstances, but form a picture in your mind of circumstances as they should be. Hold that picture, develop it firmly in all details, believe in it, pray about it, work at it, and you can actualize it according to that mental image emphasized in your positive thinking.[56]

51 Rosemary Ellen Guiley, 1991: 124.
52 Op. cit.: 283.
53 Norman Vincent Peale, 1996: 223. Peale's *The Power of Positive Thinking* was first published in 1953; is reported to have sold over fifteen million copies and has obviously been highly influential.
54 Op. cit.: 224
55 Ibid.
56 Ibid.

Although not unique to Peale, the procedure he describes accurately illustrates the basis of what has occurred at many such sessions I have attended at New Age workshops.

With regard to the relationship between healing and visualization techniques, like Peale, Shakti Gawain believes that 'Conscious creative visualization is the process of creating positive thoughts and images to communicate with our bodies, in place of negative, constrictive, literally "sickening" ones.'[57] Gawain stresses the importance of self-responsibility for healing and suggests that

> One of the basic principles of holistic health is that we cannot separate our physical health from our emotional, mental, and spiritual states of being. All levels are interconnected and a state of 'dis-ease' in the body is always a reflection of conflict, tension, anxiety, or disharmony on other levels of being as well. So when we have a physical disorder, it is inevitably a message for us to look deeply into our emotional and intuitive feelings, our thoughts and attitudes, to see what we can do to restore natural harmony and balance to our being. We must tune in and 'listen' to the inner process.[58]

Furthermore, Denise Linn – who, it can be remembered, was the most mentioned person who has been influential through direct or personal contact with participants – leads themed visualization workshops in many countries. One workshop attended by this writer, entitled 'Attuning to the Planet's New Frequencies Through Cellular Regeneration', involved imagining oneself shrinking in size and entering the body through the mouth. In my case, I travelled into my body shrinking to such a small size in various stages that I was able to 'see' my DNA/RNA helix as a ladder made of light. I had visualized myself to be so small that I could climb up the helix to polish any dark areas in order to allow all of its energy to be activated. It felt a little like changing light bulbs in Piccadilly Circus! The point here is that in the visualization process I was actually attempting to heal myself.

Visualization techniques, as have been noted, do not necessarily require the assistance of a therapist for their enactment. In fact, many books and cassette tapes are available to guide individuals through

57   Shakti Gawain, 1985: 57f.
58   Ibid.

their own visualization processes.[59] By following these or similar methods, it appears possible to develop visualization processes suited to almost any requirement. In fact, in this regard, ground-breaking work has been carried out in the treatment of cancer by, among others, the Bristol Cancer Help Centre. This centre includes visualization among its therapies to allow individuals to help 'influence events and our physical and mental state' (brochure).

My survey findings have shown that visualization techniques play an important part in healing processes, whether these were used towards more spiritual or more therapeutic ends. However, the survey was not constructed in such a way that it would be possible to determine whether these techniques were more important than any other healing activity in the New Age, although they appear to be the most frequently practised. The techniques can be used wherever and whenever an individual wishes, as no external material accessories are necessarily required; and it can therefore play a part in participant's daily meditations, in even more frequent positive affirmations, or be used more expansively in conjunction with healing workshops or spiritual gatherings.

Healing and the paranormal

There appears to exist a strong relationship among participants I have surveyed between healing practices and the paranormal; and various forms of psychic, occult, and spiritualist healing (especially the former) seem to be fundamental New Age practices. In fact, my survey findings demonstrated a great deal of activity in this field, although

59   With regard to affirmations, Louise Hay (1988) and Shakti Gawain (1985 and 1993), demonstrate a variety of approaches, and other visualization processes can be found in many areas of spiritual empowerment, for example, in the Tibetan Buddhist teachings given at Samye Ling Tibetan Centre in Scotland by Dharma-Ayra Akong Rinpoche (1987), and in those of Osho (Bhagwan Shree Rajneesh), 1995.

prior to reporting these it is relevant to describe briefly what might be entailed.

Psychic and occult healing practices are described as being comprised of extremely diverse methods, and tools include pendulums, crystals, and dowsing rods as well as hands.[60] What this type of healing involves is that

> Like Christian healing, psychic and occult healing is based upon a notion of a transcendent healing power – something outside and greater than the individual. Thus, healers in the psychic tradition, as in Christian healing, view themselves as mediators of that healing power to others who need it. Unlike Christian healing, however, psychic and occult healing groups emphasize that healing power may be readily tapped by any knowledgeable or spiritually developed person.[61]

Here further evidence is provided that the New Age is seen by some to comprise of both immanent and transcendent qualities, in that the healing power – which, those involved report, can be engaged in various forms including channelling, visualizations, and distance healing – is claimed to be a universal energy which pervades every thing and every place.

Turning more specifically to my survey results on paranormal activities, it was found that the influence and use of divinatory arts among participants – in the form primarily of astrological, palm, tarot, and numerological readings – was not particularly extensive. Although most participants reported having had at least one reading at some point in their lives, only a very small minority claimed to have frequent readings. However, the experience of paranormal phenomena was found to be considerably greater, as over 80% claimed experience of at least one type, and two-thirds claimed more than three such types of experience.[62]

---

60 Meredith McGuire, 1988: 147. Further descriptions can be found, for example, in Daniel J. Benor; 1995, Larry Dossey, 1989, 1993, 1994; and Robert Fuller, 1989.
61 Ibid.
62 The mean average of types of paranormal phenomena experienced was 4.33: the number of actual experiences across all types is not known 'although it is thought to be considerably higher.

While the content of the paranormal phenomena does not appear to overtly involve healing, a number of such activities are claimed to include healing properties. For example, past-life recall is reported to be used by some to discover and heal emotional 'blocks', and in the occurrence of meaningful coincidences – as are claimed to be experienced in synchronicity – participants suggest this can point to a healing requirement or be in itself healing. Moreover, several individuals whose writings were reported to be influential in the New Age combine involvement with the paranormal and with healing. Most noticeably, these include Edgar Cayce and the work of White Eagle Lodge.

Therapists in New Age healing practices

In Chapter 3 it was noted that among participants were a substantial number of New Age individuals – over 20% – who reported that their occupation was to do with healing practices. Almost without exception, as would be expected, this subgroup demonstrated the highest usage levels of healing ideas and activities out of all participants. The fact that such a large number has been encountered highlights the notion that in complementary therapy as a whole there must be a substantial number of therapists, although it is impossible to say to what extent they may also consider themselves to be involved in the New Age. In either case, it is extremely difficult to estimate accurately how many there might be.[63]

---

63   In 1982 a survey identified that there were 'a total of 30,000 complementary therapists practising in the United Kingdom' (cited in Margaret Emslie et al., 1996: 39); and one later estimate puts the growth in the number of complementary therapists at more than 10% annually (The Guardian, 25 June 1996: 16). If this is the case, and given that complementary therapy as a whole has grown significantly since the early 1980s, it can be anticipated that the number of therapists has now doubled or even trebled from the 1982 estimate. In fact, there would need to be a very large number if, as Margaret Emslie et al. suggest, in the region of 25% of the general population have used complementary

Information given in my survey relating to the occupation of these individuals sheds light in three ways on the mix of therapists who can be encountered in the New Age. Firstly, types of the therapists' claimed occupations can be divided into broad categories which stem from osteopathy (which can be considered as one of the complementary therapies that has become most widely accepted by allopathic medicine) to various types of psychic healing. The largest group of therapists (36%) appear to be found in the skills relating to bodywork practices.

The second way in which studying individuals' occupations helps to understand therapists was that they reported the practice of 63 different therapies, and the ten most mentioned of these (in descending order) were healers, counsellors, aromatherapists, psychotherapists, astrologers, masseurs, reflexologists, undefined therapists, workshop facilitators, and acupuncturists. What this finding confirms is that there appears to be no single type of therapy or activity which is practised significantly more than any other. For example, my survey demonstrated that there were about as many aromatherapists as psychotherapists claiming to be practising in the New Age.[64]

Thirdly, many practitioners listed more than one therapy which they practised. In all, almost 300 healing occupations were given by

therapies (1996: 41). It must be added that not all these people would necessarily require the services of a therapist. However, a 1985 estimate of the number of therapists by Stephen Fulder and Robin Munro of the Research Council for Complementary Medicine suggests that 'the mean number of therapists was 12.1 per 100,000 population, equivalent to 26.8% of the number of general practitioners' (1985: 543), which is a considerably smaller number than Margaret Emslie et al. found, although their definition of a complementary therapist was narrower. With regard to the comparative number of therapists and general practitioners, Fulder and Munro point out that consultation times with therapists are considerably longer than with general practitioners and represent 'only 8% of general-practitioners consultations' (1985: 545). These authors also point out that complementary therapists therefore see far fewer patients and that the principal reason for this is because the average consultation time is six times the length of those given by general practitioners (Ibid.).

64　It should be noted that a great many therapies practised by therapists include variations of creative visualization, the most widely used healing technique, although no therapists reported that they specialized in this activity.

this subgroup, which meant that the average number of therapies practised by each person was 1.4. Similar evidence was found in another
survey, which reports that 42% of therapists practised more than one
therapy.[65] Furthermore, in the region of one-third of therapists recorded in my survey listed non-healing occupations in addition, which
demonstrates that for some healing activities were part time or not
seen as their prime source of income. In fact, half of all the practitioners surveyed claimed total earnings of less than £10,000 per annum.

With regard to practitioners of healing techniques, a number of
well-known individuals have been identified. Clearly Deepak Chopra,
Gill Edwards, Shakti Gawain, Louis Hay, Denise Linn, M. Scott Peck,
and Stuart Wilde (all influential through their writings and/or workshops) are key figures in Britain and America, and indeed further
afield. However, the survey has brought to light literally hundreds of
names of practitioners who, it is thought, practise locally – both with
individual clients and by running healing workshops – and who have
not necessarily ventured into the national or international healing arenas or into the field of publishing.

Finally, several categories of practitioners appear to exist. Firstly,
there are those who have established professional practices – either on
an individual practitioner basis or in the form of, for example, group
practices such as natural health clinics; secondly, there are accredited
practitioners who practise informally; and the third group is comprised
of practitioners who are not professionally accredited but, nevertheless, are skilled in particular healing or therapeutic techniques. In addition, there is likely to be a fourth category containing individuals
who are neither professionally accredited nor even particularly skilful
at the therapies they purport to practice. Again, the findings of Fulder
and Munro's survey broadly support this matrix.[66] This situation reflects the types of training involved. For example, kinesiologists or
psychosynthesis counsellors need to train for some years to obtain accreditation, but touch for health therapists or aromatherapists, or even
reiki masters, for example, need only train for a few weekends or the
equivalent. It can be added that many people who undertake training

65   Stephen Fulder and Robin Munro, 1985: 543.
66   Ibid.

in one or more disciplines do not necessarily do so with the intention of becoming professional practitioners.

Efficacy in healing practices

Nowhere are problems of efficacy more apparent than in the domain of healing practice. This is because a large number of specific claims are made with regard to the beneficial nature of its ideas and activities. Many of the practices used in New Age healing – which form a substantial part of the range of complementary and alternative healthcare as a whole – have not been assessed with regard to whether they might conform to any standard or whether, in fact, they may or may not work. This, in turn, has created widespread criticism both from the allopathic medical professions and from the media.

With regards to the media, typically one or two incidences of failure in a particular field or therapy have been used to argue that alternative and complementary methods as a whole are suspect. An example of such journalistic criticism was published in a national newspaper under the headline 'In sickness, there is no alternative', reporting that

> conventional and alternative medicines are not equivalent, equally viable, choices. Whatever its flaws, conventional medicine is based on research, submits to scientific scrutiny and is practised by those bound by strict ethical codes. The other is less proven. It surfs along on assertions that natural is safe, and that it is ecologically friendly, even though areas of Chinese medicine have extravagant ways with endangered species. Alternative medicine puts itself above rational investigation, encouraging a climate where voodoo doctors flourish.[67]

67 *The Guardian*, 21 August 1995. Rosalind Coward, the author of this article, previously wrote a study on complementary health, *The Whole Truth*, which is referred to elsewhere.

In this article, which features one case of psychotherapy and one of homoeopathy, the journalist by implication links Chinese medicine (which was not mentioned in the main text) and 'voodoo doctors' to all practitioners of non-conventional medicine, thereby apparently damning the lot.

When conventional medicine and the media join forces the results can be highly damaging. An illustration of this relates to the Bristol Cancer Help Centre where incorrect and negative research was published by *The Lancet* and reported in depth by the media. The result caused substantial financial difficulties for the centre which had been, in fact, achieving notable successes in the fight against cancer using complementary methods, including creative visualization;[68] and the publication of the flawed research 'did serious damage to the complementary approach for cancer in this country, highlighting the rift between conventional and alternative medicine'.[69]

The allopathic medical professions generally demand verification of the efficacy of complementary healthcare methods; and this is required by using the same scientific methods as those applied to conventional medicine. However, in total, the issue which relates to what methods of 'proof' are required by whom in order to assess whether a particular practice is efficacious is not yet settled and involves many difficulties. Six problems have been identified which complementary therapists experience in executing clinical trials using standard allopathic methodology. These are problems involved in evaluating the all-inclusive nature of holistic treatment which, in the main, concentrates on the causes of illness rather than its effects; the problem of 'blind' tests, for example in regard to use of creative visualization and reflexology where placebos cannot be used; the role and result of the therapist as healer; and gauging the interaction between the mind and the immune system.[70]

68   Michael Weir, 1993.
69   *The Times*, 11 January 1994: 13. This debacle is chronicled at length by Martin Walker (1993), and his study as a whole highlights the conflict of interest that exists between the large pharmaceutical companies which dominate allopathic medicine and alternative methods of treatment where such pharmacology is frequently avoided.
70   Honor Anthony, 1987: 762.

The issue relating to efficacy is beginning to be addressed and the first stage of the process appears to be that complementary health practitioners are starting to introduce their own forms of legitimization through professional accreditation and, where feasible, acceptance of tests for the efficacy of particular therapies. However, this process is a lengthy one and it has been pointed out that only since the 1970s has more widespread use of complementary healing practices occurred and therefore it is 'not surprising that the full panoply of professional bureaucracy is not all in place'.[71] Nevertheless, there are numerous studies published concerning the efficacy of some of the practices involved – for example, a review of over one hundred trials of homoeopathy has been published by the *British Medical Journal.*[72] What is more, professional associations for some of the main therapies have been established.[73]

The more considered view with regard to the legitimacy of 'new' forms of healthcare appears to be that the conflict between complementary and orthodox systems is slowly on the wane as it is becoming apparent to the medical mainstream that some or many complementary methods provide a beneficial addition to healthcare overall. In this respect, a study of Californian holistic practices reports that 'orthodox medicine will not necessarily steadfastly stick to its own current identity – especially if consumers (that is, patients) demand a greater emphasis on holistic health.'[74] That the conflict between the two seems to be declining is confirmed in the survey referred to above carried out by Stephen Fulder and Robin Munro. These authors found that

> The evolving complementary systems of medicine are not in direct competition with conventional medicine even if historically they may have appeared to be so. The highest levels of complementary consultation we found were in [geographical areas] which are well served medically. Other reports have established that complementary medicine does not thrive in regions where conven-

---

71   Simon Mills, 1995: 3.
72   Reported in *The Guardian*, 25 June 1996.
73   Some examples are given above; see also Sara Cant and Ursula Sharma, 1996, with regard to the professionalization of accrediting associations.
74   Jane English-Lueck, 1990: 159.

tional medicine is poorly represented [...] Most complementary medicine patients are within the middle of their lifespan, whereas more of those of the general practitioner are towards the beginning or end of it. A third of complementary medical patients were seeking simultaneous help from doctors.[75]

There is a very wide range of practices which go to make up complementary and alternative healthcare – many of which are involved in New Age healing – and some of these have already become substantially adopted by the mainstream allopathic medical professions – for example, osteopathy, homoeopathy, and acupuncture. However, many practices have not been accepted in this way but are, nevertheless, practised with what appears to be a widening interest – for example, creative visualization and yoga. What is plain is that there now exists a thriving healthcare industry operating outside of general medical practice which has been spurred into growth – as New Age participants have reported – by the perceived limited capabilities of medical science. With regard to the origin of this situation in general, one commentator pinpoints the damage caused by the use of the sedative Thalidomide by pregnant women in the 1950s (that is, just prior to the counter-culture) which, he reports, 'more than any other event, marked the turning point in the public perception of modern medicine [...] New drugs could harm, and harm seriously.'[76]

Additionally, for many respondents to a study of healing in suburban America, 'alternative healing involves more than merely alternative "techniques"; rather it entails an entire belief system';[77] and, similarly, a journalist has suggested that complementary medicine sheds light on the '"spiritual bankruptcy" of orthodox medicine'.[78] This journalist believes that,

> For many, the notion of being alternative is considerably more than just doing it differently from orthodox medicine. It is also a symbolic activity. It is a profound expression of a new consciousness which individuals have about health and the body. It involves a commitment to finding a new life style, to pursue a new well-being, and to finding 'natural' ways of achieving this well-being.

75   Stephen Fulder and Robin Munro, 1985: 545.
76   Simon Mills, 1993: 24.
77   Meredith McGuire, 1988: 187.
78   Rosalind Coward, 1989: 11.

Above all it is a new consciousness of the importance of the individual in achieving health.[79]

And an American social researcher talks about the body being central to healing experiences and suggests that the 'body figures predominantly in contemporary spiritual quests [...] bodily involved rituals structure spiritual awareness and transform individual identity'.[80]

Clearly, as these commentators suggest, there is a strong interrelationship between the body, healing, and spirituality, so strong in fact that they each become inseparable parts of the overall process of developing personal well-being.

However, the question of what degree of conventional proof of a treatment's efficacy is required specifically by those involved in the New Age is not settled. My survey has revealed participants who report that forms of inner wisdom or guidance, intuition, and personal experience might be more important generally in their lives and this may well mean that the same 'authority' is sufficient in determining the legitimacy of particular therapies – that is, on an individual's own need-by-need basis. External forms of verification with regard to the efficacy of their practices may not be as highly valued.

Regardless of technical and other problems involved, some sort of legitimization appear to be increasingly required for most healing practices, not just by the allopathic medical professions but by therapists themselves. Indeed, one study of complementary medicine believes this to be a fair demand.[81] The fact that these problems are now being aired will, it is anticipated, lead to a more profound and comprehensive understanding of the pros and cons of many types of healing involved in the New Age in the future. Doubtless this will entail an expansion of complementary practices in society at large, although this does not necessarily mean that participation in New Age ideas and activities will be expand to the same degree.

79   Ibid.
80   Wade Clark Roof, 1999: 103ff.
81   Ursula Sharma, 1992: 207.

Summary

Healing practices, both ancient and new, have been found to play a very important part in participants' lives, although this is not such an important part as spiritual concerns appear to play. There is no doubt that healing therapies are widely used and that it is now possible to pinpoint which are the most popular. With regard to activities and practice in the domains of healing and spiritual empowerment discussed in this and the previous chapter, it can readily be seen just how great the overlap and connection between them is. Healing through bodywork therapies, especially for women, can be seen as one of the paths – in some cases, the principal path – that participants have adopted which, wittingly or unwittingly, enables a spiritual transformation.

8. Community Activity

The richness of reality is becoming even richer through our specific human endowments; we are the first kind of living beings we know of which have the potentialities of living in community with all other living beings. It is our hope that all these potentialities will be realized – if not in the immediate future, then at least in the somewhat near future.

Arne Naess[1]

The domain of community activity has two distinct aspects – that of kinship[2] and that of sustainable living. The reason that these aspects are not separated into distinct domains is simply because the high degree of their interconnectedness prohibits any meaningful separation. The two can be distinguished by saying that kinship primarily concerns relationships with other people, while sustainable living concerns the ways in which those involved with the New Age relate to their surroundings. This aspect of sustainable living incorporates an extremely wide spectrum of social activity which includes economics, environmental issues, and politics. Overall, ideas and activities in this domain appear to operate in close harmony with the two domains described in the preceding two chapters, in that many spiritually empowered and healed individuals appear to relate to other people and their surroundings in similar ways as will now be shown.

---

1   Arne Naess, 1995: 239.
2   The term 'kinship' is not used here in its strict anthropological sense of blood relationship but in the broader sense of ideological kinship and membership of a wider 'family'.

Kinship

In my first chapter it was suggested that in the New Age 'All life [...] is interconnected energy.'[3] This energy is thought to be creating a new consciousness and a new understanding of life and, because of this, 'we are currently in the process of evolving a completely new planetary culture.'[4] This new culture, it is anticipated, is likely to affect all aspects of human life both at the individual and group levels. It is also suggested that there will be a resulting myriad of changes to the status quo which are likely to include 'the way we use power, openness to experience, capacity for intimacy, new values, lowered competition, [and] greater autonomy in the face of social pressures'.[5] However, the sphere upon which transformation in New Age culture will have the greatest impact – and the first impact – will be that of relationship.[6]

These ideas describe the effects of transformation in similar ways and are summed up by the suggestion that

> our private awareness of spiritual realities becomes a shared public reality and, with this experience, we change our whole perception of society. Instead of seeing it as made up of savage and competitive humans, we recognize that it consists of fellow creatures of spirit, sharing the same difficulties and challenges and the same spiritual purpose.[7]

What is pointed to here amounts to a peaceful, yet complete, revolutionary change or transformation of the way in which we go about our lives. In Bloom's view, gone will be the attempt of each individual to struggle against other individuals; the resulting discord to be replaced by cooperation and harmony – not with sameness, but with unity in diversity.

There has been little sustained argument against the principles of this change – primarily, it seems, because it appears to represent, first

3   William Bloom, 1990: 13.
4   Op. cit.: 14.
5   Marilyn Ferguson: 1982: 429.
6   Ibid.
7   William Bloom, 1990: 9.

and foremost, a change of heart and direction toward a much improved future for all. The characteristics of the transformation would mean there would still be those who are better off and those who are less well off in terms of all the benefits and happiness that life can contain, although the extremes of poverty, waste, and hoarding would naturally disappear. Bloom's concepts are clearly idealistic, although he believes the opportunity to realize the goal exists if – and it is a big if – sufficient desire is there to create such a change. Bloom's thesis is that, in the New Age, the desire *is* there, and the prime agent which might bring this new state of being into fruition is love.

We have seen in earlier chapters the crucial importance love holds in the New Age, and nowhere is it more important than in the relationship between people. This can be described not as a romantic or familial love, but as a compassionate love of all life, between all people, and from all people to other forms of life. It is a love which has a strong spiritual focus – in fact, some of those involved have described this love as being or emanating from God, or from similar concepts such as Energy or Light.

One of the leading exponents of this philosophy in the New Age is an American teacher and physician, Deepak Chopra. Chopra believes that 'When love and spirit are brought together, their power can accomplish anything.'[8] Chopra describes how all the main historical religious figures – Buddha, Krishna, Jesus, and Mohammad – have taught this message and through their teachings the world has been changed for the better. Through Ayurvedic principles, Chopra considers that this power can be found and developed in all people. He suggests that

> Restoring the spiritual dimension to love means abandoning the notion of a limited self with its limited ability to love and regaining the Self with its unbounded ability to love. The 'I' that is truly you is made of pure awareness, pure creativity, pure spirit. Its version of love is free from all memories or images from the past. Beyond all illusion is the source of love, a field of pure potential. That potential is you.[9]

---

8   Deepak Chopra, 1997: 29.
9   Op. cit.: 33.

From this description, we can clearly see a non-dual basis to Chopra's ideas, in that the 'I' is God (Brahman) and beyond space and time although, paradoxically, present now – both transcendent and immanent. Chopra has divided his path into seven spiritual 'laws' to success, to being affluent, here meant as 'the abundant flow of all good things',[10] and not necessarily solely laws of wealth production, which he sees to be negative when practised in isolation. The laws he outlines include those of pure potentiality, of giving, of *Karma* or cause and effect, of least effort or efficiency, of intentionality, of detachment, and of *Dharma* or purpose.

Chopra's ideas are, at heart, similar to those of many other New Age writers including William Bloom, Louise Hay, and David Spangler and, as Chopra himself points out, they are not dissimilar from most religious teachings. The recurring theme behind their beliefs, and behind the New Age as a whole, is that world society has, over hundreds of years, lost its spiritual and loving nature and become dysfunctional and dis-eased through unbridled individualism and separatism. This point is taken up by Marilyn Ferguson who found that, in the New Age, 'Many old friendships and acquaintances fall away; new friendships, even a whole new support network, take their place. Based as they are on shared values and a shared journey, these new relationships are perhaps more intense.'[11] Ferguson's findings, as has already been demonstrated, echo what was found in my survey where not only friendships were ended, but families and marriages were affected in what can be described as a clash of the old paradigm with the new at the individual level. In fact, like Chopra, Ferguson sees that

> Whatever the cost in personal relationships, we discover that our highest responsibility, finally, unavoidably is the stewardship of our potential – being all we can be. We betray this trust at the peril of mental and physical health. At bottom, as Theodore Roszak observed, most of us are 'sick with guilt at having lived below our authentic level'.[12]

10   Deepak Chopra, 1996: 2.
11   Marilyn Ferguson, 1982: 426.
12   Op. cit.: 430f.

However, a sociologist has argued that evidence[13] of personal relationships in the New Age demonstrates that there is little difference between such relationships and those that occur within mainstream society; therefore, it is contended, the New Age itself is fundamentally a failure and, moreover, incorrect in perceiving present society as flawed.[14] This argument is based on the notion that the stability of traditional authority (in this author's case, conservative Protestantism) is a vital foundation for any society. However, in condemning three decades or so of the New Age, in comparison to the several centuries of conservative Protestantism, this commentator misses an important point. The problem with conservative Protestantism, according to those involved with the New Age, is that it has lost its loving spiritual content, and the *raison d'être* of the New Age is to develop ways to reintroduce spirituality, firstly into individuals' lives and then to let that filter up to influence greater numbers of people. Such a process is likely to take considerable time, and so it is perhaps a little early to pronounce that the New Age itself has failed. What is more, kinship in the New Age is not so much about personal relationships on a one-to-one basis which, it can be anticipated, will always have its ups and downs, but represents a wider point of view which transcends old group definitions. According to Marilyn Ferguson, the

> discovery of our connection to all other men, women, and children joins us to another family. Indeed, seeing ourselves as a planetary family struggling to solve its problems, rather than as assorted peoples and nations assessing blame or exporting solutions, could be the ultimate shift in perspective.[15]

According to those involved in the New Age, this transformational process has only just begun. Unlike the Protestant Reformation, the process is from the bottom up, not from the top down, which may mean that its progress, if it occurs, could be slower.

Turning to a related topic, it must be added that the New Age does not necessarily support the notion of communal living. In the

---

13 Steve Bruce bases his argument primarily on two biographies of New Age people, those of Peter and Eileen Caddy and Judith Boice (1998: 26).
14 Op. cit.: 23ff.
15 Marilyn Ferguson, 1982: 442.

1960s, innumerable communes were founded, although many did not last long. The most notable exceptions include The Farm in America as well as the Findhorn Community in Scotland[16] which, given several ups and downs, still appears to thrive. Paul Heelas[17] describes the problems which have occurred at the community still being established at Auroville in South India and suggests that for communities to flourish there needs to be authority, structure, and tradition, none of which the New Age has or, as William Bloom points out,[18] desires. The New Age, as we have seen, is about the transformation of individuals, but not for them to live together in separate communities – the New Age, it appears, is for a transformation of the world, of all individuals.

It is important to note here that while the subject of human relationships may not be widely discussed in commentaries on the New Age, a number of psychotechnologies which have been influential to some of those involved offer a variety of means to bring about transformed relationships. These include, for example, encounter group therapy and transactional analysis. Furthermore, of more particular interest to the New Age are Fourth Force transpersonal psychotechnologies. An example of this type is Psychosynthesis, developed by Roberto Assagioli, which, while primarily based on the self-realization of the individual, 'may also be considered as *the individual expression of a wider principle, of a general law of inter-individual and cosmic synthesis*' (Assagioli's emphasis).[19]

A final identification of the depth of change the New Age advocates with regard to kinship is given at length by Fritjof Capra who, in concluding his synthesis of theories and models of system thinking, sees that

> The origin of our dilemma lies in our tendency to create the abstractions of separate objects, including a separate self, and then to believe that they belong

16   The Findhorn Community is described by Carol Riddell (1990), and Steven Sutcliffe (2002).
17   Paul Heelas, 1996a: 207f.
18   William Bloom, 1990: 12.
19   Roberto Assagioli, 1980: 30. These examples represent yet another illustration of the interrelatedness of the domains of ideas and activities in the New Age.

218

to an objective, independently existing reality. To overcome our Cartesian anxiety, we need to think systematically, shifting our conceptual focus from objects to relationships. Only then can we realize that identity, individuality, and autonomy do not imply separateness and independence. As Lynn Margulis and Dorion Sagan remind us, 'independence is a political, not a scientific, term'.[20] The power of abstract thinking has led us to treat the natural environment – the web of life – as if it consisted of separate parts, to be exploited by different interest groups. Moreover, we have extended this fragmented view to our human society, dividing it into different nations, races, religious and political groups. The belief that all these fragments – in ourselves, in our environment, and in our society – are really separate has alienated us from nature and from our fellow human beings, and thus has diminished us. To regain our full humanity, we have to regain our experience of connectedness with the entire web of life.[21]

The New Age, according to these writers, demands a comprehensive overhaul of the way in which individuals relate to other individuals, both in a family situation and more widely, and in the way individuals relate to the world as a whole. This latter aspect in the domain of community activity is now considered.

Sustainable living

For a widespread sustainable community to exist, New Age ideas point to a radical shift towards a new paradigm in public policies, social norms, and the way of life of community members. The basis of this new paradigm appears to be primarily founded upon spiritual and ecological principles although, inescapably, it also involves a high degree of social, political, and economic influences. In fact, three uses of the term 'sustainability' have been suggested from the Findhorn Community: 'It may refer to the ecological sustainability (and hence safety) of the planet; social sustainability, which implies that we all coexist on an increasingly crowded planet; and economic sustainabil-

20   Lynn Margulis and Dorion Sagan, 1995: 26.
21   Fritjof Capra, 1997: 287f.

ity, so that there is always enough to go around.'[22] The interrelated nature of what sustainability implies means that one of these issues cannot be changed without influencing the other two. Furthermore, as can be imagined, the result of this shift towards a new paradigm is also likely to engender related effects in terms of cultural development.

However, the concept of sustainable living appears at this stage in its development to be very much more a theoretical notion than a practical one, although there are exceptions as will be shown. Its application in mainstream society faces major obstacles because its creation – the creation of a totally sustainable society – requires a radical change to existing social organization. Those involved in the New Age do not appear to accept the idea of New Age communities living alongside capitalistic communities. They feel that the two simply do not mix. Ideally, and in the longer term, according to some writers, New Age ideas will replace capitalistic ones. If this occurs, it would mean that the change would incorporate methods and types of agriculture, capitalism's method of ownership, and the existing system of representative democracy. An academic commentator on the New Age sums up the New Age view of what these changes might entail by suggesting that those involved believe 'Humanity must become one large family, *but* one which honours diversity among its members; global wholeness implies some kind of spirituality is needed, *but* one which is compatible with a diversity of traditional religions; and some kind of world government may be needed, *but* not a totalitarian world order which can overrule regional governments and individual freedom.'[23] Furthermore, with regard to capitalism, William Bloom holds that 'Our current financial and economic policies are not working in a creative and beneficent way.'[24] According to Bloom, the knock-on effect of what is now termed as 'new economics' will require substantial changes – in fact, nothing short of a transformation. Bloom believes that

---

22   Jeremy Slocombe, 1998: 22.
23   Wouter Hanegraaff, 1996: 340.
24   William Bloom, 1995b: 6.

a new economic theory needs to incorporate the emerging realities of size, scale, complexity and decentralization; auditing real costs and wealth other than simple cash values; and a change in the general framework of understanding away from savage competition for scarce resources to a more realistic appreciation of natural cooperation. The most basic supposition of mainstream economics – that we are savage beings competing for scarce resources, and that demand and supply reach equilibrium – will be replaced by other more creative and co-operative assumptions.[25]

Also looking at the concept of sustainable living from an economic viewpoint, an ex-Director of Policy Research at the Stanford Research Institute gives what he calls 'clues' to what the characteristics of the new paradigm might include: he lists wholeness, ecological awareness, peace and common security, decentralization to a human scale, gender balance, wisdom and compassion, cultural pluralism, non-violent change, and the empowerment of people.[26] Without exception, these notions are all implicit in New Age philosophy and, what is more, it is argued that business needs to take a pivotal role in bringing about change, although it is thought that the impetus has to come first from the individual taking responsibility for bringing about such change.[27] And an early voice demonstrates the continuity in the New Age of these ideas. In the mid 1970s Mark Satin's view of New Age politics was that he believed a change in scale was vital. Satin argued that

The New Age position suggests that the basic problem has partly to do with the scale of our society: the human scale is beautiful and nearly everything we have now is much too big (and powerful and speedy) [...] Accordingly, the New Age solution does not call for a top-down bureaucratic government, but for much more local autonomy than we have at present, with local cooperation on the regional and planetary levels. Similarly, the New Age solution does not call for socialism or capitalism (that kind of question would be decided on by the individual communities), but for an economy of life-oriented, mostly human-scale enterprises. Finally, the New Age solution would replace many of our 'monolithic institutions' with their biolithic equivalents.[28]

25   Op. cit.: 229.
26   Willis Harman, 1993: 284ff.
27   Ibid: 287.
28   Mark Satin, 1978: 18.

Like others, Satin points to the role of the individual because, he suggests, society is in the state it is because of its people: 'with us: with what we have become';[29] and he goes on to list New Age social values which might correct the 'unkind' nature of life in mainstream society. His list, which is not dissimilar from the Stanford director's above, includes: enoughness, stewardship, diversity, desireless love, reverence for life, and being kind to yourself.[30]

However, not all commentators on the New Age in the economic and political fields agree on a particular way forward. According to one economist, if change is left to market forces, change will not happen. This economist argues that the notion of sustainable development in capitalist philosophy is nothing more than political and economic rhetoric for the continued onward and aimless march of financial growth for the sake of financial growth alone, that is, without a broader responsibility or social criterion.[31] This view is echoed by David Spangler who fears that 'Limitless consumption without consequence or just plain limitless without boundaries is having a devastating affect upon our moral, social, and ecological landscapes. It is part of the modern attitude that the New Age is trying to change.'[32] This view also appears to be that of a network of over 30 leading non-government organizations (NGOs), the Real World Coalition, that includes Christian Aid, Friends of the Earth, Oxfam, and the World Wide Fund for Nature and which claims to represent the views of over two million people whose particular concerns include 'international development, environment, social justice, democratic renewal, unemployment, agriculture, health, poverty, pollution, transport, and community regeneration'.[33] In a report for the Coalition, the view given is that governments have to intervene and legislate internationally. Market forces

> will not generate sustainability of their own accord. Driven by short-term competition, they tend to provide insufficient investment in public goods; and they

29   Ibid.
30   Op. cit.: 86ff.
31   Richard Douthwaite, 1992.
32   David Spangler and William Irwin Thompson, 1991: 53.
33   Jonathon Porritt, 1996: 18.

are prone to generate external costs; and they generally under-value or 'discount' the future. Markets can of course be used to stimulate and achieve environmental efficiency – this is precisely the purpose of financial incentives and the eco-tax reform. But sustainability is ultimately a political choice, and it will require proactive government policy to achieve it.[34]

Nevertheless, while there is much theorizing about the best way forward to achieve sustainability, there are some New Age ideas which are already being put into practice. Robert Van de Weyer, writing from the Green political view, has identified four new general trends which he sees occurring. Although these ideas may not be New Age per se, they incorporate elements of its philosophy: the first is the shrinking factory. Through the development of microelectronics, 'Instead of sprawling cities built around huge factories, manufacturing can flourish in market towns and even villages [...] in every country.'[35] This localization is leading, according to Weyer's second trend, to a change towards a repopulation of the countryside where work will follow people rather than, as is the current practice, people following the availability of work. The third trend is a return to mixed farming and a move away from agrochemical use. According to Weyer, across the world 'We are now suffering the fate of every civilization that has tried to squeeze more from the land that the soil can give: we are turning our fields into deserts'.[36] Finally, Weyer sees that social welfare is increasing rapidly, in fact, he sees demand is outstripping supply.[37] Taken together, Weyer believes, these four trends

> point to a social and economic transformation as profound as the Industrial Revolution two centuries ago – a transformation which offers hope to our rotting civilization [...] If we can, we will not merely sail past the ecological and social catastrophe to which we are now heading; but we shall attain a new prosperity, in which we can live in harmony both with ourselves and with the natural order.[38]

34   Michael Jacobs, 1996: 38f.
35   Robert Van de Weyer, 1991: 125ff.
36   Op. cit.: 127.
37   Ibid.
38   Ibid: 128ff.

In fact, there are specific instances where New Age economic theory is to be seen working in practice. For example, in commercial organizations, Dame Anita Roddick of The Body Shop has been described as 'a prophet, often a lone voice, of enterprise without exploitation';[39] and a journalist, reporting on the activities of Ben & Jerry's Homemade Ice Cream, asserted that 'in the annals of business history, they are recorded as the first company to turn a profit while behaving like a non-profit organization.'[40] The same reporter found that there are more than 2,000 such companies. LETS schemes (Local Exchange Trading Systems, also known as 'green currencies') now exist in substantial numbers in the UK, US, Canada, Australia, and New Zealand; and there are ethical banks such as, in Europe, Triodos Bank, and in the UK, The Co-operative Bank. In America in 1971, Pax World were the first mutual to launch an ethical fund and, since the 1990s, the specialist *Green Money Journal* reports on socially responsible investing, 'from the stockmarket to the supermarket'. The New Economics Foundation is a think tank whose role is to map out new forms of economic measures based on democracy and sustainability; and the World Business Academy, with chapters in the North and South America, Europe, and Asia, has the remit to help business contribute to a future that is economically, socially, and ecologically viable for all. There are many similar examples which are now beginning to occur. Moreover, as mentioned above, various communities which demonstrate the reality of New Age sustainable living have become established, although these tend to be comparatively small and isolated, the Findhorn Community and The Farm Community probably being the largest examples.

Moreover, we can see a tremendous growth in individual and community social enterprise across the Western world, parts of which can be seen to fall within the New Age domain of community activity as it has been described, especially with regard to the environment. Examples include recycling, pollution reduction, organic farming methods, and vegetarianism and veganism. Additionally, during the same period, there has been a growth in environmental protest and

39   Walter Schwarz, 1994: 44.
40   *The Guardian Weekend*, 4 November 1995: 48.

direct-action activities – both peaceful and militant – although these often exclusively regard single issues and activists may not participate in the wider spectrum of the New Age. For example, these activities include the treatment of animals, road building, the dumping of waste at sea, and clear-cut forestry, where such organizations as Greenpeace, Friends of the Earth, and the more radical Earth First! are active.

As has already been illustrated, there has been a good deal of interest shown by some in the New Age with regard to political and economic affairs, although actual activity appears not to be very widespread. This is why it was stated above that sustainable living currently appears more a theoretical notion than a realizable one. One of the most important reasons for this is likely to be, for those involved in the New Age, that to bring about the transformation they desire would entail getting involved with mainstream politics and economics, to help bring about change from within by presenting an alternative. Very few individuals appear to do this, and those that do are often marginalized as can be illustrated by the ups and downs of the Green political movement across the world, especially in Germany.[41] Allied to this, and as reported in Chapter 3, the New Age is peopled primarily by women. In the same way as women in general, those in the New Age have demonstrated a distinct lack of active involvement in areas of interest such as Green politics, which seems to be very much a male domain.[42] To date, in no national legislature have women outnumbered men. However, this does not mean to say the those who wish to influence change do nothing. For example, it has been reported in the UK that 'almost half of organic farmers are women, compared with only five per cent of those farming "chemically".'[43] On the contrary, the approach to enacting change seems to have shifted, is now more subtle, and appears to centre on particular issues rather than on the idea of a complete transformation – that is, one thing at a time rather than total and immediate change. In this respect, it can be seen

41 The decline of environmental politics in the West is chronicled by Anna Bramwell, 1994.
42 For example, the readers of *Resurgence*, which deals seriously with ecological and spiritual issues, are predominantly male.
43 Sophie Poklewski Koziell, 1999: 36.

that much of the new activity is based specifically on ecological concerns, as it is this issue in particular where there appears to be the greatest opportunity for influence because, with or without the New Age, the degradation of the planet – BSE to ozone depletion – demands change. In fact, political and economic attention worldwide has no choice but to institute change. It is ironic that, while many in the New Age appear intensely concerned with changes in the way in which politics and economics are managed, change in this direction may occur which has little to do with a specifically New Age input.

Apart from concern for the environment, on which we concentrate below, those participating in my survey showed little enthusiasm for actual involvement in political and economic affairs. It can be remembered, again from Chapter 3, that regarding activity in Green politics, only 14% reported that they were currently involved, and those were comprised more of younger people than of older; and with regard to ethical investing, only 10% were currently active. With regards to participation in alternative political organizations, almost 50% claimed membership of or contribution to such groups – although, in the main, most of these organizations were environmental. Of non-environmental organizations, membership or contribution was highest to Amnesty International at 11%, and no other organization had more than 5% participation. Overall, nearly 140 organizations were named, the majority having one or just a few individuals claiming membership or contribution, and over 40% of these were environmental.

Several further questions were put to assess wider aspects of the New Age view of social transformation. For example, those giving a view almost unanimously felt that it was desirable to move to a sustainable society and, again almost unanimously, they felt that such a move was not possible to be brought about within the existing social and political system. With regard to political systems, and given a straight choice between two options, less than 10% thought that representative democracy (the current system in the majority of Western countries) was the best system, while more than 90% of those giving a view believed that participatory democracy (PR) was better; and most also thought PR was the fairest electoral system. However, when asked what might be the best electoral system of all, the findings were much more divided. Only 40% believed PR to be the best system and a quarter said it was not – many suggestions were made for alternative methods although none were of numerical significance. The remaining 35% did not know the answer or gave no answer. This finding suggests that, within the New Age, there is no clear idea of the means by which to bring about a transformation of society along New Age lines, although what is clear is that, whatever system is developed, it needs to allow for a high degree of local involvement. Overall, however, the vast majority (more than four out of five) were optimistic about the future of humankind on the planet, a view which appears to be in accord with the optimistic nature of the six basic New Age ideas outlined in Chapter 1, and also with the view that the New Age will take a long time to fully occur.

Turning to concentrate more specifically on environmental concerns and as deduced from the above findings, activity in this area seems to be the principal area of focus with regard to sustainable living by those involved in the New Age. It is also where the New Age and the Pagan movement – and other environmental interest groups such as ecofeminists – come into closest contact; in fact, in this area it is extremely difficult to clearly separate these groups from one another. For example, some of those involved in the New Age are also members of ecofeminist groups such as the Women's Environment Network (WEN) in the UK, who may also be Pagans; and the Pagan Federation itself asks its members to follow three principles, the first of which is: 'Love for and kinship with nature'.[44] Moreover, shamanism,[45] one of the six major Pagan traditions, draws from North American Indian traditions to describe the earth as our Mother. To muddy the issue further, many contemporary Buddhists are keenly involved in environmental concerns and, as previously mentioned, many of those involved in the New Age have been particularly influenced by Buddhist teachings.[46]

---

44   Cited in *The Pagan Federation Information Pack*, 1994: 4.
45   Outlined by Kenneth Meadows, 1995.
46   See Allan Badiner, 1990 for a number of essays on this subject; see also David Kinsley, 1995, who reviews ecological themes in Hinduism, Chinese religions, Buddhism, Christianity, and contemporary culture.

The concept of deep ecology appears fundamental to the New Age. It divides itself from shallow ecology (sometimes called 'light green') in that, according to the Norwegian ecologist and founder of the Deep Ecology Movement, Arne Naess,[47] shallow ecologists believe 'that reforming human relations toward nature can be done within the existing structure of society'[48] they avoid concern for the total picture, that is, for all species of nature and for Nature herself – for their well-being, contribution to the whole, halting species reduction, decreasing human population, reducing human interference with nature, changing policies, and enjoying quality of life rather than standard of living. The link between deep ecology and the New Age can be found in the notion that it is also a spiritual movement. As Fritjof Capra explains, 'When the concept of the human spirit is understood as the mode of consciousness in which the individual feels connected to the cosmos as a whole, it becomes clear that ecological awareness is spiritual in its deepest sense.'[49] Moreover, deep ecology is arguably against the theistic position of stewardship. In this respect, Matthew Fox, the proponent of Creation-Centred Spirituality in Christianity, suggests a shift away from the concept of the dutiful steward (shepherd) towards acceptance of a mystical cosmic ecological spirituality. It can be added that Fox's view is thought to be among the closest ideological positions to the New Age that a committed Christian can reach.[50]

However, this is not to say that all those involved with the New Age would agree with the extent to which deep ecology is fundamental to the New Age, although it is anticipated that a large number do see it in this way. As has been found in my survey, most of those involved rated themselves reasonably or considerably 'green',[51] almost half currently recycled their waste, and nearly 40% claimed to be

47   See also Bill Devall and George Sessions, 1985. For descriptions of Gaia, see James Lovelock, 1991.
48   Arne Naess, 1988: 6.
49   Fritjof Capra, 1993: 233.
50   See Matthew Fox, 1992. The relationship between the New Age, Matthew Fox, and Christianity is discussed in Chapter 10 below.
51   On a scale of 0–9, 70% rated themselves between 5 and 7 and a further 14% rated themselves between 8 and 9.

vegetarian. What is more, 25% claimed membership of Greenpeace and slightly less claimed membership of Friends of the Earth.[52] Clearly, a large number of those involved in the New Age are seriously concerned about the environment, although a sizeable number appear equally clearly not to be that much interested or not sufficiently interested actively to contribute anything towards trying to bring about change.

Nevertheless, there are many environmental writers whose ideas are influential to the New Age. Poet, farmer, and philosopher Wendell Berry, for example, gives 27 propositions about global thinking and the sustainability of cities, and argues that ecological good sense requires the replacement of all the most powerful economic entities, and that real planet-saving work will be undertaken by a multitude of small and local – humble – people.[53] Berry highlights the point that discussion of fundamental change automatically involves economics and politics. Jonathon Porritt, a Director of Forum for the Future and a key figure in environmental concerns, as with many writers influential to the New Age, draws on the life and teachings of Mahatma Gandhi[54] by seeing that materialism needs to decline and change to a more spiritual basis in order to create an ecologically balanced world. To bring this about, Porritt argues, four ideas are essential: bearing witness to and taking personal responsibility for the state our society is in, enjoying giving service to the community, showing reverence for the natural world – respect is not good enough – and celebrating all forms of life.[55] Examining these views with particular regard to a spiritual basis, biologist Rupert Sheldrake identifies three positions that individuals can take; and, clearly, those involved in the New Age

52   There was a high degree of duplication between membership of and contribution to both Greenpeace and Friends of the Earth.
53   Wendell Berry, 1991: 62f. Paul Hawken provides an eight-point plan for the design of business patterns which are sustainable and environment-friendly (1994: 16ff), and Amory Lovins, Director of the Rocky Mountain Institute, introduces four principles for what is called 'natural capitalism' (2000: 8ff).
54   See Jonathon Porritt, 1988: 6 for his argument that there should be no separation between politics and spirituality.
55   Notes from a Schumacher Lecture given at Lancaster, UK, in 1994.

would choose the third and most spiritual level. Sheldrake describes these three positions in the following way:

> Each of us, faced with the mystery of our existence and experience has to try and find some way of making sense of it. We have a choice of philosophies: the mechanistic theory of nature and of human life, with God as an optional extra; or the theory of nature as alive, but without God; or the theory of a living God together with living nature. Each of these views can be elaborated intellectually, each can be defended on rational grounds, and each is held with deep conviction by many people. In the end, we have to choose between them on the basis of intuition. Our choice is influenced by our acknowledgement of mystery, and in turn affects our tolerance of it. Those with the lowest mystery-tolerance thresholds are drawn to the mechanistic-atheistic world view, which as a matter of principle denies existence of mysterious entities like souls and God, and portrays a disenchanted, unmagical reality proceeding entirely mechanically. Those who acknowledge the life of evolutionary nature admit the mystery of life and creativity. And those who acknowledge the life of God are consciously open to the mystery of divine consciousness, grace and love.[56]

It seems that, ideally, the role (if such a thing exists) of the New Age is to transform those who advocate Sheldrake's first, mechanistic position, who simply use the environment for their own ends and short-term gain – that is, the mainstream – to the third position, which is welcoming of a transpersonal and mystical content to life. However, the New Age is not an evangelistic organization, which means that realistically ecological change is likely to be driven by the New Age only in part.

Nevertheless, as has been shown, there is underlying unanimity between 'Green' writers who are influential to the New Age and, in the same way as the survey has found, there seems to be a great optimism that, ecologically, humankind can pull back from the brink of catastrophe. Work appears to have already started and the move towards change seems to be gathering momentum, although substantial change – perhaps a transformation – has yet to take place. Joanna Macy, a Buddhist and New Science scholar, paints a highly optimistic picture by drawing attention to what she calls a time of 'Great Turning' at the end of the twentieth century. Macy points out that while the

---

56   Rupert Sheldrake, 1990: 170f.

agricultural revolution took centuries and the industrial revolution took decades to become established, she argues that the 'ecological revolution must happen within a few years'.[57] Accordingly, Macy argues that the characteristics of this Turning will mean 'we are going to have to want different things, seek different pleasures, pursue different goals' which, as indicated above, Macy sees is happening already, emerging 'like green shoots through the rubble'[58] on three levels: political, legislative, and legal efforts to slow down Earth's destruction; addressing the structural causes and creating sustainable alternatives; and that at all levels we are beginning again 'to see the world as our body and as sacred'.[59]

Macy's ideas bring us full circle, back to the notion that for a sustainable community to be brought about considerable change has to occur on all fronts – ecological, social, political, and economic. The current ecological situation demands change, although the change required may not be deep enough to incorporate all – or even many – specifically New Age ideas. The pessimistic view is that environmentally *un*friendly business is likely to try to survive by adapting and not transforming, and that governments may not be able to reach anything other than the most general agreements. Indeed, this was the case at the Earth Summit (the UN Conference on Environment and Development) at Rio de Janeiro in 1992 and the World Summit on Sustainable Development at Johannesburg in 2002. If this state of affairs continues, then for sustainable living to become a reality at some point in the future, something more than ecological influences may be needed.

Summary

Community activity is very much on the New Age agenda, and although those involved in the New Age seem to place greater impor-

---

57 Joanna Macy, 1998: 28.
58 Op. cit.: 29.
59 Ibid.

tance on their own spiritual and healing needs and not so much on the world at large, change in this direction has already been detected. Many writers, together with those surveyed, see a vital importance in transforming themselves; and little by little this new consciousness is expected to soak further into the wider fabric of world society. Those involved in the New Age believe this will be a natural occurrence, which may take a very long time to fully develop. Separation of this domain into two aspects has shown that both proceed in a similar ideological direction – a radical change in our relationships with each other and with the world at large; in fact, a new age or new consciousness. Those involved go about transforming themselves primarily through self-effort and attending spiritual and healing workshops – itself a form of transitory New Age community – and an ethnographical account of such experience is now attempted.

9. The New Age Experience

The heart is at the centre of the Circle and there are the four directions, the east, west, south, and north. And though there are four directions, there is really only one direction, the direction of greatness, or the highest potential of goodness. It is the direction by which energy is continuously rediscovering itself.

Joseph Rael[1]

Our study, up to this point, has dealt with theory and views about the New Age from a variety of sources and standpoints. The New Age is a 'lived' experience; that is, it affects many or most aspects of a participant's life most of the time. But one question still remains: what is participation like? This question needs to be answered in order to give a comprehensive insight to the New Age, and one of the best means of so doing is by giving a subjective, first-hand account of experiences at a typical long-weekend workshop. This chapter, then, is an account of my experiences of the kind of activities and events which can commonly be encountered at such events.

Whether the account of one person's experience is characteristic of the kind of experiences participants have in these workshops needs to be considered. Within the workshop now described, my experience seemed to be similar to – but by no means the same as – the majority of the other participants. Each person's journey through the workshop was unique. However, when it was over, those attending all concluded that it was one of the most beneficial they had experienced; so it may be seen as an example of a high-quality New Age event, the structure and contents of which are broadly typical of many such events.

---

1   Joseph Rael, 1993: 80.

233

'The Healing Circle' workshop

The workshop was held over five days and the venue was a large room in a building used primarily for religious purposes. The group was non-residential, convening at 10 am and concluding at 10 pm or later each evening, except on the final day which finished at 6 pm. The cost of the workshop was £95 (£70 with concessions – $150 or $110).

Membership of the group totalled ten people – seven women and three men – but some members could not attend for the full five days. One man came for the first day only and four people, two women and two men, attended all five days. The normal daily attendance was six to seven people. The age profile of the group members was broadly late twenties and early thirties to mid and late forties; at least half were single – that is, not in a partnership. With regards to the members' occupations, four were undergoing training (two in aromatherapy and massage, and two at universities), while the employment types of those in work included administrative, sales, technical, and teaching. Two of the individuals attending the workshop did not appear to be involved in the New Age and were present on the recommendation of their therapist, one of the facilitators. Of the remainder, approximately five others may only have been partially involved, and the remaining individuals appeared to be more fully involved.

All members of the group had one principal aspect in common. This was that they were all attempting to come into closer contact with – and understanding of – their inner or Higher Self. This can be described in terms of their desire to heal wounds or blockages and/or to grow in strength and purpose. Of course each person's idea of their wounds and goals at the workshop was different, but the underlying reason for attendance at the group appears to have been to work towards achieving change. At the outset, it could be argued that for the majority this change was seen as mostly to do with the psychological aspects of their lives but, as the group progressed, physical – and especially spiritual – influences became important. By the end of the workshop, for some participants the physical, psychological, and spiritual aspects had seemingly merged together and become inseparable.

There were two workshop facilitators. This was because the workshop format was designed to be both psychotherapeutic and shamanistic. William was involved in psychotherapy as a hypnotherapist and healer, with additional interests in channelling, and Brook was a shamanic teacher and healer studying under Joseph Rael,[2] a shaman and master storyteller of the Ute and Pueblo traditions living in New Mexico.[3]

The process of the workshop was divided into daily themes including inner child, past life, and soul retrieval; however, the workshop as a whole was designed as a journey around the course of a medicine wheel.[4] The shamanistic rituals, ceremonies, and journeys which occurred over the course of the five days created a sacred space within which most of the activities occurred and gave a sense of spiritual authority to the psychotherapeutic healing techniques which were enacted. The wheel itself is comprised of five points: East, South, West, North, and Centre; and each point is metaphorically symbolic – a notion which was reflected in the nature of each of the five days of the workshop. Furthermore, the importance of the use and significance of the medicine wheel grew throughout each of the workshop days, culminating with the medicine-wheel-blessing ceremony on the final day. Participants were not requested to carry out preliminary work to

---

2   Joseph Rael's North American Indian name is Beautiful Painted Arrow (see Rael, 1992).

3   The facilitators' names have been changed.

4   The medicine wheel (from North American Plains Indian origins) was used classically in the workshop 'as a vehicle for medicine power, protection, and spiritual growth. The wheel is constructed according to ritual, marked with the cardinal points, and consecrated to the spirits' (Rosemary Ellen Guiley, 1991: 355). In describing the importance of the medicine wheel, Joseph Rael suggests that 'Christians use the term "circle" of life, and others refer to it as the medicine wheel. These are all different terms for honouring, for celebration of the emotional, mental, physical, or spiritual essence of living breath' (1993: 77). For further description of medicine wheels see: Op. cit.: 90ff; Catherine Albanese, 1990: 156ff; Kenneth Meadows, 1995; and Roy Wilson, 1994.

prepare for the activities of the workshop. Instead, it was suggested that members arrived with an open mind and an open heart.[5]

Day One

We begin our journey and form the circle through ceremony, introduce our-selves and find a power animal to help us on our way. Then, we investigate what it is we need to heal over these five days. In the evening we learn about the medicine wheel as a map of consciousness.

The first cardinal point on the medicine wheel is the East: symbolized by the vowel sound A (aah) for purification; spring; sunrise; the colour yellow; wisdom and unity.[6]

I start the day in a very happy, positive frame of mind, feeling full of love and good thoughts.

The group convenes at 10am. Some people already know and embrace each other. We sit on cushions in a circle around a sacred space containing a large piece of crystal, a gourd rattle, a stick of dried leaves, an eagle's wing, a clam shell, and a candle each positioned on a metre-square cloth. The candle was lit.

William introduced the proceedings and the plan of the workshop days giving various pieces of information and requesting everyone to promise, if possible, to refrain from drink and drugs (medical or oth-

---

5   What follows is a detailed description of my journey along the course of this particular medicine wheel; however, there are elements of the five-day healing workshop processes which have been excluded from this illustration. Most importantly, in order to respect the confidential nature of the thoughts and activities of the participants, no mention has been made of any aspect of the event which might compromise participants. This illustration, therefore, represents an attempt to reveal as full a description of the writer's personal experience as possible but, even within this, the reader is asked to respect the decision that some particularly personal aspects of the workshop have been excluded.

6   Each introductory quotation consists of a description from the weekend programme notes followed by a paraphrase of Joseph Rael, 1993: 90ff.

erwise) for the duration of the workshop. Brook introduced the shamanic activities, his first words taking me by surprise. He said that he
knew everyone in the group, not that he had met us all personally before, but that each of us was known to him. I looked around the group
members one by one and realized that I too knew, or felt some kind of
familiarity with, all the people in the group. I felt that there were no
strangers there, that I was among friends. This feeling felt true but irrational. It was also warm and loving.

Brook then conducted the opening cleansing ceremony by burning aromatic sage leaves and wafting the smoke in a ritualistic manner
around each person using the eagle's wing as a fan.[7] We were each
asked to stand up while being cleansed. Brook also invited every
group member to add something personal to the sacred space.

After this ceremony, each person spoke in turn about themselves
and, as requested, talked about why they were attending the circle and
what their expectations were. I reported that I had no particular single
reason for joining the group although I had been searching for some
time for a way to move forward in my spiritual growth which, I believed, had become a little stuck.

At this point the circle began its work, with Brook leading the
first of many visualization processes which we were to undertake.
This first process was to find our power animal – our personal guardian spirit – who would guide each of us individually throughout the
workshop. This animal could take many forms, we were told, from an
eagle to a bear.[8]

Each person lay flat on their backs on the floor and were requested to relax and be as comfortable as possible. We were led into
the visualization by words guiding us to a light hypnotic trance-like

7   A process known as smudging which Kenneth Meadows describes as 'the use
    of smoke to clear away negative vibrations and to attract beneficial energies to
    oneself and others' (1995: 220).

8   Michael Harner describes power animals discovered by westerners as being
    such creatures as a 'Crane, Tiger, Fox, Eagle, Bear, Deer, Porpoise, and even
    Dragon', and suggests that 'no matter how fierce a guardian animal spirit may
    seem, its possessor is in no danger because the power animal is absolutely
    harmless. It is only a source of power; it has no aggressive intentions. It comes
    only because you need help' (1990: 67f).

state. As some of the participants had undergone hypnotherapy regularly before, getting into this state did not prove problematic. For me, however, it was difficult; and only once in the whole workshop did this happen. Nevertheless, I was familiar with visualization processes and just followed the verbal directions of getting myself into a very relaxed and open state of mind which appeared to work just as well. For this first process Brook had started drumming. The drumming was regular and monotonous and, later, Brook explained that the tone, frequency, and vibration of the drumming were known to effect key brain waves.[9]

Once the instructions for entering into the process were complete, only the sound of the drumming remained and each participant began the journey to find their power animal. I became aware that I was in a landscape, standing on the side of a hill overlooking countryside. There was a tree behind me, perhaps more than one. I gazed over the landscape reflecting on thoughts as they passed through my consciousness: that I was an insubstantial speck in this huge landscape, that I was part of the landscape and it was part of me. Many thoughts although no power animal. The drumming helped to maintain the visualization. Towards the end of the process I looked up into the nearest tree behind me and there, not far away, perched in silence, was a large brown owl. I felt a little foolish. All of the time, standing in the landscape, I must have been being observed. I smiled broadly, welcoming the contact. The owl observed me with a penetrating gaze. At about that time the process, which had lasted perhaps half an hour, was brought to a close. The drumming stopped and we were all slowly and gently brought back to normal consciousness and to the circle.

For a few minutes we were asked to draw or write about what had happened in the process, and then individually we described the images and events to the group. I found the use of this space in time between the end of each process and talking to the group to be useful to attempt to make sense of what thoughts and images had occurred.

9   The drum beats at approximately 180 beats per minute. Michael Harner suggests that drumming is fundamental to shamanic activities because it acts both as a means of transport to enter an altered state of consciousness and, subsequently, acts to sustain the journey (1990: 51).

In addition, the technique of drawing what had been visualized helped to focus on important experiences and their meanings. Returning to the circle after a few minutes, each person – if they wished – told the group what had occurred in their visualization. Surprisingly, it transpired that five members of the group (out of eight attending that day) had the same experience of an owl, although each instance differed. Brook reported that he had felt the presence of his power animal, a leopard.

The Circle broke for lunch.

The first part of the afternoon was comprised of three games. The first game involved a cushion and embraces, similar to the childhood game of 'tag' or 'it'. One person had to touch another with a cushion to pass it on, but if the other person was hugging someone else they were 'safe' – so there was lots of running around the room, hugging, and laughter.

We then went into the garden to play two more games. In the first, the group split into pairs and one person in each pair took it in turn to be blindfolded. The other person had to lead the blindfolded person safely around the garden. This game was to do with putting all my trust into the hands of the partner although, for me, it also had other meanings. I guided my partner around the garden introducing him to trees, earth, and scents. Then the process was reversed. Being led blindfold and in silence through a garden meant that complete trust for my safety had to be given to a relative stranger whose only contact was his leading hand. Without sight, the normal spatial reality dissolved into a glimpse of a completely different reality. The strangeness was acute – for instance, the feel and smell of a bluebell, or the branch of a tree. As I have problems with my eyes, this game also brought home to me what blindness might be like.

The final game was a meditation in three parts. Firstly, we were asked to imagine ourselves enacting the seed of a tree sprouting and growing. From a curled up ball in the grass, each group member uncurled slowly and grew (stood) up to become a mature tree. The second part involved choosing a particular tree in the garden and meditating or communing with it. We were asked to select a tree which might have some similarities or qualities with how we each felt about ourselves, to experience it, to feel compassion for it. We stood communing with our trees for about a quarter of an hour. The third part of the meditation took place back in the large, airy workshop room. Here, we were asked to draw how we saw the tree. When the drawings were complete, we gathered in the circle each displaying our drawings and talking about what had been represented.

My tree drawing was of a sturdy tree half of which was colourful and alive and half of which was broken and dead. The tree was drawn on its own and set against a landscape of rolling hills with woods (groups of trees) in the distance. The explanation for the drawing was that because I had multiple sclerosis, I felt that a part of my body was broken. However, the other part of my body was very much alive and strong. On the alive side of the drawing I had included birds flying. I talked about what MS has meant to me – that it was primarily physical, which left my mind and especially my heart and spirit strong. I felt full of love. In my drawing, this was illustrated in the use of contrasting bright colours. I pointed out that the tree was on its own, which symbolized that, primarily as a result of MS, I had become a solitary and sometimes lonely person. This was the first time I had spoken about MS like this and it became quite an emotion-filled experience. As I looked round at the people in the circle looking at me, I saw such compassion and warmth coming from them. The moment was quite beautiful.

After each person had talked about their tree drawing and we had some tea, one further game was played in the room. In the game, one end of the room was designated negative and the other positive. William requested each person to position themselves in the room according to how they felt about various aspects of their lives. Each time William said a word – for example, work, relationships, life, study, family, spirituality, yourself – everyone moved to the position which they believed best reflected how they felt in the different extremes between positive and negative. This game was a process of self-reflection and was carried out without regard to where fellow participants were positioning themselves. Immediately following the game, William led a guided meditation which allowed each person to focus on how they felt about themselves. This was followed by a period where participants, if they wished, could share their thoughts with the group.

The many such periods of sharing – sitting in a circle around the sacred space – were often charged with emotions. With compassionate but resolute intentions, William would listen to the thoughts and ideas that each person who had chosen to talk had expressed, and would then probe various aspects with deeper questioning. In consequence, these periods contained expressions of each participant's hidden pains, their fears and frustrations, their tears. At some points, participants found it immensely difficult, if not impossible, to talk; and for the other listening members of the group it was difficult not to be deeply affected by what was being said. I could not help but notice how solemn some moments were, and at other moments how little joy and happiness there was in some people's lives. I found myself wanting to absorb the others' pains.

After a two-hour supper break the circle came back together. Each time the circle reconvened, those present held the hands of the person sitting either side of them to form an unbroken chain around the sacred space. William (or Brook) would say a prayer to the spirits who were guiding us, asking for strength and success in our work. Then, after squeezing our hands, the chain would break and activities begin. For me, this ritual became an intensely pleasant and meaningful exchange, not only in feeling the warm emotions of fellow group members through their hands, but also feeling a higher, more powerful energy which the ritual evoked by bringing this group of people back into a remarkable communion with one another.

The first evening session was led by Brook, who talked about the meaning of the medicine wheel as a map of consciousness, about the meaning of metaphors, and about how making vowel sounds can resonate with the deeper mysteries to life.

Day Two

Today we discover the child within us. We ask what this child needs from us so he or she can feel nourished and more whole. We learn what this child can offer us to help us feel more fully alive. In the evening, Brook teaches us overtone chanting and we share this together.

The second cardinal point on the medicine wheel is the South: symbolized by the vowel sound E for the relationship of the physical and the spiritual; summer; white; the thirst for knowledge and emotional awareness.

The circle is reconvened, the candle is lit, then the group forms a chain and is sanctified with prayer. Again, I start the day in a happy, positive frame of mind, feeling full of love and good thoughts.

Each group member had been requested to bring an item from their childhood – for instance, a photograph of themselves as a child or a teddy bear – to the circle for this day. The first session was spent with each person describing their childhood, especially their relationship to parents and immediate family, evaluating it and answering questions put by William or Brook or other group members. Photographs were passed around the group.

The circle then moved outside into the garden for three games. The first game allowed a free expression of happy emotions. The group stood in a circle and individually each person was asked to move into the centre to say 'I am [their name] and I am happy.' However, each person had to express how happy they felt by the way they moved to the centre and through the expression in their voice. After each person had performed their part it was then mimicked by all group members. Some people performed twirls, some simply strolled into the middle, and one person somersaulted in. Copying each person's performance proved to be hilarious.

The second game involved touching and stroking. Everyone lined up in two facing lines. Then each person in turn imagined themselves to be a particular type of motorcar and 'drove' between the two lines of people, which became a car-wash. Dirty cars received a good scrubbing, old cars a gentle one, and sports cars went through double quick.

Finally, the third game involved more intimate and meaningful touching. In twos, in silence, and with eyes closed, the idea of the game was to say hello to your partner using only a hand.

Back inside the room, William then conducted the first visualization process of the day on the theme of the inner child.

Each visualization process took place in an altered state of consciousness which was described as a hypnotic trance or deep meditation. In fact, William stated that he thought the characteristics of these two mental states were practically identical both in their nature and in the resulting effects. William usually led the group into a semi-hypnotized trance state through a shortened relaxation process. The process had been shortened because so many of the group members had been or were currently his clients and so were used to his methods. However, I was not and would have preferred a longer beginning to the processes. The processes started with a short talk by William (or Brook) discussing what the theme and direction was to be. Once we had made ourselves comfortable lying down, William asked us to find a spot on the ceiling in order to concentrate our focus. Then we were asked to take three deep breaths and at each breath we were to find ourselves going deeper and deeper into an altered state of consciousness. William spoke gently, saying that the environment we were occupying was a safe space for healing and that we were to put our rational minds to one side to allow our creative, nonrational minds the freedom to take over. He asked us to relax our bodies completely, starting from the top of the head and down through the neck, the shoulders, the arms, the abdomen, through our legs, and down to the toes. We were then asked to count backwards from the number one hundred until the numbers had gone from our consciousness. Our eyes, William said, were now so relaxed that even if we wanted to open them we could not. To most participants (they later reported), by the number ninety-seven they had moved into a hypnotic state of mind and the ability to count had ceased although, as described above, I did not normally reach this state and just stopped counting. William asked participants to nod their heads when the numbers had gone.

Following the direction of the process theme of the inner child, an image started to appear in my mind. The image which developed was of myself standing inside my body which had transformed itself into a huge cavernous space. It was warm and dimly lit. Nothing at all happened to me in this place, but being there I felt quite happy, safe, and problem-free. Some other members of the group were having very different experiences. From one or two people came agonized sobbing, and another sounded as if he was having convulsions. I could sense William and Brook tending to those most needing help. After some time, William brought the process to a close and we were requested to spend a few minutes drawing our experience. The drawings and our experience in the process were subsequently discussed in the circle after a lunch break.

The drawing I had produced was of my body as an empty, headless cylinder, a vast safe space. I described to the group what had happened during the process. However, later that evening I realized I had misinterpreted what had occurred in the drawing.

A second visualization process followed in two parts. The group split into pairs and one person underwent the process while the other person assisted in its progress by asking pertinent questions. Then the process was reversed. Following the now usual method of relaxation, William led the visualization by asking that we should find a place in our bodies which was an area of pain to do with our childhood, and to put a hand on that place. I did not feel any such pain as I was still feeling happy and positive. I decided to put my hand on where I felt the most emotion – on my heart. From that time onwards we were to follow what was occurring in our altered consciousness, being prompted with questions from our partners. My partner asked various questions – for instance, where was I?, and what was happening? – and I described to her what I could see and feel. The image which came into view was that I was in my heart and that I felt no pain, only love. The space in my heart looked like a vast amphitheatre – womb-like and cathedral-like. It was a warm, dimly lit and lovely place.

People started to appear in my heart. My Mother appeared and I gave her a hug. Other people appeared and love flowed everywhere, into all who were there, and there was no pain. The size of my heart seemed infinite. Many people were there – my daughters, my son, friends. My process partner was there. The whole of humanity was in my heart, and the whole of nature. A liquid light was falling on me, a waterfall of light which felt to be unconditional love. It flowed into everybody. The scene I had visualized was a very beautiful picture. I was smiling. Everyone was smiling. However, at the same time sounds of great pain made by other group members could be heard in the room. Frightening, violent hammering on the floor, cries of distress, sobbing, and anger. I tried to send out my liquid light to reach and soothe the other group members but the howls of anguish and pain continued until William brought the process to a close and our roles were reversed. The contrast of emotions my partner and I had experienced during this first process, that of tremendous beauty surrounded by abject despair, was immense.

After a few minutes, William led us into the second process where I assisted my partner in her visualization. The images she described were of towering, stalking figures, mysterious, and only seen in silhouette. They were not human and did not threaten her, yet they appeared to have great influence over her life. She knew they controlled her destiny and would be instrumental in her death, so their appearance filled her with foreboding. The room was a little more calm during this process but now other members had started sobbing. The images given in response to my questions by my partner appeared to represent an underlying fear that her life span was to be cut short at any moment, that it was just a matter of time before it would happen, but exactly how much time she thought she had left she did not know. In discussions after the process, my partner reported that she had experienced the same images several times before and believed that their appearance foretold an early death.

From this time onwards, I felt there was a strong feeling of bonding throughout the group. I felt that we were all starting to become emotionally, spiritually, and physically close. There was a genuine warmth pervading the circle, both among participants and its leaders.

At this time the circle broke for supper and reconvened later to listen to Brook talking about, and demonstrating, overtone chanting. This was an astonishing and magical sound as the chanting was of two voices – one low and one high – coming from the same person. We were invited to participate in chanting vowel sounds. Unusually, I found I was unable to utter a sound and so made silent mouth movements so as to feel as if I was joining in.

What was happening in me was that my mood had changed at the end of this second day from one which was extremely happy to one of deep sadness. I felt as if I had absorbed a great deal of the pain that others had expressed in the two processes of the day and that it had overwhelmed me. Coupled with this, I discovered that what I had experienced and drawn at the first inner child meditation of the day did not mean what I had thought it to have meant. Its meaning was entirely different. I realized that the cylindrical shape I had experienced and drawn instead of representing a vast safe space in fact, metaphorically, signified a cocoon. It was later pointed out that why I had not drawn a head was perhaps because all of me was contained within this safe space. By applying this metaphor to the way in which I had led my life, I saw that I had consciously cocooned myself over the years – that is, insulated myself – from many important emotions and relationships. I realized that this had happened partly because of the effects of MS and partly because of damaging relationships I had experienced both as a child and a teenager. The cocoon I had woven enabled me to avoid having to face difficult aspects of my life. It had acted as an anaesthetic to enable me not to feel. I learnt that I needed to react to this if I was to grow.

Day Three

Going deeper, we explore our past lives and learn how these experiences relate to our present needs. William offers a full demonstration of what the process involves. Then there is the opportunity for everyone to experience their own past lives through supervised processes in pairs. In the evening we relax with massage.

The third cardinal point on the medicine wheel is the West: symbolized by the vowel sound I for awareness; autumn; black; concreteness, harmony, calling, and the process of coming into being.

As usual, the circle was sanctified with prayer to the guiding spirits, and the candle in the sacred space was lit. I start the day feeling very sad indeed.

There were two activities prior to the first visualization process of the day. Firstly, William played a disco-music tape cassette and we all danced. For the second activity we separated into pairs for a period of touching. In this period no words were spoken, we held and caressed each other's hands and looked into each other's eyes. For my partner and I (not having met before the workshop) it was a period of great emotional warmth and exchange of loving emotions. I found it remarkable that two relative strangers – without speaking – could feel and convey such deep feelings to one another. We smiled a great deal together.

The first visualization process was led by William and it prepared the way for the main activity later in the day, that of exploring our past lives.[10] William talked about the concept of past lives and how he believed it was possible that the effects of traumas in previous existences can be carried through to effect our present lives.

As we entered into the first visualization process of the day, William asked that during the process we concentrated our attention on discovering what might be ill in our bodies and minds, and on what the sensations of these illnesses could be. The results of this process would then act as the foundation for work we would carry out later in the day. As I began the process no visual images came into mind. However, following on from how I had been feeling, I began to feel

10   The practice of past life recall and, relatedly, the concepts of reincarnation and karma, according to Denise Linn, help to answer 'questions such as why we keep repeating the same negative patterns again and again; where our recurring fears and phobias come from; why we feel an instant attraction to some people and some places; and, more importantly, what our purpose is here on earth' (1994: 38). Linn suggests that 'Past life exploration has proved incredibly powerful in many cases where regular introspection into present life circumstances has failed to bring changes. Understanding our place and mission in the present can be helped through understanding what we have been in previous lives. Life is not a one-time affair; it is not a series of meaningless experiences strung together. Past life exploration can assist the process of emerging as a conscious, loving being, gradually realizing our full potential' (Op. cit.: 53f).

even more sad, not sad about any particular event or person, just utterly sad. At the end of the process the usual period of drawing or writing was given so that we could collect our thoughts. I could not draw or write anything. Instead, I quickly drew a patch of blue on a piece of paper. When it came to discussing in the circle what had happened I did not particularly want to speak.

The method of speaking in the group up until this time had been that William would open up the floor by inviting anyone who so wished to speak. Long periods of silence often followed where no one chose to speak. Then someone would start. Then silence again. In this way, each person could speak when (and if) they felt ready. Later on in the workshop a teddy bear – the 'talking' bear – was introduced to the centre of the group, which participants would pick up to signify they wished to speak and not put down until they had finished. After a period of time had elapsed since the last person had spoken, William would close the opportunity to speak and the group would move on to the next activity.

On this occasion I was one of the last to speak. I showed my blue drawing and said that I did not have much to say except that I felt immersed in a sea of sadness. There was a break for lunch, and the circle reconvened. William decided that before the work of the group proceeded he wanted to probe what I was feeling. I was asked to sit on a chair in the middle of the circle and to close my eyes. He then asked a number of questions. I reported that the blueness was a pain mostly felt in my heart and that it was not without some beauty; that it was to do with the love I felt and the pain I had absorbed from what was happening in the group – both from others' experiences (that there existed so much pain in the world) and from what I was learning about myself. Although talking in this way was difficult and painful, I was inwardly glad of the opportunity to expose what I was feeling – that although there was pain in all lives, there was also the possibility of a surfeit of love.

Then followed the main visualization process of the day, that of a journey back into our past lives. The participants split into pairs with, as before, one person helping the other through their process and then reversing the order. William led us into an altered state of consciousness in the now usual manner, and asked us to focus on that part of our

248

bodies which needed healing. We were to visualize the sensations and ask ourselves where the pain occurred and what had caused it. The role of the partner was to carry on asking similar questions. At the same time, we were to remain aware of our bodies and use them as a bridge or guide to the cause of our pain.

My immediate vision was looking down upon a pair of feet wearing leather-thonged sandals and standing on hot dusty ground. I was not sure that the feet were mine but I presumed that they were. I looked up slowly to see that I was in a hot and dry place. All around were hundreds of men clothed in traditional white Middle Eastern dress with loosely wound white turbans. Everybody, including myself, was just standing around. There was no movement to go anywhere. We were just waiting. All was peaceful. Then I could see a person I knew to be Jesus milling among the throng, and then a Roman soldier. I had no idea whether what I was seeing was in any way real or was, in fact, images drawn from picture books I might have seen earlier in my current life. I did not know why this particular picture had come into my consciousness. Brook had joined my partner and several questions were asked to try to probe the relatedness and meaning of what was going on. I had deliberately changed the warm, bright scenes in my mind to be bleak and dark. William also asked me questions. Why did I want to blacken the images? In discussion after this process, Brook suggested that what I had seen and talked about might not have been an actual past-life experience but my unconscious surfacing in the form of a metaphor – the message to me being that it is possible to learn to forgive ourselves for our thoughts and deeds which we know now to have been wrong. At that moment in the discussion I spontaneously remembered the Christian concept of forgiveness as it is written in the Lord's Prayer.

The process was reversed and I assisted my partner through his sequence which was also very painful. He was a tall, strong man and he became very physical, writhing about on the cushions and angrily hammering on the floor. It became obvious that he was experiencing violent and heart-breaking emotions, all the time yelling Why?, Why?. I stayed close by him listening to his sobbing and trying to protect him from hurting himself.

Following on from the past-life visualization processes there was no group discussion, but from talking with fellow group members later that evening I gathered that the experiences which occurred were diverse. One person was slain with a sword on a medieval battlefield, and another had died through being left alone tied to a bed while having an epileptic fit.

Following the break for supper, the circle reconvened for an evening of massage. First of all, a demonstration was given on how to massage using oils blended with essential essences. The room was lit very dimly and gentle music was played. The group then split into pairs, each person stripping to their underwear and taking turns to massage and be massaged. The experience was sensual but also trusting and caring. No sexual boundaries were crossed. A tremendous sense of intimacy and sharing combined with playfulness and sheer pleasure developed between my partner and I as we massaged each other from head to toe over the next three hours.

Day Four

Using the Shamanic technique of Soul Retrieval we search for aspects of our Self that have been lost or suppressed and seek inner help to bring those parts of our Self 'home' to our being. We invoke contact and support from our inner guides and teachers so we can gain greater purpose and meaning to our lives. In the evening we share the experience of Spiritual Healing.

The fourth cardinal point on the medicine wheel is the North: symbolized by the vowel sound O for innocence, clarity, and the infinite void; winter; the colour red; truth, completion, and knowing our path.

Again, the circle was sanctified with prayer and the candle lit. We all linked hands to form an unbroken chain around the sacred space.

The first activity of the day was the playing of a game whereby the female participants lined up facing the (outnumbered) male participants. The women were to say yes and the men were to say no, and each had to be persuasive in terms of volume. The game became a screaming contest which many participants found to be negative, gendered, and unnecessarily confrontational. This game was followed by a period of dancing to a tape cassette of rock music which, again, felt uncomfortable.

The circle reconvened and Brook talked in some depth about the day's principal activity – a shamanic journey of soul retrieval.[11] However, before the journey could begin, Brook reported that it was necessary to ascertain what it was exactly that we were going to search for on the journey. To find this out, a visualization process was enacted whereby we were asked to look into our bodies to identify a place which felt empty. It was this empty space which would later form the focus of the journey of retrieval, the objective of which was to find what was needed to fill the space. Filling the empty space, it was said, acted as a form of healing in that we could become more complete and, therefore, stronger, more balanced, and power-full beings.

After this first visualization process had ended, the usual few minutes were set aside in order to illustrate where the empty space in our bodies might be. These drawings were then discussed in the circle. In my process I had visualized not one but two empty spaces in my body – a large one in my abdomen and a small one in my forehead, which I drew. Visualization of more than one space, as it turned out, was not unusual. Additionally, I had written down some of the thoughts which occurred during the process and which, in some way, described the feelings which related to the empty spaces I had experienced. These thoughts also closely characterized what I felt I wanted to achieve from my shamanic journey, ideas which (as I came to realize) linked in with what I had been learning about myself over the previous three days. The thoughts included:

- take back my power lost in childhood
- fill in the emptiness or void inside me
- take that power
- put it back in myself
- find my intuition
- know who I am.

11   For further information on shamanic journeying and soul retrieval see Michael Harner, 1990, Chapter Five.

The first four thoughts I saw as being more to do with healing, but the last two related to my spirituality. I had been thinking prior to the workshop that learning more about how to free intuitive thoughts from overpowering rational ones – and how to accept them – would be a big step forward. And I had been working with a number of spiritual teachings which all pointed to the phrase 'Who am I?'.

Following a break for lunch a final discussion was held before the group began the shamanic journey. This discussion centred on the method of the journey. Brook described how his drumming at a particular beat-rate would be used to call our power animals and carry us through our journey. We would need to await the arrival of our power animals and to follow their lead. The process commenced with Brook carrying out a cleansing ceremony. Brook, himself, was wearing North American Indian sacred vestments. Again, sage leaves were ritually burnt and each participant was cleansed by the smoke which was wafted around them by using the eagle's wing. Throughout this part of the activity Brook was chanting and appeared to be offering prayers to the group's guiding spirits. Brook had earlier described his views about the importance of ritual in life. It was his belief that the same ritual needs to be repeated frequently and, in this way, he believed the practice of shamanic rituals could be compared with other meditational practices such as prayer and t'ai chi.

When the cleansing was complete, we were asked to find a comfortable place (lying down) for the journey. To start the journey we were told to keep aware of the purpose of the activity – to find what we would intuitively know to use to fill our empty spaces. We were led into the process in the usual way. Once in trance – and this was the first and only process where I felt I reached a deep meditative trance state – we were asked to place ourselves in a favourite or meaningful place to await the arrival of our power animals. My first thought was of a beautiful and much-visited broad riverless valley near where I lived in Lancashire. I was building a picture of this when, for an unknown reason, I suddenly switched my vision to the top of a low cliff at Rhossili Bay at the tip of the Gower Peninsular in South Wales – a place which I had visited often in the past and had been planning to revisit. The monotonous, vibrant drumming effected the calling of the power animals.

I was standing on the low cliff top about fifty feet above the sea. The wind was blowing warm and hard, making the long grass wave and my hair sweep back off my forehead. I was waiting. I did not know what to expect. I had forgotten the previous episode with an owl, and occasionally I looked around the cliff top half expecting a snake or tiger or the like to join me on the cliff. Then an eagle swooped down from the sky, and immediately I knew I had to climb on its back. Sizes and proportions were not a problem – I sat astride the eagle's neck (in approximately the same scale as if I was riding an elephant). We flew up into the sky. High up. And then out of the sky over a land or place made of huge blue crystals. Flying and flying. Then into blackness, like deep, starless space, or a tunnel. All of a sudden the face of my ex-wife appeared and we flew like a speck through her forehead, then in the same way through my paternal grandmother's forehead, my mother's, and through the forehead of a great aunt who had died thirty years before. We flew on. We came upon a bluish castle-like structure which was a cavernous labyrinth of different spaces. Flying through. Finally, we arrived at a fossilized forest comprised of towering green stone trees. On one of these trees was the eagle's nest, and this was where we landed. In the nest there were many large eggs. I dismounted. I looked at the eagle for guidance. Could I have some of the eggs? I did not know what to do. I felt my abdomen swelling. I felt I wanted to put an egg (or eggs) into my abdomen and my forehead – exactly the spaces I had identified earlier. It seemed this was the right thing to do, what I had come for. But I felt stuck. I did not know how. As I lay on the floor, I lifted my shirt and arched my back so that my abdomen was raised into the air. Then the eagle (now about six feet tall) landed on my abdomen and laid several eggs into me. I felt them fill my abdomen and I needed to push them around inside me to get them in the right place until the space felt tight and full. Then the eagle (now about eighteen inches tall) landed on my forehead and filled that space with eggs. I asked what the eggs were to hatch as. Telepathically, I was told that the eggs were my seeds that were to act like a new beginning and that I was to know they were there and nurture them. I came back to Rhossili, to the wind and the sea. I said 'thank you' to the eagle, who disappeared. A change in the drumming signified the end of the process. The drumming ceased. All was quiet. Brook's voice brought me back from the cliff top into the workshop room.

I returned to normal consciousness slowly. My abdomen ached, my shirt was drawn up over my chest. We were asked to draw or otherwise illustrate what had taken place on our journeys. I could not draw what I had experienced but wrote down what had happened. When the circle reconvened I read out the account of my journey. At that time I found that it was impossible to discuss or analyse what had happened as I felt too exhilarated by the events; but in the following days and weeks I came to understand more about the meanings of some of what had happened. I had, indeed, filled the empty spaces in my 'body' and felt more complete and stronger. I understood the metaphor of the eggs as seeds to represent a vibration and energy which was sacred (in that it was given to me and is precious and fragile – in fact, all that I have) and that I have the seeds (the germs of potential) which, if I nurture them, will grow into what I want them to be. This, I felt, is now all within my power. I understood the image of the eagle to symbolize my connection to the source of all that is.

After a two-hour break for supper (when I rested but did not eat), William introduced the group to spiritual healing. In his opening discussion, William again described his view that each of us had the guiding help of spirit beings throughout our lives. In fact, he told us of his experiences in channelling two particular spirit beings – Sojah and Dagmar. What was most interesting to me was the notion that almost any person can be a healer. This was because we were told that the individual acts only as a channel (or conduit) of healing 'energies' which are given freely by the spirit world when requested. William described the most normal actions a healer uses, that of following the position of the seven principal chakras.[12] William suggested that healing could also be applied to specific areas or, in fact, be spread all over the body. The method we were to use was simply to lay our open

12 The term 'chakra' is the Sanskrit word for wheel and these points are 'said to be shaped like multicolored lotus petals or spoked wheels that whirl at various speeds as they process energy. Chakras are described in Hindu and Buddhist yogic literature' (Rosemary Ellen Guiley, 1991: 86f; see also Richard Gerber, 1988, and Shirley MacLaine, 1991).

hands either on the subject's body or at a distance – perhaps two or three inches away or further – wherever and for however long it felt right so to do. At some points, William reported, heat might be felt by one or both parties.

Following a short meditation, the group split into pairs so that one person would enact healing on the other, and then the roles would be reversed. The lights in the room were dimmed and soft music was played. Each healing session lasted for approximately three-quarters of an hour. My partner in this activity was William and, after the session healing me, he reported that he had felt most heat at my heart chakra. In my session of being the healer, I found it remarkable that having travelled all over William's body with my hands at a close distance, I had felt a distinct heat emanating between my hand and his body both at the heart and solar plexus chakras – and nowhere else. William later explained that healing did not necessarily affect the human physical plane but, more likely, the etheric plane.[13]

By the end of the day's proceedings (at around 10pm) I felt the need of physically earthing myself – in this instance, spending a little time out in the countryside. After the healing session finished I drove out of the city into nearby moorland and sat in silence on a farm gate under a bright moonlit sky and scudding clouds, listening to the sound of owls hooting, and sheep gnawing at the grass.

Day Five

Today we want to bring together the experiences of the previous four days. We consider our next steps and engage in an extended Medicine Wheel Blessing Ceremony. We share what we have gained together, giving thanks and then we release the circle.

---

13 The etheric plane is said to be one of the constituent parts of the aura which surrounds all life forms and which contains a number of different planes. For a full description, see Rosemary Ellen Guiley, 1991: 40ff.

The fifth cardinal point on the medicine wheel is the Centre: symbolized by the vowel sound U and the notion of carrying. The Centre is an empty place – part of all existence which is full of nothing. The Centre bonds all four directions and is the position of highest awareness.

For the final time the circle came together in group prayer, holding hands in a chain of unity. The candle was lit.

We started the day with a period of paired gentle touching and massage. This was carried out fully clothed and in silence with one person sitting on a chair being touched by the other, and then reversing roles. This exercise became a very moving expression of giving and receiving love, a compassionate sharing of each other's suffering, of humility, of building our trust in each other, and of deepening bonds which had developed over the previous four days. The experience of giving the massage and of touching evoked feelings in me of the flow of positive emotions to the partner, of trust and respect; and the experience of receiving was immensely pleasurable – full of wonderful, warm sensations. The exchange was emotionally intimate and completely silent.

The group reconvened in the circle and commenced the first of two periods of talking in the day. Each person, when they wished to talk, picked up the 'talking' bear from the centre. In many instances, ideas and problems were spoken of and developed. Some people found it extremely difficult to talk, and there were many anguished and tearful periods. By this stage in the life of the group the bond which had developed between all of the participants was at it strongest – so much so that I felt I could almost 'see' the compassion for each other that everyone was experiencing and sending out across the Circle. This period of talking continued after a break for lunch.

The final trance meditation process was then held. In this period, we were requested to direct our focus onto our futures and our potentials. William led us through the now familiar steps and left us in the trance-like state to develop our visual images. When the process was ended we illustrated what we had experienced in drawing and then came together in pairs to discuss what had occurred. In my process, which was not in trance, I had visualized a vista of never-ending rolling hills across which my road (my path in life) traversed – up hills and down hills. The road I had subsequently illustrated was comprised of three words which were repeated over and over again – TRUTH, BALANCE, NATURALNESS. In the explanation of the drawing to my partner I suggested that the notion of truth entailed keeping intuitively true to myself and others; that the notion of balance entailed living in harmony with all and everything, in equanimity; and that the notion of naturalness described the way the road flowed most true. I saw this to mean that untruth, imbalance, and unnaturalness were all negative influences which I needed to recognize and avoid. When asked by my partner what was the largest cause of negative influences I replied that it was my ego or, rather, ego-driven directions. While I realized that there was nothing new in these thoughts, I found the thought of them at this particular moment in time to be both poignant and relevant.

The group came back together in the circle to enact a rite of passage based on the idea of taking the first step into the future which we had experienced in the final visualization process. An imaginary gate was positioned at one point of the circle, at which William stood. Each person in turn stood before the gate and described to the group what had occurred to them in their process with regard to what the future might hold. At my turn, I described the essence of how I had seen the road ahead. William asked how I felt about it and I replied that I was excited and ready to get going. I was then asked to take a ritual first step through the gate of my future which I did with enthusiasm and which was witnessed by the group members. Not all participants showed as much enthusiasm; in fact, several were hesitant, and one participant had great difficulty stepping through the gate into their future. However, eventually each member of the group passed on through the gate – albeit, in some instances, after renegotiating the terms of their passage.

The final event of The Healing Circle was the Medicine Wheel Blessing Ceremony. For this, Brook built a more formal medicine wheel which comprised of four gates at East, South, West, and North. Four spaces were created between each gate. At the Centre was the sacred space. Brook now wore a Pueblo Indian headband and necklace together with moccasins on his feet. When the wheel was completed we were asked to sit at the point around the outside perimeter of the

257

wheel to which we were drawn or which we felt was particularly appropriate for whatever reason. One swift look at the wheel drew me instinctively to a point just west of the South Gate where I went and sat down, waiting for everyone to do the same.

Brook consecrated the wheel and cleansed each participant with smoke from smouldering sage leaves which had, for this ceremony, been mixed with juniper. During the cleansing, Brook was chanting under his breath. The first part of the ceremony entailed 'reading' the position of each group member sitting around the wheel. Where we had sat had a symbolic meaning which Brook proceeded to determine. Brook identified the position I had sat at on the wheel to mean that I would 'become a teacher but not yet'.

The main activity of the blessing ceremony was a dance. This dance was carried out individually to the beat of the drum. Each person was to leave their position on the perimeter of the wheel and walk or dance clockwise around to the East Gate. Entry to the gate was made by turning full circle while walking forward through the gate. Visiting each gate in turn from the inside of the circle, the dance involved turning through 360 degrees with one hand held up with its palm facing the sky and the other hand held down with its palm facing the earth. Facing outwards, both hands were raised to the sky, and then the participant bowed down so that both hands pointed to the ground. At this point, all group members would sing the vowel sound appropriate to the gate at which the dancer was standing. This was continued for each of the five gates. At the final gate, the sacred space, each dancer additionally knelt to place their hands over the flame of the candle and then metaphorically cleansed the top of their head and their heart with the fire. The end of each participant's dance was an exit from the medicine wheel via the East Gate, touching the shaman's drum. Once that person had returned to their place the next person repeated the process, and so on until everyone had passed through. The effect of the dance – shuffling to the beat of the incessant drum and the rituals which were enacted – I found surprisingly uplifting and symbolically meaningful. The dance became a process of thanking the spirit beings for watching over us for the five workshop days and of releasing them from their responsibilities.

The final event of the workshop was a talking session. Here, the 'talking' bear was passed in turn to each person in order that they might say what they wished about how they felt. Each person expressed warmth and good wishes. There was much laughter. Finally, the group stood in a tight circle around the sacred space with arms around each others shoulders to sing a song:

I am a circle
I am healing you.
You are a circle
You are healing me.
Unite us
Be one,
Unite us
Be as one.

Then we all blew to extinguish the candle and the Circle was released.

PART THREE

CRITICAL RESPONSE

Introduction

Souls of a day, a new generation of men shall here begin the cycle of its mortal existence. Your destiny shall not be allotted to you: you can choose it freely for yourselves. Let him who draws the first lot be the first to choose his next life which shall be his irrevocably. But virtue owns no master: as a man honours or slights her, so he shall have more of her or less. The responsibility lies with the chooser: Heaven is blameless [...] it was a truly amazing sight to watch how each soul selected his life – a sight at once sad, and ludicrous, and strange, for the choice was largely governed by the habits of their previous life.

Plato[1]

The advent of new or renewed cultural, social, and spiritual ideas and activities which has been shown to be incorporated in the contemporary New Age have attracted critical attention from a number of quarters; yet, in total, this attention has not been particularly great. Criticism of the New Age has been primarily from Christian writers, although more objective critical analysis is starting to emerge from other sources, as we shall see. One of the main reasons for this lack of analysis is because of Western society's general acceptance of many of the attributes and benefits which are inherent in New Age ideas and activities. Some of these have been explored in earlier chapters – for example, adoption of complementary and alternative therapeutic practices, methods of increasing a person's potentiality through humanistic and transpersonal psychotechnologies, ecological philosophies, and aspects of counter-cultural social values. Of course, there was a great deal of critical activity during and immediately after the counter-culture – what might be called the 'shock of the new' – although this abated as many of the new ideas started to be taken up into the mainstream. The extent of this absorption has been quantified to some de-

---

1   Plato, 1980: 210.

gree.[2] This is not to say that all New Age ideas and activities have been accepted, nor is it to say that criticisms of certain aspects have been – and still are – valid.

The final part to this examination of the New Age is divided into three chapters. The first deals specifically with the Christian response, while the second assesses a number of separate (though related) areas of its ideas and activities which have attracted specific critical attention. The final chapter summarizes what has been discovered about the New Age and then engages with the principal consistencies and inconsistencies which have been found to exist between commentaries and as revealed by participants. A brief summary view is then given of what the New Age, at its centre, can be seen to represent.

2   See Daniel Yankelovich, 1981.

10. The Christian Response

every individual soul is a centre of consciousness which is open to every other and to the universal consciousness itself. In its final fulfilment it participates in the consciousness of the supreme being and reflects the other centres of consciousness in itself, but it does not cease to be a unique centre of consciousness.

Bede Griffiths[1]

There is a wide range of styles that different Christian groups adopt in their approaches to the New Age although, as a whole, significant similarities exist in the principal issues involved in their response. With regard to styles, these primarily reflect the degrees of either the conservatism or liberalism of particular groups. Overall, the conservative Christian sectors are more strident in their criticism, whereas the liberal sectors are more charitable; however, few fully endorse what the New Age has to offer. As is to be expected, Christian criticism is primarily directed at the spiritual concerns of the New Age and less at its healing or other practices.

To survey the overall Christian response three approaches are used. Firstly, a review of the range of responses is analysed and, secondly, basic New Age ideas are assessed with regards to criticisms by Christian groups. Finally, notable exceptions to the majority Christian response exist and these are reviewed.

1   Bede Griffiths, 1982: 98.

The range of Christian response to the New Age

By studying the approaches that different, primarily Protestant, Christian groups have taken in their engagement with the New Age, there appears to be a wide spectrum of views. Almost without exception, and not surprisingly, the vast majority of groups are, in the end, critical of these ideas and activities, although it is in the range of criticism which makes up the spectrum that there occurs much variation. This variation can be described as being, on the one hand, an outright and often vitriolic condemnation of the majority of New Age ideas and activities (described as the 'antichrist approach'[2]) to, on the other hand, a much more mild – even accommodating – positions: these two extremes are respectively exemplified in the writings of Constance Cumbey and Michael Perry. This broad range will now be reviewed in more detail.

The Christian response to the New Age did not start in earnest until the early 1980s. This was when Christian groups – especially those with a fundamentalist or conservative focus – started to perceive the New Age as posing a threat to Christian society. However, according to literature research,[3] the first evangelical response to the New Age in monograph form was written by Gary North and published in 1976, although it was not until 1983 that Constance Cumbey and Dave Hunt woke 'the Evangelical subculture from its dogmatic slumber to the existence of the New Age movement'.[4] Both of these authors made apocalyptic claims against the New Age, Cumbey's being the more vitriolic.

Constance Cumbey,[5] an American lawyer, opened her fundamentalist attack with the following statement: 'It is the contention of this writer that for the first time in history there is a viable movement – the New Age Movement – that truly meets all the scriptural requirements for the antichrist and the political movement that will bring him on the

---

2   Martin Palmer, 1993: 90.
3   Carried out by Irving Hexham, 1992: 154.
4   Ibid.
5   Constance Cumbey, 1983.

world scene.'[6] Participants in the New Age, according to Cumbey, are mainly comprised of 'the lonely, the confused and bewildered, the young and naïve'[7] who, in her view, do not realize that its teachings are 'deeply anti-Semitic',[8] and promote genocide.[9] Cumbey suggests that participants are generally unaware that they have been 'manipulated by extremely sophisticated forms of mind control'.[10]

Cumbey and Hunt are not alone in attacking the New Age in this way. For example, ex-US presidential candidate and TV evangelist Pat Robertson, speaking at the 1990 annual convention of religious broadcasters,

> lowered his voice to a throaty whisper as he looked into the future and issued a dark prophecy: 'There is something coming from the East,' he warned. 'It's a modified version of Hinduism. It's called the New Age. It's sweeping into American businesses, the classrooms of America, infiltrating into Europe. It's even in the Soviet Union.' He went on to denounce it as 'blatant demonism', and called for a Christian crusade against it.[11]

Another American fundamentalist Christian reports that 'New Age methods are not only attracting the unchurched but are treacherously finding their way into the Christian community';[12] and that 'The serpent as described in Genesis chapter 3 [...] clearly applied to Eve many of the methods which are used in today's pseudopsychological cults, self-help therapies, and other New Age programs.'[13] This critic also cites Constance Cumbey and Dave Hunt with regard to the parallels both these authors drew between the New Age and Nazi philosophy.[14]

Yet Cumbey's main concerns are those which are also the concerns of the majority of all Christian groups. Principally, these include

6   Op. cit.: frontpiece.
7   Op. cit.: 186.
8   Op. cit.: 188.
9   Op. cit.: 190.
10   Op. cit.: 189.
11   John Drane, 1991: 207.
12   Caryl Matrisciana, 1985: 21.
13   Op. cit.: 22.
14   Op. cit.: 216.

firstly what they consider to be the monistic nature of the New Age, on which point Cumbey argues that 'stating that man himself could be as God was also one of the original lies of the Eden serpent';[15] secondly, the New Age notion of the existence of an inner or Higher Self, against which Cumbey suggests that the 'inward journey is usually achieved through a variety of psychotechnologies virtually guaranteed to induce demonic control';[16] and, thirdly, the notion that all religions are essentially very similar, about which Cumbey reports that 'nearly all non-Judeo/Christian religions are extremely similar because, as the Bible indicates, they are from *one* source, the "god of this world" – Satan himself.'[17]

While Cumbey's writings have been criticized by one commentator for their lack of academic credibility[18] – and by another who suggests that her 'thesis is riddled with mis-handled facts and logical fallacies'[19] – evangelical critics of the New Age are generally supportive of her basic concerns. In fact, the overriding value of Cumbey's work as been praised by the same commentator, who suggests that she

> has made several valuable contributions to the Christian church [...] By her own report, many New Agers have become Christians through her efforts. Certainly, she has alerted many Christians to the subtle dangers of programs like the Forum, Silva Mind Control, *A Course in Miracles*, and so forth [...] Her warnings against such men as Matthew Fox, Rodney Romney, Thomas Merton, and Robert Schuller have no doubt saved many believers from deception.[20]

However, Douglas Groothuis has been acknowledged as providing the 'first really serious, semischolarly Evangelical critique of the New Age movement'.[21] The approach Groothuis takes is to confront New Age ideas with biblical evidence as to their 'counterfeit' value. Groothuis reviews nine prominent New Age ideas – including monism, pantheism, transformation (which he describes as a counterfeit

15   Constance Cumbey, 1983: 170.
16   Op. cit.: 173.
17   Op. cit.: 189.
18   Irving Hexham, 1992: 154.
19   Eliot Miller, 1990: 197.
20   Op. cit.: 206.
21   Irving Hexham, loc. cit.

form of conversion), and ideas aimed at building human potential –
and demonstrates why he believes they are all false. Overall,
Groothuis suggests that 'Rather than being a mere fad, the New Age
movement is a substantial cultural trend that is not destined quickly to
blow away in the wind. It offers Christians a deep challenge to un-
mask and lovingly confront a very potent spiritual counterfeit.'[22] Here,
Groothuis's message is caged in more conciliatory terms although it
nonetheless includes all the arguments laid against the New Age by its
more vociferous fundamentalist opponents.[23]

There are many examples of evangelical organizations and publications which argue against the New Age. A representative example
can be seen in the Worldwide Church of God's magazine, *The Plain
Truth*,[24] which published an issue attacking the New Age entitled:
'The New Age: Subtle Seduction'.[25] Elsewhere, particular ideas or
teachers have been singled out for critical attack, and James Sire's
pamphlet on Shirley MacLaine is a typical example. Sire describes
MacLaine as a 'pop guru'[26] and, following the pattern of other conservative Christian authors in his dissection of the New Age, believes
that 'MacLaine's own experiences are hers alone. The possibility of
self-deception, let alone demonic deception [...] is clearly present
[Her] experiences might well be pure fantasy.'[27] Sire accuses
MacLaine of 'frequent distortion or misunderstanding of religious
texts'[28] which may well be the case, although this distortion is precisely the fault that has been found to exist in the majority of Christian
literature which attacks the New Age.[29]

---

22 Douglas Groothuis, 1988: 32.
23 Georg Feuerstein argues the opposite, that 'from the vantage point of authentic
    spirituality, conventional religion is counterfeit spirituality' (1992: 190). Au-
    thentic spirituality, according to Feuerstein, is only found in esoteric and not
    exoteric religion.
24 The publishers estimate that 2.5 million copies are published monthly in a total
    of seven languages.
25 Vol. 58, No. 8 (September 1993).
26 James Sire, 1988: 8.
27 Op. cit.: 20f.
28 Op. cit.: 22.
29 Irvin Hexham, 1992: 158.

It is not just Protestant churches which fundamentally oppose the New Age. The Vatican, for example, views the advent of the New Age as a 'resurgence of an ancient heresy in modern guise. The ancient heresy is gnosticism, and its modern guise is that constellation of practices and teachings commonly referred to as "New Age".'[30] His Holiness Pope John Paul II also warns that

> We cannot delude ourselves that this [New Age] will lead towards a renewal of religion. It is only a new way of practising gnosticism – that attitude of the spirit that, in the name of a profound knowledge of God, results in distorting His Word and replacing it with purely human words. Gnosticism ... [is in] conflict with all that is essentially Christian.[31]

And according to another Catholic critic, Cardinal Joseph Ratzinger, the New Age represents a 'pernicious syncretism'.[32]

Adding to this Catholic response, an academic commentator gives the view that the New Age appears to have become a contemporary repository of long suppressed, discredited, and discarded Christian sects. He suggests that

> We see today the New Age as a partial reconstitution from the flotsam of rejected Christian and quasi-Christian ideas of a competing theological position. In many respects, the condemned heresies of Arianism, Monophysitism, Monarchianism and Sabellianism as well as the various forms of Gnosticism (the Valentinians, the Basilidean sect, the Ophites) and also the Marcionites, the antinomian practices and the wisdom literature of the Jewish and Christian pseudepigrapha are resurfacing yet again within the variations and permutations embraced beneath the New Age umbrella.[33]

In support of this view, findings shown from my survey demonstrate a strong conviction among many participants that the New Age in part represents a re-assessment of what is collectively known as ancient wisdom teachings. In fact, some participants listed the influ-

---

30   *Inside the Vatican*, November 1994.
31   Pope John Paul II, 1994: 90.
32   Cited in Isotta Poggi, 1992: 285.
33   Michael York, 1994: 17.

ence of various sects which originate in the theistic traditions including, for example, the Essenes.

Turning to the opposite side of the spectrum, liberal critical approaches to the New Age appear to be more accommodating in their stance although, in the end, even liberal Christianity cannot fully endorse all the core New Age ideas. An American liberal approach is illustrated in Ted Peters, an American who is described as having a Lutheran background and whose critical analysis is based on 'the world [seen] through the eyes of the Californian romance with the New Age'.[34] Peters reports that he is sympathetic to what he sees as the wholesome values incorporated in many New Age teachings although, overall, he is critical of the basic ideas. The principal reason that Peters gives is that he finds, in the same way as the Catholic's, that 'the new age has inadvertently fallen into a gnostic form of spiritual quest.'[35] Peters's conclusion incorporates four 'theses':

> First, modest dabbling in new age spirituality is probably harmless; it may even be helpful [...] Second, the new age vision is a noble and edifying one [...] Third, pastors, theologians, and church leaders should take the new age movement seriously [...] Fourth, the gnostic monism at the heart of new age teaching is dangerous because it leads to naiveté and to a denial of God's grace.[36]

What Peters sees of value in the New Age is where it 'speaks a religious language in areas of life and learning from which religion was once banished',[37] and where it is characterized by 'peace, harmony, and fulfilment'.[38] However, according to Peters, the New Age ultimately poses a threat to the Church because he sees that large numbers of people are involved and that core theological issues are being threatened.

Peters's arguments have attracted criticism not for his theological position (the critic in question is also a liberal Christian) but for his method of attack. Peters, he suggests,

34 Martin Palmer, 1993: 87.
35 Ted Peters, 1991: ix.
36 Op. cit.: 194ff.
37 Op. cit.: 194.
38 Op. cit.: 195.

relies on buzzwords like *monism, pantheism, reincarnation,* and *eschatology* which he does not define and which mean one thing in his theological universe and several others among various representatives of New Age thinking. This semantic carelessness can easily degenerate into a kind of sophisticated name-calling [...] Also, Peters misses the point of a great deal of New Age teaching about Jesus. Jesus is more than a teacher or mystic. He is the cosmic Christ, the transformer and revivifier, and the true Self of each finite person. Peters may not like these teachings either, but he owes it to his readers to get the distinctions right.[39]

Nevertheless, this critic also finds that 'Peters is correct in declaring [the] New Age naive and unrealistic.'[40]

Even a decade or more later than Cumbey, Groothuis, and Peters, and even though a considerably more accepting attitude is generally seen to be taken of New Age ideas and activities as a whole,[41] the American evangelical Christian response appears not to have changed. This is illustrated in John Newport's 600+-page comparison of the New Age with biblical teachings. Newport, an evangelist and academic, writes another Christian antagonistic apologetic designed, as he states, as 'a basis of study for churches, colleges, seminaries, and lay people'[42] particularly, it seems, for those 'unfortunate' Christians who are caught up in the New Age without realizing it.[43]

Although using more subtle language than Cumbey, Newport follows directly in her footsteps by seeing the New Age as satanic. His sixty-page penultimate chapter 'Modern Satanism and Black Magic'[44] incorporates barely a mention of the New Age; nor does it cite any New Age writers or commentators to any meaningful degree. Instead, Newport works his way through the history of Satanism, Aleister

---

39   Lowell Streiker, 1991: 29.
40   Op. cit.: 30.
41   For example, reports of US First Lady Hillary Clinton's consultations in 1996 with the paranormal through 'sacred psychologist' Jean Houston met with fairly mild reactions by the press and American society, according to Wade Clark Roof (1999: 288f).
42   John Newport, 1998: xv.
43   Ibid.
44   White magic Newport deals with in a separate chapter (Chapter Six), together with Neopaganism and the Goddess movement.

Crowley, Charles Manson, Hitler, and various other 'miscreants'. It can safely be anticipated that those involved in New Age ideas and activities would be incensed to see that a comprehensive study of the New Age incorporates such clearly non-New Age material. They would also argue that this type of approach to alternative, non-Christian, forms of spirituality betokens a negative and combative stance which, as we have seen, is opposite to that which the New Age takes. In fact, the reverse seems to be true: the New Age welcomes dialogue with all religions and celebrates what has been called 'unity in diversity' – a harmonious acceptance that different people are free to build their own spiritual pathways in whatever direction.

Much of Newport's (and fundamentalist Christians' as a whole) opposition to the New Age centres on – or as Newport puts it, radically opposes[45] – ideas about God. The primary trait of the New Age, he states, is its denial of God as creator and healer. With regard to health, Newport continues:

> In the New Age worldview, God is not necessarily a person, and God is not separate from humanity and the universe. The authority shift – from without to within – is related to New Age 'selfism'. Healing comes from within, from one's own body – as spiritual energy [...] In other words, the religious point of view embodied in the New Age health movement is an integral part of the occult/mystical worldview that is making its way into every aspect of our cultural consciousness. It is not a fad. It will not go away. And it is fundamentally hostile to biblical Christianity.[46]

Through Newport's long arguments on the many topics he raises, it can be seen that, at least for evangelical Christianity, the meeting points between it and the New Age are still far apart. Newport sees Christianity as a 'dynamic and superior alternative to the New Age'[47] which 'cannot embrace' it.[48] However, he urges Christians to seek out those who have turned to the New Age in order to demonstrate to them that their religious needs 'can be satisfied only by biblical reli-

---

45   Op. cit.: 324.
46   Op. cit.: 324f.
47   Op. cit.: 607.
48   Ibid.

gion'.[49] The subtitle of Newport's book – *Conflict and Dialogue* – therefore seems partly inappropriate: conflict, certainly; but dialogue, perhaps not.

Much the same arguments as those of the American evangelist tradition have been put by two British liberal responses to the New Age. John Drane, for example, a Religious Studies lecturer and evangelical preacher, additionally sees that the Christian Church can learn from New Age ways of overcoming three hundred years of rationalist reductionism by becoming much more experiential. Drane gives the example of the thriving non-Western Christian ministries and suggests that by adopting some of their methods of worship the Church may be able help those involved in the New Age to rediscover Christianity.

Michael Perry's approach to the New Age is much more liberal – but no less purposeful – than that of Constance Cumbey, in that he states the aim of his writing is to bring participants of the New Age 'to a knowledge of Jesus, the Christ whose service is perfect freedom'[50] – which he describes as a 'more excellent way'.[51] Perry, a Canon in the Church of England and, like Drane, an academic, ends his study not with a criticism but with a description of how he sees a reformed Christian Church acting as a replacement for the spiritual ideas of the New Age – and 'of every religious quest'.[52] It can be noted that, throughout his study, Perry takes every opportunity to use negative language in describing the New Age, albeit in a more subtle way than many of the Christian fundamentalists. For example, in describing the complexity of its ideas and activities, Perry believes the New Age is 'ill-organized',[53] 'a kind of DIY religion',[54] and 'an uncoordinated medley'.[55] He also compares transformation to drug addiction[56] – there are many other such examples.

49   Ibid.
50   Michael Perry, 1992: 7.
51   Ibid.
52   Op. cit.: 160.
53   Op. cit.: 19.
54   Op. cit.: 22.
55   Op. cit.: 29.
56   Op. cit.: 145.

Turning to the subject of religious experience, a marked difference of views can be noted among the various Christian groups. Those groups which incorporate a greater degree of experiential forms of worship appear to give a blanket denial that there is anything of value to be gained from contact with the New Age. On the other hand, those groups which incorporate less experiential worship in their religious practices intimate that there is at least some benefit to be gained by engagement with its ideas. Michael Perry, for example, believes that 'The most serious accusation [by those involved in the New Age] – and there is some truth in it – is that the Church is embarrassed by religious experience. It has domesticated the holy, and only made it acceptable if it is expressed in certain stylized ways.'[57] M. Scott Peck, a psychiatrist, Christian, and author widely read in the New Age, also believes that 'The sin of Christianity has not been the sin of doctrine. It has been the sin of practice – a failure to integrate its behavior with its theology.'[58] Moreover, Ted Peters suggests that the Church needs to recognize that a 'spiritual thirst'[59] exists and is, to some extent, being satisfied by New Age spiritual practice. Peters argues that to quench this thirst

> may mean dipping into the reservoir of the Christian tradition and retrieving spiritual practices that have been set aside, practices such as meditation and contemplation. It may mean encouraging people to pray for an outpouring of the Holy Spirit so that they can experience the power of transformation toward a God-given wholeness.[60]

In some respects, concerns which the New Age has raised among the more liberal Christian critics – for example, Michael Perry – are seen as being 'legitimate'[61] and able to be incorporated into Christian doctrine. Among these Perry lists concern for the environment, equality for all human beings, countering 'barren and loveless material-

---

57   Op. cit.: 154.
58   M. Scott Peck, 1993: 200.
59   Ted Peters, 1991: 196.
60   Ibid.
61   Michael Perry, 1992: 153.

ism',[62] and some aspects of questioning authority. M. Scott Peck, while arguing on the one hand that the New Age has created 'a considerable amount of [...] spiritual confusion'[63] sees, on the other hand, that its virtues are 'absolutely enormous'.[64] The New Age, according to Peck, is a movement in the direction of 'integration and integrity'[65] which he sees as particularly realized in holistic medicine, ecology, aspects of global activities, and greater cooperation among people. Ted Peters, too, supports much of what Perry and Peck suggest, and adds 'It seems to me that Christian faith and the striving for integrative wholeness are natural complements of each other, and that the new age has much to teach us in this regard.'[66] John Drane goes further by suggesting that in some respects 'many New Agers are a lot closer to God's Kingdom than some of their Christian critics'.[67]

These views, of course, are not intended to demonstrate that any of the above mentioned authors fully supports the New Age – far from it. What this review of the Christian response to the New Age illustrates is that, on the whole, the Church appears to consider that New Age spirituality represents a competitive threat. What is more, the Church – whether in the form of conservative or liberal groups, in

62   Ibid.
63   M. Scott Peck, 1993: 198.
64   Op. cit.: 216.
65   Ibid.
66   Ted Peters, 1991: 92.
67   John Drane, 1991: 215; see also Colin Slee, 1999. Slee, provost at Southwark Cathedral in London, who, in his discussion of new religious movements as a whole which he sees to include the New Age, identifies several 'threats' these movements pose to mainstream religions, not just to Christianity. Firstly, a threat posed by the implied criticism that traditional religions do not teach the truth – or teach it inadequately – about God; secondly, the threat to membership numbers; and thirdly, the bringing of all religion into disrepute, thus damaging its cultural standing (op. cit.: 169). However, Slee outlines four ways in which he has found that the mainstream Christian Churches have failed people who have moved to or joined new religious movements. These he describes as their failure to provide teachings which equip people to question newer doctrines, the insufficient spread of information about Christian practice, possible lack of sufficient demands on church members, and of their inability to provide clarity for those who seek a clear, direct and uncomplicated solution to their enquiries or problems (op. cit.: 171ff).

America, Britain, or elsewhere – albeit in a variety of ways, believes that there are significant faults inherent in New Age spirituality.

The Christian view of basic New Age ideas

As has been shown, there is a range of Christian approaches to the New Age between conservative and liberal critics, although there appears to be an underlying agreement on their major points of argument. In fact, John Drane summarizes what he sees as being fundamentally wrong with the New Age in a list with which he believes the majority of Christians would agree:

> It is wrong when it affirms that we are all God, or all equal with God [...] It is wrong when it suggests that 'going within' will solve all our problems [...] It is wrong when it refuses to recognize the reality of undeserved suffering and the presence of evil in our world. And it is wrong when it denies that there can ever be absolute values and beliefs, emphasizing instead what seems 'right for you'.[68]

These four points – which show considerable similarities with another Christian academic's view of the four ways that New Spirituality differs from the Christian tradition[69] – involve interrelated issues which are now discussed in more detail.

Drane's first point relates to the basic New Age idea that all life is interconnected energy and that there is no separation between God[70] and the Higher Self – which, accordingly, enables an individual to have a direct experience of God. The Christian Church fiercely contests this view because, as Ted Peters argues, the New Age

---

68 John Drane, 1991: 215.
69 Linda Woodhead, 1993: 173.
70 The concept of God in the New Age is different from the traditional Christian view and has been discussed in Chapter 5 above.

fails to accept the plain fact: although we humans were created for union with God and with one another, we are estranged from God and neighbour because of sin. It rejects the message of the gospel, that God is the one who takes action to overcome this estrangement by granting us forgiveness of sin and the gift of eternal life.[71]

Michael Perry gives a similar argument,[72] as does Douglas Groothuis who cites the biblical view that God brought about 'a wondrous diversity of created things [which are] not reducible to a mystical oneness'.[73] In this respect, Groothuis believes that the 'New Age takes the truth that we are all made in God's image and warps it to mean we are all gods'.[74] Moreover, Groothuis draws a distinction between what Christians conceive of as unity and New Age interconnectedness in that 'Jesus taught the unity of his followers as the body of Christ (Jn 17), as did Paul (1 Cor 12:12–31), and yet this unity is not the undifferentiated oneness taught by the New Age.'[75]

Exploring the argument further, another scholar suggests that 'revelling in how godlike we are, even affirming that in principle we are God, looks past pervasive sin and evil in ways that make the New Age appear shallow indeed.'[76] Sin and salvation lie at the heart of Christianity, according to this critic, and the fact that neither of these concepts exist in this manner in the New Age is the one issue which he argues 'most deeply troubles church people'.[77]

With regards to the interconnected nature of God, another view from academe suggests that a parallel can be drawn between the New Age concept of Universal Energy and the Pentecostal/charismatic view of the Holy Spirit – the latter is described as 'the divine force moving behind the miraculous events of healing, prophecy, glossalalia, and exorcism'.[78] In many ways, it can be argued that the character-

---

71   John Drane, 1991: 170.
72   Michael Perry, 1992: 156.
73   Douglas Groothuis, 1988: 21.
74   Op. cit.: 23.
75   Op. cit.: 22.
76   Harmon Hartzell Bro, 1993: 192.
77   Ibid.
78   Philip Lucas, 1992: 195. Christopher Lasch (who we will meet in the following chapter) also draws comparisons between the New Age and Christian funda-

istics of Universal Energy and Holy Spirit appear to have common properties, although the principal difference between the two seems to relate to the authority behind this energy. Here, Michael Perry argues that 'The New Age conception of God [...] is very different from the Christian. There is a basic and universal spiritual energy, but this is not the personal God of Christianity.'[79] According to another, the Pentecostal belief is based on biblical authority, in that while accepting the principle of Christian duality, Pentecostalists argue that 'God is pouring out the Holy Spirit on his elect [and] is thus a divinely given pre-taste of the heavenly realm.'[80] From my survey, it is likely that many participants of the New Age would have little trouble in accepting the basic Pentecostal description of the Holy Spirit as being one of a number of ways of describing God, although the key differences between the two views appear to lie in the description of the source of this power and the means of its accessibility and availability.[81]

Moving to Drane's second point on the New Age view that 'going within' can help solve human problems, he suggests that in fact the opposite is true. Drane argues that looking within has been the cause of most of humankind's problems in the first place.[82] Here, Drane considers that making contact with what is called the Higher Self represents a turning away from God. Similarly, Ted Peters points out that it is not up to the Christian individual to initiate their own salvation, as he believes that this can only come from God's grace.[83] Michael Perry, too, agrees and further suggests that the New Age contact with the Higher Self does not occur in the way William Bloom de-

mentalism in that he believes they share a literal understanding of sacred mythology and both see spirituality as being therapeutic – Lasch believes 'it is no accident that miracle cures and faith healing figure prominently in both' (1987: 180).

79   Michael Perry, 1992: 147.
80   Ibid.
81   A further comparison can be seen in the apparent close relationship between spiritualist and psychic healing with regard to the source of the healing power (see Chapter 7 above).
82   John Drane, 1991: 215.
83   Ted Peters, 1991: 177.

scribes it[84] – as a spiritually imbued activity – but argues it is merely an 'inner conviction of the value of the self'.[85]

The Christian position with regard to the notion of the Higher Self is that there is a separation between God and people, that God is not contained within the person – He is seen to be wholly transcendent and wholly Other. The difference between Christianity and the New Age on this point can be expressed as a matter of seeing where the onus of responsibility for 'salvation' lies, and here an academic suggests that 'The New Age is Self-directed; [while] conservative Christianity is in the hands of God. The conservative Christian believes that salvation ultimately lies with external agency.'[86]

Drane's third point particularly regards the significance of evil, which he believes is played down in the New Age. Drane's belief here is that lack of concern about evil leads to moral weakness.[87] Michael Perry, too, puts forward a similar argument. Extending from what he believes to be the doctrine of pantheism in the New Age[88] is the concept 'that the Cosmos is seen as basically good, and there is no such "thing" as evil. Evil is due to ignorance, and is banished by the acquisition of knowledge – knowledge, not of brute facts [...] but of one's true nature and its relationship to Reality.'[89] Perry argues that no Christian theology denies the existence of evil or would agree that it is simply a manifestation of ignorance which can be eradicated by knowledge.[90] Peters continues Perry's argument by suggesting

What the new age teaches is clearly naive, almost blind, to the reality of human sin and the existence of evil in the world. Perhaps this is a voluntary naiveté [It] is very appealing to be able to think only positively, only in terms of essential goodness [which is] already within me – so that all I have to do is execute the right psychotechnique and I can bring it to full flower [...] The paradox is that

---

84 See Chapter 1 above.
85 Michael Perry, 1992: 145.
86 Paul Heelas, 1996a: 38.
87 John Drane, 1991: 227.
88 For a review of the Christian response to New Age pantheism see David K. Clark and Norman L. Geisler, 1992.
89 Michael Perry, 1992: 149.
90 Op. cit.: 158.

God's presence shows us that he loves us 'while we still were sinners' (Rom. 5:8) while at the same time transforming us through spiritual power.[91]

The heart of this Christian argument is that to deny the existence of sin denies the whole purpose of Christ's suffering and sacrifice and, therefore, denies Christianity itself. Douglas Groothuis pinpoints the division with a play on words by suggesting that 'The New Age substitutes its monistic idea of "at-one-ment" for the Bible's revelation of Christ's atonement for sin [...] The New Age promises infinite potential through self-discovery. Christ promises eternal life through self-abandonment.'[92]

Finally, John Drane's fourth point particularly relates to the New Age view that each individual is free to choose her or his own spiritual path. For a Christian, obviously, there is only one direction to follow – that primarily outlined within the religious texts – and the many paths within Christianity all head in the same general direction. Here, the Christian critics are likely to agree with other commentators that the New Age is 'amorphous' in that it appears to have no leadership, no clear direction, no unifying dogma, and no institutional hierarchy.

There are many more differences between the New Age and Christian ideas although the four described here represent the most important. As has been shown, some points of agreement can be found between the two although these are, in the main, peripheral to the very real central differences which exist and which are summarized in the suggestion that

> Until saved, the self of the conservative Christian is fallen; the Self of the New Ager is intrinsically good. Theistically envisaged, the Christian God is infinitely more than *anything* we can hope to be (at least in this life), rather than being what, in essence, we *already are*. The orthodox Christian lives in terms of a religion whose God transcends human comprehension; the New Ager follows the dynamics of the human and the natural. The Christian, valuing knowledge of texts, heeds Biblical commandments; the New Ager, valuing experience, heeds the voice within.[93]

91   Ted Peters, 1991: 196f.
92   Douglas Groothuis, 1988: 124.
93   Paul Heelas, 1996a: 37.

With regard to similarities, a number of parallels have been drawn between the New Age and Pentecostal and charismatic Christian groups.[94] The description here relates to the similar concept of a universal healing energy, and the suggestion is made that further parallels exist. These, it is argued, can be seen in the New Age notion of transformation compared with becoming 'born again' into the Christian Church, and a similarity in the decentralized and non-hierarchical nature of both New Age and Pentecostal movements. These parallels, however, do not suggest any form of mutuality or even similarity between the beliefs of the two groups.

It can be seen that there are many profound objections that Christianity – especially its more conservative wing – has made against the New Age. However, there are notable instances where the New Age has become more acceptable to some Christian groups, and these are now reviewed.

Christian acceptance

Within the overall criticism of the New Age by Christian groups, as has been stated, there is no complete endorsement of its basic ideas; and this is primarily because of fundamental differences between the basic beliefs outlined above. However, it can be argued that if the New Age incorporated its own spiritual doctrine and created a degree of structure, then more significant levels of mutual concerns and compatibility might be found to exist between the two. In fact, there are spiritual associations whose remit is to seek out and develop ways in which different religious groups can develop a cooperative harmony with one another. The most notable of these – and the first interfaith organization – is the World Congress of Faiths, founded in 1936 by Sir Francis Younghusband. In 1987, the Inter Faith Network for the UK was founded with the following declaration:

94   Philip Lucas, 1992.

We meet today as children of many traditions, inheritors of shared wisdom and of tragic misunderstandings. We recognize our shared humanity and we respect each other's differences. With the agreed purpose and hope of promoting greater understanding between the members of the different faith communities to which we belong and of encouraging the growth of relationships of respect and trust and mutual enrichment in our life together, we hereby jointly resolve: that the Inter Faith Network of the United Kingdom should now be established [...][95]

This organization includes a membership of representative bodies drawn from all three principal Western theistic traditions together with Baha'i, Buddhist, Jain, Hindu, and Sikh traditions and other related groups. The point being made here is that, in comparison to the objectives of the Inter Faith Network and given the description of New Age already outlined, if the New Age had its own representative body there does not appear to be any ideological reason why such a body could not become part of this network.

In reviewing the basic principles of the Inter Faith Network,[96] certain key similarities seem to exist in New Age ideas. For example, in relation to the New Age claim that 'All religions are the expression of [the] same inner reality',[97] the Inter Faith statement reports that 'Our traditions make different claims about the sources of their values and ethical principles. But in their varied ways they all point to the value of human, animal and natural life, and to a Reality which infinitely transcends all that we can see, touch, smell, taste, and hear.'[98] By this statement, it can be seen that the Inter Faith network refers to a single ultimate transcendent reality which is not necessarily different for each tradition, nor is it completely different from notions proposed in the New Age.

Moreover, in relation to the New Age claim that 'All souls in incarnation are free to choose their own spiritual path',[99] the Inter Faith statement reports that 'We recognize the need to respect the integrity

95   Pamphlet.
96   Published in their pamphlet entitled *Statement on Inter-Religious Relations in Britain*, 1991.
97   William Bloom, 1990: 13.
98   Pamphlet.
99   William Bloom, op. cit.

of each other's inherited and chosen religious identities, beliefs and practices [...] To be able to live by our traditions, share our convictions, and act according to our consciences are freedoms which we all affirm.'[100] Here again, there appears to be very little difference between this particular Inter Faith principle and a core New Age idea.

Further expressions of the acceptance of New Age ideas specifically by Christian groups also exist. These can be found most particularly in the way in which some Christian Churches accommodate other spiritual groups, especially with regard to the physical sharing of their facilities. A prime example of this is St James's Church in Piccadilly, London. Apart from a full Anglican Christian ministry, this church also houses the following non-Church of England groups: Centre for Creation Spirituality, Health and Healing Centre, Sufi Healing Order, Dunramis (a group which discusses problems involved in national and international defence and security), Alternatives (probably the largest and most active New Age organization in the UK), The Blake Society, an Edgar Cayce group, Alcoholics Anonymous, a music ministry, and other smaller groups.

Donald Reeves, the former Rector of St James's, suggests that this fragmentation of activities accurately reflects the late-twentieth-century state of Christianity, which he believes does not provide a coherent and unifying focus for the church community. In his ten-year plan for the church, what Reeves believed could come to exist at St James's is a 'community of the seekers of God's truth [of] women and men who are ready to face up to, to embrace, and to absorb the chaos [...] so that a community of grace and vitality will be born.'[101]

St James's is not an isolated example. In a great many towns across the world some churches now permit different faiths and non-traditional organizations to share their facilities and, by implication, their communities. This does not in any way mean that the host organization necessarily endorses all of the activities which these organizations might engage with although, importantly, they appear to be acceptive of the differences.

100   *Statement on Inter-Religious Relations in Britain* pamphlet, op. cit.
101   Donald Reeves, 1990: 3f.

Probably the most comprehensive accommodation offered by a Christian 'Church' to other spiritual groups – including groups which can be considered as New Age – is given by the Religious Society of Friends (Quakers); and there are a number of parallels which can be drawn between the beliefs of the Quakers and the New Age. For example, the Quaker view of God is described as 'a creative, loving power in all people and in the world around [...] Everyone can become aware of it by listening to its promptings in their hearts.'[102] Because of this, 'Quakers believe the spirit that inspired the early church [...] is not bound to any one religious tradition.'[103] Moreover, because the Quaker faith is founded upon 'a direct personal experience'[104] of God's power, there is no requirement for a hierarchical Church. Quakers since their foundation have 'stressed that their faith is something they live rather than put into particular words'[105] and, in consequence, believes that organizational structures and formal creeds are, in the end, divisive.

This philosophy has resulted in Friends' Meeting Houses becoming a focus for non-traditional spirituality in many communities. For example, the Meeting House at Lancaster, UK, provides space for various weekly meditational activities including the New Kadampa Tradition of Mahayana Buddhism, Serene Reflection Meditation (Soto Zen), Sufi Dances of Universal Peace, t'ai chi ch'uan, Osho (Bhagwan Shree Rajneesh) meditation groups, together with occasional spiritualist or New Age healing groups and channellers, along with other non-spiritual community activities including a men's group, a drama factory, the philosophical discussion group Dialogues, and children's playgroups.

Throughout all of these examples given so far it is clear that there are Christian groups and factions which are not necessarily antagonistic to the New Age; and there are more which could be reviewed here: for example, Don Cupitt's 'Sea of Faith' Network[106] and Peter Spink's

102 Harvey Gilman, 1994: 8.
103 Op. cit.: 18.
104 Op. cit.: 8.
105 Op. cit.: 7.
106 Don Cupitt, 1984, 1993.

Omega Order.[107] Moreover, in some areas the gap between Christianity and the New Age appears to be narrowing. Evidence for this is illustrated by the suggestion that 'there are many New Agers who fully identify as Christian – many, even, who still regularly or otherwise continue to attend church services';[108] and by another which notes that 'New Age ideas may be bound up with Christianity, but it is a Christianity that can absorb aspects of other faiths and philosophies.'[109] Furthermore, this view is reinforced by the report that 'There is plenty taking place, under the rubric of Christianity, which is remarkably similar to what is going on in New Age quarters. Spiritual retreats have proliferated; many forms of Christianity – including Unitarians and Quakers – emphasize the immanence of God; there are now over 100 "rave churches" in Britain; and so on.'[110]

Finally, from my survey, Christianity has played a significant part in a large number of participants' lives (albeit not necessarily in a positive way), and at least 15% claimed Christianity was one of the spiritual disciplines which had the greatest affect on their lives. Some participants claim to be practising members of Christian churches.[111] Among individuals who listed names of those who have been important through contact, a few mentioned either the Cosmic Christ or Jesus Christ himself; and, in answer to my question regarding individuals whose ideas have had an important influence through their writings, the seventh most-mentioned name, given by 5% of participants, was the Bible.

Two particular Christians warrant individual attention as not being antagonistic to the New Age because it seems that the difference between their ideals and those of the New Age are, in many respects, insignificant. The first instance is the Benedictine monk Father Bede Griffiths, who helped to establish the Saccidananda Ashram in Southern India. This ashram has become a place of pilgrimage which

107   Peter Spink, 1983.
108   Michael York, 1994: 17.
109   Eileen Barker, 1989: 191.
110   Paul Heelas, 1996a: 149.
111   Peter Spink reports finding New Age participants who claim to also be practising Christians (1991: 38).

draws thousands of people to what is described as a 'powerhouse of meditation and prayer'.[112] Griffiths's teachings are described as bringing together immanence and transcendence in that 'while he sees Christ as perfectly revealed in Jesus and takes no issue with orthodox definitions of Christology, he is equally insistent that this same Christ is active at every stage in history and in the hearts of human beings, regardless of religious boundaries',[113] an ideal, it is reported, which has particular appeal among young people who are disaffected with the Christian Church.[114] This contemporary spirituality has been described as a 'new consciousness' which, as reported in an earlier chapter, is an epithet used in place of the term 'New Age' by some participants.

The second instance regards a Western-based group of people whose ideology is founded on the notion of a creation-centred spirituality developed by Matthew Fox. Fox, a Dominican priest in California until ejected from the order by Papal decree for alleged heresy, now heads the Institute for Culture and Creation Spirituality at Holy Names College in Oakland, California.[115]

What is remarkable about this group is Fox's insistence that spirituality – in this case, Christian spirituality – 'begins with original blessing instead of original sin'.[116] Fox argues against the mainstream Christian view that human beings start their spiritual lives with sin but suggests instead that 'religious experience begins with awe and wonder'.[117] As demonstrated above, this argument is almost identical to one of the major criticisms levied by the majority of Christian groups against the New Age idea that the world is ostensibly good. Moreover, Fox argues against traditional Christian dualism, that is, the complete Otherness of God. Instead, he puts forward a panentheistic view where 'everything is in God and God is in everything'[118] which, again, is closely compatible to the New Age idea of an interconnected Supreme

112 Peter Spink, 1990: xi.
113 Op. cit.: xiiif.
114 Ibid.
115 For a description of creation-centred spirituality, see Matthew Fox, 1991.
116 Matthew Fox, 1992: 25.
117 Op. cit.: 26.
118 Ibid.

Consciousness. Fox provides a comprehensive list of the differences which he sees to exist between the traditional 'fall/redemption' concepts which form the heart of traditional Christianity and those of a creation-centred spirituality[119] – and again, none of these appear in principle to be at odds with the New Age.

However, it must be added that Fox has a number of critics: not least Michael Perry,[120] who himself suggests that Fox overstates the case for a shift from original sin to original blessings.[121] Also critical of Fox's division between traditional Christianity and creation-centred spirituality is another academic, who suggests that Fox's ideas have the 'defining characteristics of a fundamentalism'.[122]

Fox himself discusses the strengths and weaknesses of the New Age, and it is relevant to review these in the light of the overall Christian response to the New Age. With regards to New Age strengths, Fox believes these include its 'mysticism and the quest for the experience of the Divine [...] our need for a *cosmology* to live our lives in [and] its explorations into body consciousness',[123] the latter point relating specifically to therapeutic massage used as a meditative experience. With regards to its weaknesses, Fox argues that the New Age needs to accept the existence of 'dark' aspects in human life, and believes 'It is necessary to enter into the darkness not cover it up with excessive light energies. This is where the fact of and archetype of the crucifix of Jesus can play a truly redemptive role.'[124] Moreover, Fox claims that the 'New Age can be notoriously indifferent to the suffering of others and to issues of injustice [...] New Agers are often self-centred'[125] and are 'open to trivializing the spiritual journey'.[126] Overall, however, Fox believes that the traditional Christian Church has much to learn from the New Age and he lists ten 'lessons' for Christians to consider which include expanding the mystical content of

119   Matthew Fox, 1983: 316ff; 1993: 206.
120   Michael Perry, 1992: 77.
121   Ibid.
122   Linda Woodhead, 1993: 175.
123   Matthew Fox, 1993: 207f.
124   Op. cit.: 209.
125   Ibid.
126   Op. cit.: 210.

Christianity, decreasing its anthropocentrism, renewing forms of worship to make them more participatory, and to rediscover the premodern era.[127]

Summary

This chapter has demonstrated that few, if any, traditional Christian groups agree with the principal New Age ideas, although there appears to be a growing acceptance of the New Age as an increasingly significant spiritual concern in its own right. There are obvious difficulties involved in this acceptance because there is no formalized New Age doctrine or any organizational structure with which Christian groups can meaningfully engage. To the more conservative factions of Christianity, the New Age remains an anathema, although this is no different than these groups' attitudes towards any form of spirituality which is not wholly Christian. However, to the more liberally oriented Christian groups the New Age may well be starting to become recognized as a valuable form of spirituality – one which some commentators have suggested may provide part of the impetus for change which has been noted to exist or seen to be desirable within the Christian groups themselves.

Moreover, participants of the New Age itself report that they have had significant Christian influence in their lives, and some appear to claim that they experience little or no conflict between practising New Age ideas and activities while remaining members of a Christian Church. Spiritualism, also, appears to play a part in the healing activities of the New Age. Certainly, in the reverse situation, New Age ideology does not appear to preclude the additional tandem practice of any religious tradition of an individual's choice – and that includes Christianity.

127   Op. cit.: 211ff.

11. Social and Cultural Responses

The first thing to be done is laughter, because that sets the trend for the whole day. If you wake up laughing, you will soon begin to feel how absurd life is. Nothing is serious: even your disappointments are laughable, even your pain is laughable, even you are laughable.

Bhagwan Shree Rajneesh[1]

Apart from the Christian response, there has been little serious criticism of the New Age and probably the main reason for this is that many of its core ideas have appeared to be eminently sensible and practical. However, through analysis of the relevant literature (the majority, but not all, from academe), five often interrelated ideas – or problems – are found to have attracted particular critical interest and each of these is examined in turn. The first is the problem of the efficacy of spiritual empowerment. Second, Ken Wilber argues that the New Age trivializes its spiritual concerns, and his views are examined from the point of view of his notion of a spectrum of consciousness. Third, Christopher Lasch argues that the New Age represents a culture of narcissism caused, he suggests, by the disintegration of traditional values in society and religion. However, other commentators, such as Theodore Roszak, do not agree with Lasch. Fourth, some critics have argued that the New Age represents just another form of consumerism and fuels, as Paul Heelas and others contend, the prosperity ideals of Western capitalism and spiritual materialism. Finally, the criticisms that New Age participants are self-centred are examined. In each case, responses to the problems are given so as to provide, overall, a balanced view of the principal critical responses to the New Age.

1   Bhagwan Shree Rajneesh, 1983: 17.

Problems regarding the efficacy of spiritual empowerment

Many criticisms of the New Age, according to Paul Heelas,[2] arise from problems associated with the substance and efficacy of its claimed spirituality. The criticisms he cites range from 'the (supposed) absurdness of New Age beliefs'[3] to concerns about the New Age's apparent lack of solid spiritual foundations. Regarding the latter problem, Heelas suggests that participants are

> engaged in a perpetual struggle, combating the 'pull' of the ego by practising disciplines to make contact with the Self itself. Depending on the state of play of this struggle, the Self – assuming it exists – is in control; or, conversely, the ego is in command. Successful activity in everyday life thus depends on how the Self-ego contest is resolved at any particular moment. In sum, the New Age is not – in its own terms – secure and permanently *grounded*.[4]

Because of this insecurity Heelas sees the New Age itself to be a 'precarious undertaking'[5] which arguably requires the addition of external authority to provide balance[6] – a view also held by Christopher Lasch (although for different reasons)[7] and by Steve Bruce,[8] but not by

---

2　It needs to be remembered from previous chapters that Heelas views the New Age primarily as a form of humanism (1999: 56), and its methods and activities as a means of perfecting what he calls 'Self-spirituality' which he sees may well be a deviant form of genuine Self-spirituality (op. cit.: 99). Heelas's descriptions, often made only as suppositions, do not sit comfortably with the findings of my examination of the New Age. What Heelas terms as New Age might be better described as the Human Potential Movement (examined in Chapter 2 above) and therefore largely beyond the scope of this volume.

3　Paul Heelas, 1996a: 201.

4　Op. cit.: 206.

5　Op. cit.: 212. Discussing the Human Potential Movement, although applicable to the New Age as a whole, Roy Wallis and Steve Bruce describe this precariousness as being 'a consequence of its diffuse belief system [where] authority is seen to lie with individual members of the movement' (1986: 177).

6　Paul Heelas, 1996a: 214.

7　Christopher Lasch's arguments are reviewed later in this chapter.

8　See Chapter 8 above.

Robert Wuthnow, who sees a need for a third dimension.[9] For some participants of the New Age, Heelas believes that the Higher Self is viewed as being insufficiently enduring to become any more substantial than it already is; and accordingly, the predicament faced by the New Age, argues Heelas, is to find a way to incorporate the authority of 'external voices' without 'becoming too traditionalized or hierarchically authoritative'.[10] Not having such external voices of authority, Heelas maintains, anarchy could well reign.[11]

With regard to spiritual authority, we have seen participants claim that guidance comes from within, although Heelas points to the possibility that

> New Agers might think that they are listening to their inner voices or are drawing upon their intuitive wisdom; in practice, however, they are listening to internalized renderings – by way of socialization – of what they have read about the Buddha or Gurdjieff [...] New Agers might think that they are arriving at their own values; in practice they are adopting those which have become *established* as a set of variations on the theme of Self-spirituality. Supposedly inner-directed truth acquisition is, in fact, routinized.[12]

The possibilities that Heelas outlines appear to be very real problems concerning how individuals verify their spiritual influences and experiences in the New Age, and my survey findings go some way to confirm that Heelas's suggestions may have some truth. For example, while the authority of individual teachers appears not to be very strong (a point also found in Marilyn Ferguson's survey), participants most frequently claim to have been influenced by many teachings and, what is more, report that they are widely read in New Age subjects. Collectively, this could form the basis to what Heelas sees as a tradition.[13]

There is no way of verifying Heelas's ideas, which he puts forward only as unsupported possibilities: and in any case, participants

---

9   Robert Wuthnow suggests there needs to be a rediscovery of practice-based spirituality as an alternative to what he calls 'dwelling' (traditional) and 'seeking' spirituality (1998: 16).
10 Roy Wallis and Steve Bruce, 1986: 214.
11 Op. cit.: 206.
12 Op. cit.: 206f.
13 Op. cit.: 207.

would argue, there are other equally valid sources of authority. For example, in response to Heelas's suppositions, participants appear to suggest that they do not believe their inner guidance to be isolated or disconnected; instead they describe their spirituality as being part of a much greater whole. In this sense, it can be argued that participants see themselves as having what might be considered as external author-ity, although this is in the form of a connectedness to their notion of God. These views were expressed in various ways by survey partici-pants describing their spirituality and the New Age itself, and is also expressed in the first and second basic New Age ideas put forward by William Bloom.[14] For many participants, their spiritual security ap-pears to be much more dependent on an individual connectedness to God than on any more worldly forms of connection and, moreover, they report that they find direction and spiritual fulfilment through being guided by their intuition.[15]

Discussing Heelas's suppositions at the end of the twentieth cen-tury, American sociologist Wade Clark Roof sees a distinct change in spirituality over the previous twenty years among baby boomers. Roof finds that, 'identity is still a powerful theme, but its mode of expres-sion is now different: the energizing forces arise out of quests not so much for group identity and social location as for an authentic inner life and personhood.'[16] Roof finds that personal meaning is where re-ligious energies are now focused.[17] Additionally, what Roof has found is that

> Even if some people flit from one small group or spiritual experience to an-
> other, and levels of spiritual understanding are shallow and inconsequential –
> flaky, some would say – the majority are inclined to stick with a particular

---

14   Discussed in Chapter 1 above.
15   Marilyn Ferguson has described the importance of intuition as a means of inner
      guidance and authority among Aquarian conspirators and has found many who
      believe that 'if we give up the need for certainty in terms of control and fixed
      answers [...] we begin to trust intuition' (1982: 114). The subject of intuition is
      discussed more fully in Chapter 4 above.
16   Wade Clark Roof, 1999: 6f.
17   Ibid.

group or spiritual discipline over a period of time long enough to benefit from those experiences in ways that often do affect their outlooks and identities.[18]

Further evidence for different kinds of authority have been found again in my survey where, for example, four out of five participants reported that they had experienced various kinds of meaningful psychic phenomena (which are difficult to prove by any rational formula),[19] some participants also reported that spirit guides offered help and direction which they claim could be received (channelled) either consciously or unconsciously, while others even argue that they are spiritual beings having a human experience. In these cases, the locus of spiritual authority appears to be quite different from some of the scenarios that Heelas appears to suggest. Hence, the 'pull' of the ego, as Heelas describes, although it may be thought by many participants to be strong and continuous, nevertheless appears to be against what they might consider to be a grounded interconnectedness.

Added to this argument, psychologist Peter Russell believes that 'the pure Self can in no way be affected by the ups and downs of the outside world.'[20] Although Russell is describing the claimed existence of enlightened or Self-realized people, he points to what he sees as a possibility of not being dominated by the ego[21] – which means that

> Since he is no longer psychologically dependent on his experience, the enlightened person is not kicked around by the world. Personal criticisms, loss of a job, or other events which before would have been a source of anguish are still very real, but they are no longer perceived as personal threats. This is borne out by the experience of many people, who, though not enlightened, are nevertheless already making progress in this direction. They often remark that it is not so much the sense of oneness that first becomes noticeable, but the experience of being at ease with themselves, combined with an increasing sense of inner security and invulnerability.[22]

---

18 Op. cit.: 306.
19 Rupert Sheldrake (1994) suggests ways in which some psychic phenomena can be tested.
20 Peter Russell, 1982: 138.
21 Ibid.
22 Ibid.

Russell appears to suggest that through continued effort the ego is able to be contained and, by so doing, other aspects of life – notably love – become 'simultaneously [...] less conditional'.[23] Moreover, similar arguments have been made by a number of commentators in their descriptions of connectedness given in Chapter 5 above, not least by Fritjof Capra with regards to the influence that he sees the Eastern world view has had on framing New Age ideas in this respect.

Problems are likely to occur among New Age participants in their attempts to maintain contact with what they claim to be their inner authority, as Heelas suggests, although these may be seen as not being unique to the New Age but similar to problems encountered in many other forms of spirituality and religious beliefs. These problems as a whole concern the contrasting relationship between a person's ego-driven desires together with the conflict between their need to live in society and the demands of their spirituality.

Related to the problems outlined concerning spiritual efficacy in the New Age are the questions regarding the power that some charismatic teachers may hold over their followers – although, as no individual teacher is reported by participants to hold sway over any large part of the New Age, this may not be such a widespread problem.[24] With regard to teachings in general, Ken Wilber argues that 'authentic religious experience must be differentiated from mere emotional frenzies, from magical trances, and from mythic mass-enthusiasms'[25] which, in his view, can only be accomplished when 'knowledge claims are based [...] not on belief, faith, or transitory experience, but on actual levels of structuralization, cognition, and development'[26] which can be tested, ultimately, through gnosis.[27] However, Dick Anthony et al. (including Wilber) describe what they see as four types of spiritual guides and highlight the difficulties individuals face in making such differentiations. These authors believe that seekers are 'not capable of distinguishing *for certain* among the four kinds of guides,

23   Ibid.
24   A spectrum of spiritual teachers is outlined by Georg Feuerstein (1992: 131).
25   Ken Wilber, 1983: 68.
26   Op. cit.: 73.
27   Op. cit.: 134.

let alone among the different kinds of help they offer'[28] unless they themselves attain a degree of spiritual insight equal to that of their teacher. This view, it appears, adds further substance to Heelas's idea mentioned above that the New Age is a precarious undertaking.

It is not possible to come to any firm conclusions over the idea – stated only as a possibility – that Heelas raises regarding whether participants arrive at their own conclusions or internalize renderings of existing teachings. However, as Marilyn Ferguson has found, it is possible to argue that participants appear to give much greater credence to intuitive wisdom than to any particular teachings[29] and to the changes of perception that she believes a transformed awareness can create.[30] Yet there is no doubt that certain New Age teachers have a wider influence than others – for example, Louise Hay and Carl Jung – which means that many of those involved share the same influences. Moreover, particularly with regard to the New Age, participants claim that sources of authority and guidance may also arise through other forms of external influence than tradition, in this case by means of channelled teachings from what they call discarnate spirit beings. In this situation, it can be argued, there may be little difference in principle between New Age spirituality and spirituality encountered in religious mysticism, at least in terms of its verification.

Additionally, Heelas's suppositions may not apply equally to all New Age participants, as there exist variations in the levels and categories of association individuals can have. Some individuals, it can be argued – for example, those who are likely to participate more at the 'glamorous' or lower levels of partial association, or mainstream-empowerers (that is, those who, according to Heelas, place a higher value on the institutions of mainstream society)[31] – could well adopt more in the way of established traditional forms of inner direction. Whereas, in respect of participation at the full level or world-rejecting category of association – described by David Spangler as 'an incarna-

---

28   Dick Anthony *et al.*, 1987: 6; see also Georg Feuerstein, 1992: 325.
29   Marilyn Ferguson, 1982: 325.
30   Op. cit.: 72.
31   Paul Heelas, 1996a: 31.

tion of the sacred'[32] whereby individuals become 'more fully at one with the presence of God'[33] – the need for such traditional forms of authority may be much reduced. As is the case with most if not all religions, in the New Age it appears that it can only ever be possible to study the efficaciousness of established voices of authority, and not of those which are claimed to be inner directed.[34] The New Age, in the same way as many religions, may never have completely solid foundations and is likely therefore to remain spiritually precarious.

Problems concerning trivialization

Ken Wilber is one of the New Age's most outspoken critics, but also in many respects one of its ardent supporters; and in a number of works written since the 1970s his criticisms of its principal activities have remained consistent. Overall, as reported in Chapter 6 above, Wilber has found that approximately 80% of those involved in the New Age have what has been described as unwitting or partial participation in its ideas and activities. It is against these individuals that Wilber, in the main, levies his criticism that core New Age ideas and activities have become trivialized. In fact, he traces the roots of this trivialization to the counter-culture where, he argues, mysticism all

32   David Spangler, 1984: 80.
33   Op. cit.: 81.
34   James Martin has remarked that 'Any account of religious experience must recognize the fact that all experience is to some extent theory laden' (1987: 324), and its study is, he believes, most appropriately engaged through analysis of a religious tradition. Martin cites William James (1952) and Alister Hardy (1979) as agreeing that there can be no precise analysis of what might be contained in spiritual experience (1987: 330). In fact, even the definition of spirituality appears to vary according to particular studies, some examples of which (although by no means a comprehensive selection) can be found in: general studies, Geoffrey Ahern, 1990, Ken Wilber, 1995a, and Stuart Rose, 2001b; ecological studies, Jonathan Porritt and David Winner, 1988, and Charlene Spretnak, 1986; feminist studies, Katherine Zappone, 1991; and humanistic studies, David N. Elkins *et al.*, 1984, and Joel Kovel, 1990.

too easily became 'subverted into pre-rational, narcissistic, and competitive ends'[35] and he agrees with the American sociologist Robert Bellah who argues that the counter-cultural approach to Eastern religions was based 'on a "cafeteria model" – namely just something else to purchase, something else to try'.[36] This trivialization of what he considers to be fundamental aspects of spirituality – much of which he describes as being brought about by confusion – is Wilber's main concern with the New Age, and the different aspects of this criticism will now be reviewed in depth.

The basis of Wilber's argument is founded on his concept of a 'spectrum of consciousness' which was explored in detail in a work of the same name[37] and which he has subsequently developed in a number of essays and books.[38] The spectrum needs to be briefly explained here in order that Wilber's criticism can be clearly revealed.

The principle of Wilber's spectrum is that it divides human consciousness into ten levels which are deployed in three groups.[39] Wilber describes these groups as important stages in the growth of human consciousness that commence with 'developmental stages [which] are prepersonal, in that a separate and individuated personal ego has not yet emerged. The middle stages of growth are personal or egoic. And the highest stages are transpersonal or transegoic.'[40]

Bearing this model in mind, Wilber identifies two fundamental ways in which he sees the New Age becoming trivialized. The first of these relates to the growth of consciousness which reaches – but halts at – the middle group of levels, particularly level 6 (existential); and the second relates to a confusion between the first and third groups – which Wilber sees as a confusion of the 'pre' and the 'trans'. These criticisms are interrelated and will be explored together.

35 Ken Wilber, 1987: 12.
36 Ibid.
37 Ken Wilber, 1977.
38 For instance, Ken Wilber, 1981, 1996.
39 Wilber's spectrum includes nine actual levels. The tenth level, unity consciousness, is non-dualistic and thereby in itself incorporates all levels in the one.
40 Ken Wilber, 1993: 189. The world views at each level from the lowest to the highest respectively are described as: 'archaic, magic, mythic, mythic-rational, rational, existential, psychic, subtle, and causal' (1993: 199).

The level of consciousness reached at the culmination of the middle position of the spectrum is portrayed as the growth of a fully developed ego. This growth Wilber sees as an essential process in order that a person can proceed with further development in the trans-egoic levels of consciousness. The criticism with the New Age here is that, in comparison to mystical notions – primarily of Eastern origin but including some aspects of Western mysticism – at this point,

> The modern West has specialized in all the stages of growth and development leading up to the mature ego. And it has spotted all the psychoses and neuroses that can and will occur if this growth is disrupted or traumatized or derailed. But it aggressively and vehemently denies any higher stages of growth beyond ego.[41]

Problems which dominate this level of growth and development (which Wilber calls 'the Centaur' level[42]) are 'existential problems, problems inherent in manifest existence itself, like mortality, finitude, integrity, authenticity, meaning of life [...] And therapies that address these concerns are the humanistic and existential therapies, the so-called Third Force [psychotechnologies].'[43] It can be noticed here that Wilber makes little mention of spirituality, and this is because he believes 'genuine spirituality is transrational'[44] – that is, in effect trans-egoic.

Wilber argues that different ways of developing an individual's consciousness are required at different levels and that 'far from being conflicting or contradictory, [they] actually reflect the very real differences in the various levels of the spectrum of consciousness [thereby representing] complementary approaches to different levels of the individual.'[45] Wilber does not deny the importance of psychotechnologies to the New Age. In fact, he believes they can 'heal the split between the ego itself and the body [whereby] the vast potentials of the

41   Ken Wilber, 1995b: 47.
42   Ken Wilber, 1993: 194.
43   Ibid.
44   Ken Wilber, 1995b: 47.
45   Op. cit.: 11.

total organism are liberated and put at the individual's disposal'.[46] By contrast, the role of transpersonal therapies is seen to add to the work of humanistic types of therapies and is 'deeply concerned with those processes in the person which are actually "supra-individual", or "collective" [which] transcends the boundaries of the individual organism'.[47] Ultimately, according to Wilber, continued growth through the levels of the spectrum leads to the attainment of the highest level of consciousness – unity consciousness – which he suggests is found in more formalized spiritual disciplines primarily of Eastern origin.

The point Wilber is making here is that the vast proportion of what are taken to be New Age ideas and activities effectively fall short of what he sees they need to entail if they are to bring about a true new age. For Wilber, it is essential that the New Age incorporates the transpersonal or what he calls the trans-egoic levels of consciousness, as well as the personal or egoic levels, in what is described as a 'marriage' between psychotechnologies and spirituality[48] which can then lead on to what he sees to be the highest of all levels – that is, humanity's ultimate goal of unity consciousness. Halting this growth at the Centaur or existential level – that is, without genuine spirituality – blocks further development and, it follows, is unlikely to create a sufficiently comprehensive transformation to bring about his concept of what a new age could be.[49]

Following on from this argument, it seems that Wilber might consider the attainment of all such levels in the spectrum, except unity consciousness to be more or less trivializations, that is, 'partial – i.e. less than comprehensive – states of consciousness'.[50] In Wilber's view, therefore, what a 'real' new age might be seems to have marked differences from much of what has been described in this study. Wilber describes the spiritual content of a new age as being substantially more all-encompassing than by all but a few participants might

---

46   Op. cit.: 12.
47   Ibid.
48   Ken Wilber, 1995b: 47.
49   David Benner (1989: 27) and Paul Vitz (1983: 27) also point to the limited and often non-spiritual nature of existential psychotechnologies.
50   Ken Wilber, 1981: 141.

achieve – much of which, he intimates, appears to be incorporated in Zen Buddhism.[51] However, he sees the accounts given by participants to my survey as a very important start which 'has its heart in the right place [and suggests that] maybe, hundreds of years from now this whacked out new-age movement, grown up and sober, will turn out to have been the seeds of an actual and genuine new age.'[52]

The second fundamental criticism of trivialization that Wilber levels at the present New Age relates to a confusion which he sees to exist between the pre-egoic and trans-egoic levels of the spectrum of consciousness. Wilber argues that in the New Age much pre-egoic activity is falsely elevated – and given unwarranted mystical and spiritual significance – to the trans-egoic levels; a situation he calls the 'pre/trans fallacy'.[53] This confusion relates to the idea that because both the prepersonal and the transpersonal states of consciousness he describes are, each in their different ways, non-rational, 'they appear similar or even identical to the untutored eye.'[54] According to Wilber, this elevationalism appears to have been occurring, perhaps in varying forms, since the 1960s and is

> exemplified by, but by no means confined to, the New Age movement. All sorts of endeavors, of no matter what origin or of what authenticity, are simply elevated to transrational and spiritual glory, and the *only* qualification for this wonderful promotion is that *the endeavor be nonrational. Anything* rational is wrong; *anything* nonrational is spiritual.[55]

Here, Wilber believes that a large proportion of the individuals involved in the New Age trivialize its spiritual content through their regression to magical and narcissistic levels of consciousness.[56] These levels, he believes, were developed in what he calls the hyperindividualistic American culture which reached its zenith in the 'me dec-

51   Ken Wilber, 1987: 12; 1995b: 45ff.
52   Ken Wilber, 1987: 12.
53   Ken Wilber, 1995a: 206.
54   Ibid.
55   Op. cit.: 207.
56   Narcissism in the New Age is assessed in the following section.

ade'.[57] Wilber sees this regression to be 'one of the major problems with the new age movement'.[58] Furthermore, the problem appears to be compounded by the fact that, according to Wilber, the small percentage of those who are more fully involved in the New Age[59] 'have attracted a huge number of prepersonal, magical, and prerational elements [who] then claim [...] that they have the authority and the backing of a "higher" state, when all they are doing, I'm afraid I have to conclude, is rationalizing their own self-involved stance.'[60]

Hence, Wilber reports that a great deal of confusion arises in at least two areas of the problems involved in the efficacy of New Age spirituality discussed in the first section of this chapter. On the one hand, many participants are faced with the difficult problem of having to appraise the value and authenticity of their teachers. On the other hand, participants can come to believe that their spirituality is authentic and transpersonal whereas, in reality, they may well be deceiving themselves or are being deceived by others. It is Wilber's argument that these two confusions can also act in concert and, as a result, perpetuate a false sense of security with regard to the perceived level in the growth of consciousness among many individuals.

Participants in my survey did not raise many of Wilber's concerns, although some pointed to the fact that their spiritual effort and progress was not an easy or smooth path;[61] which, again, can be seen to relate to Paul Heelas's ideas surrounding the supposed 'pull' of the ego discussed in the first section above. However, Wilber raises three important points which help to identify patterns in the different levels

57   Ken Wilber, 1993: 266.
58   Op. cit.: 267.
59   Regarding the ideas of these individuals, Wilber suggests that 'You can usually find the transpersonal elements because they don't like to be called "new age". There's nothing "new" about them; they are perennial' (1993: 268), a view which has some similarities with William Bloom's basic New Age ideas described in Chapter 1 above.
60   Op. cit.: 267f. In much the same way, Maurice and Jane Temerlin have identified the existence of a psychotherapy cult mentality which they believe may be widespread (1982: 132, 139).
61   This finding reflects the limited nature of quantitative studies, and further qualitative research is required to establish whether or not participants share Wilber's views.

and categories of association individuals can have with the New Age. Firstly, he marks out a framework for the existence of levels of association individuals could have through his 'spectrum of consciousness' and, in so doing, points to confusions which are likely to occur among participants, not least because of the existence of unscrupulous – and possibly not New Age – teachers, and of excessively zealous students. Secondly, the New Age (as described in William Bloom's six basic ideas) is not seen by participants as being easy to adopt fully, a situation which can also lead to partial engagement – what Wilber might see as halting at the Centaur level that he believes to incorporate little in the way of spirituality, or at lower transpersonal levels. Thirdly, he points out that such substantial changes which the New Age suggests may not be achievable overnight (if they can ever be fully achieved), and he presents a strategy for identifying partial and/or trivialized elements of the New Age which are likely to be present if, as he argues, humankind is currently in such transition.[62]

It is not at all certain what comprises Wilber's New Age in detail. He indicates that he aspires to what he calls unity consciousness – a notion of complete nonduality embedded in Zen Buddhism and Advaita Vedanta in Hinduism and taught, for example, by Sri Ramana Maharshi[63] – and which he believes to be the ultimate goal for humanity. This itself appears to represent a clearly defined religious path which, although of influence to the New Age, has not been shown by participants in my survey to be a central feature of its ideas and activities. In the end it may well be that Wilber's idea of a new age is not the same as that envisaged by many participants and described in earlier chapters; although this does not necessarily mean that his criticism of the trivial nature of much of the New Age is invalid, or that he has not made a significant contribution to its literature.

---

62   With regard to the notion of transition, Peter Russell suggests that 'If there is one lesson that has been learned since the rush for enlightenment began in the 1960s, it is that enlightenment doesn't follow as rapidly as many of the pundits would have us believe [...] we are still pioneers – and pioneers make mistakes' (1982: 151).

63   See also David Godman, 1985, and Arthur Osborne, 1978. Sri Ramana Maharshi, 1969, is described by Ken Wilber as 'perhaps the brightest light, East or West, in the modern era' (pamphlet).

Problems of narcissism

In two essays[64] Christopher Lasch, social and cultural historian and, to some 'a neo-conservative untouchable',[65] argues that Americans have misplaced their sense of self-value. The self has become technologized, commodified, and has lost its sense of purpose. Contemporary individuals do not now develop a deep character of their own according to Lasch, rather they identify themselves through their activities, for example, with what they buy and what groups they join or empathize with. The cause of this situation, Lasch believes, is that 'people have lost confidence with the future [and have executed] a kind of emotional retreat from the long-term commitments that presuppose a stable, secure, and orderly world.'[66] What has developed Lasch describes as a 'culture of narcissism', which he portrays as

> not necessarily a culture in which moral constraints on selfishness have collapsed or in which people released from the bonds of social obligation have lost themselves in a riot of hedonistic self-indulgence. What has weakened is not so much the structure of moral obligations and commandments as the belief in a world that survives its inhabitants. In our time, the survival and therefore the reality of the external world, the world of human associations and collective memories, appears increasingly problematic. The fading of a durable, common, public world, we may conjecture, intensifies the fear of separation at the same time that it weakens the psychological resources that make it possible to confront this fear realistically. It has freed the imagination from external constraints but exposed it more directly than before to the tyranny of inner compulsions and anxieties. The inescapable facts of separation and death are bearable only because the reassuring world of man-made objects and human culture restores the sense of primary connection on a new basis. When that world begins to lose its reality, the fear of separation becomes almost overwhelming and the need for illusions, accordingly, more intense than ever.[67]

Viewed in this way, Lasch believes that many of the ideas which comprise contemporary society are intellectually lightweight and full

---

64   Christopher Lasch, 1979, 1985.
65   Russell Jacoby, 1995: 122.
66   Christopher Lasch, 1985: 16.
67   Op. cit.: 193.

of narcissistic forms of life which are aimed at satisfying this craving for illusory security. Lasch sees that parts of this craving can be fulfilled by New Age ideas and activities, although this does not mean to say that he is critical of the New Age as a whole. In fact, in a later essay he points out what he sees to be its positive ideological features. Lasch suggests that

> The intuition underlying New Age movements, the bedrock feeling, hard to put into words but scarcely inchoate or confused, deserves better than ridicule: that mankind has lost the collective knowledge of how to live with dignity and grace; that this knowledge includes a respect not just for nature but for the nurturant activities our society holds in such low esteem; and that man's future depends on a renewal of prematurely discarded traditions of thought and practice.[68]

Yet what Lasch believes to be missing in much of New Age thought (and, for that matter, in contemporary society as a whole) and, by inference, one of the prime causes of the narcissistic predicament, 'is spiritual discipline – submission to a body of teachings that has to be accepted even when it conflicts with immediate interests or inclinations and cannot constantly be redesigned to individual specifications'.[69] The New Age, argues Lasch, employs 'a lax standard of truth'[70] because it allows individuals to develop idiosyncratic beliefs which in his view lack substance and are illusory – a view which has been expressed by several commentators above.

Lasch concludes – in the same way as the Christian response outlined in the previous chapter – that the New Age is a form of Gnosticism.

> The New Age movement is best understood, then, as the twentieth-century revival of an ancient religious tradition; but it is a form of Gnosticism considerably adulterated by other influences and mixed up with imagery derived from science fiction, flying saucers, extraterrestrial intervention in human history, escape from the earth to a new home in space [...] Where second-century Gnostics

68   Christopher Lasch, 1987: 82.
69   Ibid.
70   Ibid.

306

imagined the Savior as spirit mysteriously made flesh, their twentieth-century descendants conceive him as a visitor from another solar system.[71]

In the end Lasch appears to advocate a conservative, apologist position in favour of traditional values – especially the more formalized, traditional religions and most particularly those of a Judeo-Christian nature whereby, in his view, ultimate meanings are more secure – against those of the New Age. 'In a dying culture [argues Lasch], narcissism appears to embody – in the guise of personal "growth" and "awareness" – the highest attainment of spiritual enlightenment'[72] which he considers as being insufficient for the maintenance of a stable society.[73] Moreover, Lasch believes the New Age seeks

> the shortest road to Nirvana. Whereas the world's great religions have always emphasized the obstacles to salvation, modern cults borrow selectively from earlier mystical traditions in the West, from ill-digested Oriental traditions, from mind-cure movements and various expressions of 'New Thought', and from an assortment of therapies in order to promise immediate relief from the burden of selfhood.[74]

Lasch sees much of the New Age as a kind of 'quick fix' idea shaped on a 'degenerate form of an ancient tradition [Gnosticism]'[75] which has been reduced to therapies offering spiritual 'highs'. In response to its advent, Lasch believes that 'The only corrective to the ersatz religions of the New Age is a return to the real thing.'[76]

Lasch is not alone in raising this particular critique of the counter-culture and the New Age; but many commentators do not agree with his conservative approach. In his survey of the 'antinarcis-

---

71 Op. cit.: 85.
72 Christopher Lasch, 1979: 235.
73 Ken Wilber has also criticised aspects of the New Age as being narcissistic. As has been shown above, Wilber refers to a confusion of levels in his spectrum of consciousness between the prepersonal (level two is described as mythic and narcissistic) and the transpersonal.
74 Christopher Lasch, 1985: 165.
75 Christopher Lasch, 1987: 180.
76 Ibid.

sistic literature of the seventies',[77] Theodore Roszak – who contests Lasch's thesis – lists David Bell, Peter Marin, W. W. Norton, Robert Nisbit, Harvey Cox, and Edwin Schur as providing similarly conservative views.

Roszak argues that there are positive aspects to narcissism. For example, he suggests that 'for all its suspect qualities, [narcissism] may be a necessary stage in the creation of an authentic personal identity',[78] a healthy attribute without which, Roszak reports, 'we could not invest our unique self-representations with the positive feelings necessary for self-esteem and self-assertion'.[79] Roszak describes the quality of what is new in contemporary society as the

> willingness of so many to lay bare their confusion and self-doubt before the world, to reveal themselves as the antiheroes most people have always been. Even when, for lack of better means, they resort to 'psychobabble', they are telling us a great deal about weaknesses and inadequacies that may deserve more mercy than they have received from critics who would have us believe they share no such frailties.[80]

Roszak is critical of commentators such as Lasch who discredited the counter-culturalists by accusing them of being immature and frivolous[81] while not crediting the same people with doing 'a reasonably effective job of stopping the Vietnam war, unseating a corrupt president, raising issues of justice in every mainstream American institution, and in general authoring the most sweeping indictment of the nation's moral failures since the days of the muckraker'.[82]

Moreover, Roszak himself is not alone in his criticism of Lasch. Peter Clecak, for example, suggests that Lasch 'focuses primarily on the interplay between an idealized past and the fallen present'.[83] Clecak views Lasch's critique of American society as presenting a 'powerful if nearly always exaggerated characterization of the worst fea-

---

77   Theodore Roszak, 1993: 350.
78   Op. cit.: 267.
79   Op. cit.: 268. Here, Roszak is citing James Masterson.
80   Op. cit.: 272.
81   Op. cit.: 273.
82   Ibid.
83   Peter Clecak, 1983: 254.

tures of contemporary culture ... [which confuses] the vices of the times with the virtues, the peculiar excesses with the norms'.[84] By commenting on one extreme as if it were the norm, Clecak (in a similar way to Roszak) accuses Lasch of refusing to see – or, at least, failing to report[85] – the rise of many positive activities between the 1960s and 1980s, of which Clecak gives several examples including significant growth in activities to do with service to the community in American society which is, as noted in earlier chapters, a particular feature of the New Age.

Drawing on Alexander Solzhenitsyn's idea that 'Western society is outraged if an individual gives his soul as much daily attention as his grooming', Marilyn Ferguson, too, argues that critics of the New Age like Lasch who call participants narcissistic do not clearly understand the thoughtful nature of their inward search.[86]

Moreover, a social researcher criticizes Lasch for making arbitrary and incohesive descriptions of what he sees as the narcissistic personality of contemporary Americans, and notes that Lasch fails to provide any evidence that the culture of narcissism actually exists to any meaningful extent. He believes that Lasch 'is surely correct in noting a preoccupation with self as a sign of the times, but he is wrong to reduce the American quest for self-fulfilment to the pathology of narcissistic personality disorders'.[87]

While Lasch appears to be correct in highlighting the existence of narcissistic activities which developed in the counter-culture and still exist today, much of his writings refer more directly to those in American society who were at the forefront of the capitalistic boom of the 'me' decade and not, to such a great degree, with those more fully involved with New Age ideas and activities which, as Lasch himself points out in his later essay specifically on the New Age,[88] has a heightened spiritual content. My survey participants, for example, while reporting the employment of many therapies which can be used

84   Op. cit.: 252.
85   Ibid.
86   Marilyn Ferguson, 1982: 399.
87   Daniel Yankelovitch, 1981: 35.
88   Christopher Lasch, 1987.

for narcissistic – and hedonistic – purposes (aromatherapy, for one) do not consider playfulness and pleasure as a significantly important benefit of their practices, whereas they believe that heightened spirituality and meaningfulness are much more vital. In New Age healing, the concept of nurture is an important part of the spiritual process and, in this sense, pleasure itself can be therapeutic and transformational.

Nevertheless, Lasch's criticism of the counter-culture – and hence the New Age – as being narcissistic has stuck. Clearly, some of the activities and a proportion of participants may well be self-absorbed and narcissistic, although these individuals appear more likely to be associated less than fully with the principal ideas and activities. As has been outlined in Chapter 5 and again by respondents to my survey, love, not narcissism, is a key factor in the New Age; and love of one's self is seen as being a vital part of a fully inclusive and unconditional love. Without loving oneself many argue that it is not fully possible to love others – and the thought that this love might be narcissistic is one of the 'blocks' which participants would argue needs to be removed to enable a greater engagement with the basic New Age ideas. In sum, Lasch appears to want to hold on to the institutional pillars of Western society including its religious traditions for meaningfulness, security, purpose, and continuity and considers any reliance on the Higher Self to be (negatively) narcissistic, while New Age participants want to replace what they see as outmoded institutions and harmful materialism which negatively affects their lives with a more positive and heightened experiential spiritual focus.

Problems of consumerism and prosperity

a. Consumerism

Several criticisms which relate to consumerization in the New Age have been identified by Paul Heelas. One of these Heelas sees to be the commercialization of ancient wisdom teachings – for example, where 'New Agers are seen as engaging in cultural imperialism or theft [...] speeding [the teachings] up [...] and arriving at something which is user-friendly'.[89] This kind of activity also appears to occur in what some see as the inappropriate use of sacred symbols, e.g. the marketing of Celtic trinkets and bric-a-brac. From the commercial viewpoint, 'Somewhat ironically, given the elevated place of money in contemporary society, the most general way the sacred is desacralized is to turn it into a saleable commodity.'[90]

The most common criticism Heelas encounters relates to the perceived high cost of participation in New Age activities and therapies.[91] In a number of the more critical studies of the New Age, including some by Christian authors, cost of the activities is frequently mentioned as a prohibitive – and hence negative – factor in their assessment. It seems as if these authors believe that the cost of these events or activities should somehow be lower or even free. The idea of making a profit or an income out of the New Age, it transpires, is an anathema to these critics. There are examples where some fees appear high, although study of New Age magazines and leaflets shows that the average fee for a workshop is usually pitched at an affordable level – and frequently this level is one which is unlikely to make the workshop leader a rich person. Bursaries or discounts are also often available to help the less-well-off to attend. Some teachers take no fees for themselves but support particular charitable ventures – for example, Ram Dass raises funds for the Hanuman (educational) and Seva (care for the dying) Foundations.

There are, however, some workshops for psychotechnologies which are pitched at a higher price, although these, in the main, concentrate more on personal development (Human Potential Movement) than spiritual empowerment. Wade Clark Roof has found that this may have been the case previously, but now people have moved on. He argues that

---

89   Paul Heelas, 1996a: 202.
90   Russell Belk *et al.*, 1989: 23.
91   Paul Heelas, 1996a: 202.

spiritual yearnings are leading many Americans beyond the self-centered, therapeutic culture in which they grew up. Self-fulfillment as a cultural theme in the 1960s and 1970s set in motion a powerful quest, but now for a generation older and more mature that quest has moved beyond the solutions that were promised in consumption, materialism, and self-absorption.[92]

Among these psychotechnologies now can be found most management training seminars, including those held by Landmark Education International (formerly est), Jack Black,[93] and Anthony Robbins. The latter American management-training guru and entrepreneur – whose seminars include 'Unleash the Power Within Weekend' (£622/c.US$930 per person), and the one-day 'The Tools for Strategic Influence, the Power of Personal Marketing' (£293/c.US$440 per person)[94] are attended by approximately two thousand people at a time – clearly is in business to make money. It can be added that, from personal experience, the majority of fees for this type of seminar are paid not by the attendees but their employers and are tax-deductible as a business expense. Moreover, the spiritual content of some of these activities is low or even non-existent and, in this respect, they fall outside of the remit of what is considered as New Age.

Those involved in my survey, when asked to raise any negative aspects about their activities, did not view the costs involved as prohibitive. In fact, the cost of attending some New Age events was considered excessive by only five out of over 900 participants. In this case, therefore, criticisms regarding the high cost of participation and excessive consumerization that Heelas reports are unfounded.

b. Prosperity

Related to the above, Paul Heelas has also encountered criticisms which he describes as 'the way in which inner spirituality has been put

---

92   Wade Clark Roof, 1999: 9.
93   Jack Black is described by *The Guardian* as a business evangelist, Britain's number-one motivational speaker for businesses and organizations who charged £350/c.US$525 per person for a one-day seminar attended by three hundred delegates (*The Guardian Weekend*, 25 May 1996: 22ff).
94   *Changing Times*, September 1994 – February 1995: 9.

to work for the purposes of outer prosperity'[95] and builds his argument on the thesis that 'One of the great and most widely held certainties of our times is [...] that prosperity is a good thing.'[96] Moreover, Heelas suggests that 'given the undoubted importance of teachings and practices which treat inner spirituality as a means to the end of material acquisition, and given the undoubted cultural value attributed to wealth acquisition, it can safely be concluded that many get involved in the New Age for reasons to do with prosperity.'[97] Heelas believes that prosperity is mostly associated with financial wealth, yet there is no convincing evidence that many participants from my survey or who can be encountered at New Age events would go along with the view that they have become associated with the New Age to improve their material standing. On the contrary, people involved have suggested that their association is more to do with spiritual empowerment together with finding greater meaning in their lives.

Heelas suggests that there are two groups of people who become involved with the New Age and both of which are comprised of what he describes as 'middle class or higher class people whose lives are not working well'.[98] The first of Heelas's groups is comprised of those 'who have lost faith in the certainties of the capitalist mainstream',[99] while the second group is comprised of those who 'are intent on pursuing the utopian vision provided by the capitalistic system itself'.[100] There is, as has been demonstrated in Chapter 3, substantial evidence that the first group which Heelas describes is indeed New Age, although there is little evidence to suggest that the second group is at all characteristic. In fact, looking at the income levels of participants and the number of years of their involvement, it seems clear that many if not most of these individuals did not become involved with the New Age to become financially prosperous. Additionally, as has been shown, many participants work in healing or in areas of service to the

---

95   Paul Heelas, 1996a: 202. It is not specified from where most of these criticisms have arisen, although some are of Christian origin.
96   Op. cit.: 147.
97   Op. cit.: 147f.
98   Op. cit.: 137.
99   Op. cit.: 138.
100 Ibid.

community where prospects for higher than average material prosperity are poor.

It is possible that there is some confusion between activities to do with personal development and those to do with New Age spiritual empowerment. Regarding the former, some psychotechnologies are used more for commercial or utilitarian reasons, for example 'to improve relationships among employees and to step up sales'[101] (which are likely to include seminar training sessions similar to those convened by Anthony Robbins, described above) and those identified as 'new wave management tries to engineer the souls of its workers, encouraging them to see initiative and self-direction as a part of their personal identities, make them "enterprising" subjects in every sense of the word, linking their expressions of individuality with the aims of the company.'[102] The difference is marked by one academic who sees that 'the commitment of New Age humanism to unlimited personal growth, by whatever appropriate technological means, excludes the more organic view of coexistence with the natural world.'[103]

It is from capitalism that the notion of competitiveness is introduced into New Age discourse in that, as has been suggested, the company is there held to be paramount and responsibility for anything beyond its success is given scant consideration. In the New Age, it is the notion of cooperation which is all important – as highlighted, for example, by Marilyn Ferguson in her comparison of the old and new paradigms of power and politics,[104] and by Matthew Fox in his comparison of fall/redemption spirituality with creation-centred spirituality.[105] With regard to the content of seminars given by individuals such as Anthony Robbins, these are clearly based on competitive and not cooperative notions. Robbins's seminars are based on his research where

> he has set out to identify the most successful people in many walks of life and has analyzed the reasons for their success [...] His insights and convictions op-

101 Marvin Harris, 1981: 146.
102 Pat Kane, 1996: 25.
103 Andrew Ross, 1991: 70.
104 Marilyn Ferguson, 1982: 299ff.
105 Matthew Fox, 1983: 316ff.

314

erate at the very root of human motivation, giving you the determination and power to master any goal you have set yourself, whether that is losing weight, giving up smoking or making a million'.[106]

It is plain to see that there is not much that is New Age involved in what is on offer here.

With regard to New Age engagement with capitalist society, there is a movement among New Age circles to review the relationship with work and money, and hence with re-identifying what prosperity might entail. Noticeably, Alternatives in London have established a series of workshops based on the theme of 'Alternatives at Work'. Workshops have been held with such titles as 'The Money Game',[107] 'The Spiritual Laws of Success', and 'Work as an Expression of Who We Are'. The central theme of the workshops is expressed in the following way:

> One of the challenges and opportunities facing many of us is integrating the qualities of the human spirit – creativity, love, joy, inspiration, abundance, support – into our work and working lives. The Alternatives in Work programme has been created to provide training, information, ideas, inspiration and, in time, a forum for those of us interested in enjoying a feeling of greater success and harmony in work, and new definitions and success and happiness in work.[108]

William Bloom, who is also involved in the workshops, seeks a new way of looking at money, one 'which encompasses both wealth and economic justice together'.[109] Bloom finds that 'Our current financial and economic policies are not working in a creative and beneficent way [...] New ways of conceptualizing – new worldviews and paradigms – are emerging in many different arenas [which] challenge and dismantle old ways of thinking about money and economics.'[110]

---

106 Gina Lazenby, 1994: 9.
107 For purposes of comparison with illustrations given in the preceding section, the cost of this nonresidential weekend workshop was: £110 or c.US$165 average waged, £80 or c.US$120 low waged, and £45 or c.US$70 unwaged.
108 Pamphlet.
109 William Bloom, 1995b: 6.
110 Ibid.

315

Furthermore, the new thinking about money is encapsulated in the writings of Gill Edwards and Andrew Ferguson. Gill Edwards, a teacher and healer in the British New Age, summarizes what many participants might consider to be the New Age approach to prosperity. Edwards suggests that

> limiting our own wealth does not help [those living in poverty] in the slightest. It merely adds to the deprivation in the world. But if we change our own scarcity belief [...] we have reduced – by one – the number of people in the world who struggle over money; and we might choose to use some of our wealth to help others – not out of guilt, but out of love [...] I came to see the world as an abundant and joyous place to be. I no longer linked money with struggling, coveting, fearing and grasping; instead, words such as bubbling, enjoying, giving, welcoming and channelling came to my mind. My free associations about wealth changed dramatically: 'Prosperity flows through my heart as a channel of pure light – the Light of the universe, which offers me its vast abundance. It is a key which opens the doors to the wondrous possibilities in life. It is a stepping stone in my spiritual growth. Money is coming into my life easily and joyously. The more I have, the more I can enjoy and share.'[111]

Moreover, another New Age author has written at length about how the New Age transforms ways to view prosperity and to manage abundance. Like William Bloom, he argues that

> The old way clearly does not work. And a new spirit is coming through that clearly *is* working. This new spirit is more self-aware, more inclined to take personal responsibility, more concerned with personal inner growth than with monetary outer growth. It is less materialistic, less obsessed with the old definitions of success, less hostile and aggressive. And it is not nihilistic or self-effacing. It is not into poverty consciousness, vows of abstinence, turning its back on the world and the hard-won comforts of modern living. It seeks to find a correct balance between having and hoarding, power over and care for, giving and receiving, success and inadequacy.[112]

111   Gill Edwards, 1991: 66f.
112   Andrew Ferguson, 1992: 19.

The source of abundance, for this author, is the heart,[113] and he gives a forty-nine-step checklist for the practical application of his ideas.[114]

Nevertheless, words of warning regarding material improvement have been made by those influential in the New Age, thereby demonstrating that the question raised has some truth. For example, allied to the relationship between prosperity and spirituality is the idea of spiritual materialism – a notion first voiced by Chogyam Trungpa, the Tibetan teacher who founded Samye Ling in Scotland in the 1970s before moving to America – whereby spiritual ideas and activities become devalued. On this point, one writer has suggested that Trungpa's concept of spiritual materialism

> is a major contribution to the vocabulary of religious discourse [because] it cuts away the endless fog of 'human potential' speculations by which we put off being simply who we are. The term describes any form of spirituality that is practised for personal gain and self-improvement, whether through money, power, attention, purity, or bliss.[115]

In a similar vein, the poet Allen Ginsberg, who believes the New Age to be 'basically a very good thing', sees its main problem as 'accumulating experiences as "credentials for the ego"'.[116]

In summary, there appears to be little evidence from my survey to support Heelas's account of consumerism or capitalistic prosperity, and much of the literature on the subject describes prosperity as involving significantly more than purely an improvement in material standing. However, the problems involved in spiritual materialism do exist, and the whole subject links with criticisms raised by Ken Wilber with regards to trivialization and with assessing the efficaciousness of spiritual ideas and activities, both engaged with in earlier sections. The final area of criticism now addressed also links with this theme.

---

113 Op. cit.: 162.
114 Op. cit.: 182ff.
115 Stephen Butterfield, 1994: 39.
116 Allen Ginsberg cited in David Jay Brown and R. M. Novick, 1993: 269. It will be remembered from Chapter 2 above that Ginsberg was one of the influential Beat writers.

Problems of self-centredness

Paul Heelas raises one further criticism that he finds the New Age has attracted. This is to do with a self-centredness he sees to occur among some participants, where they 'are basically concerned with healing and perfecting themselves, rather than with the community or other aspects of public life'.[117] In this criticism, Heelas believes there is a strong case to argue in that 'one would expect New Agers to be doing more to improve or "transform" the quality of life at large'[118] than they actually do – and, as evidence, he points to the paucity of New Age communities which currently exist.[119]

Heelas's criticism is supported in part by evidence from my survey, although it may not be the case that the increase in the number of New Age communities – such as Findhorn in Scotland to which Heelas refers – applies in this instance. Two points arise. Firstly, my survey findings show that participants' active involvement in social concerns is low. However, a strong desire for social change has been noted although, among the three domains of ideas and activities in the New Age which have been assessed, participants appear to be more involved with their individual spiritual growth and well-being than with community concerns. Secondly, the reason why Heelas's evidence of the paucity of communities does not necessarily help his premise is because New Age activity, as I have pointed out in Chapter 8, is not in itself necessarily also a community activity – rather, first and foremost, such activity is reported by participants to represent an individual's quest for an increased spiritual and meaningful content to their lives. Furthermore, those involved would argue that if all people undertook such activities there would automatically be unity and, hence, no need for separated communities.

Where activity that might dispel the criticism of self-centredness occurs is with regards to compassionate action and service – that is, individual activity at a local, neighbourly, and family level – and some

117 Paul Heelas, 1996a: 203.
118 Ibid.
119 Op. cit.: 208.

evidence for this has been shown by my survey. In this regard and as noted above, firstly, participants' employment groups are strongly biased to the 'caring' professions and, secondly, the degree to which love and compassion in general is thought to imbue New Age ideas and activities as a whole is substantial. With regard to the latter, Peter Russell suggests that 'the enlightened person experiences a deep and universal compassion, and his life usually becomes one of service, not just service to humanity but to the whole world.'[120] While many New Age participants may not be 'enlightened beings', there does appear to be a degree of acceptance of Russell's view in the basic New Age ideas put forward by William Bloom, where he suggests that 'we are jointly responsible for the state of ourselves, of our environment and of all life.'[121] While Russell's and Bloom's ideas do not wholly answer the criticisms outlined by Heelas directly, they do point to an awareness among participants that service to the community (rather than joining a community) is part of New Age philosophy.

However, it is clear to see that the response to Russell's and Bloom's ideal is mixed. One commentator (writing in the 1970s), for example, sees that those involved in the new consciousness movement primarily come from the middle classes who, it was believed, have the time, energy, and money to devote to self-exploration and, as a consequence, be 'diverted from the more serious social problems that plague our society'.[122] In the 1980s another writer reports that

> some New Age groups teach that since people are 'responsible for' and 'create' their own reality, there is no point in giving to charity. During the massive 1985 Live Aid campaign, at least one New Age group staunchly refused to contribute any money. Although some of today's New Agers are active campaigners on issues which concern them, many have decided that a meditation or a dance will work just as well.[123]

120 Peter Russell, 1982: 140.
121 William Bloom, 1990: 13.
122 Edwin Schur, 1977: 7.
123 Rachel Storm, 1992: 194. Regarding Storm's latter point, many participants believe that distance healing is a powerful force which can be used to help transform society – Transcendental Meditation adepts use Siddhis power (the 'Maharishi effect') to much the same ends – and her use of this illustration could be misconstrued. With regards Transcendental Meditation's theories of

And Ken Wilber (writing in the mid-1990s) adds to the views given by the two writers above, in that he believes the

> 'Higher Self' camp is notoriously immune to social concerns. Everything that happens to one is said to be 'one's own choice' – the hyperagentic Higher Self is responsible for *everything* that happens – this is the monological and totally disengaged Ego gone horribly amok in omnipotent self-only fantasies. This simply *represses* the networks of communions that are just as important as agency in constituting the manifestation of Spirit.[124]

The time span of these three authors' comments demonstrates, on the one hand, a consistent criticism of the New Age since at least the end of the counter-culture with regard to its self-centred emphasis and, on the other hand, the inability of the New Age itself to dismiss such criticisms.

Summary

To sum up the criticisms discussed in this chapter, the dilemma New Age participants face has been epitomized by a group of mainly academic writers who suggest that 'more and more the meaning of human life is taken to be something that can be evaluated only by the person living the life, and this evaluation most often is based on an experiential sense of self-fulfilment or lack of self-fulfilment'[125] which they believe represents a 'strong continuity with the value shifts of the 1960s'.[126] This group points to the transference of authority from a paternalistic to an autonomous basis – to epistemological individualism – where spiritual seeking since the 1960s has primarily been

social development, the Natural Law Party – which fields candidates in political elections across the democratic world – seeks to bring about world peace and harmony through meditative activities. See also Peter Russell, 1979.
124   Ken Wilber, 1995a: 546.
125   Dick Anthony *et al.*, 1987: 7.
126   Op. cit.: 29.

320

'within one's own experience, rather than having meaning conferred externally'.[127] The result of such self-centred searching, according to these authors, is that 'autonomous authority is often extremely shallow'[128] because it lacks guidance and direction from teachers – and here it can be seen that the problems outlined above come full circle again. It seems that because there is no New Age 'institution', no observable concrete structure, its ideas and activities are particularly open to criticism relating to the difficulties incurred between what is described as the Higher Self and an individual's outer personality, the efficacy of New Age teachings, its trivialization, narcissism, and more. In fact, many leading individuals in the New Age – from Bhagwan Shree Rajneesh to Ram Dass – have emphasized the necessity of spiritual teachers, although they warn of the problems of becoming too attached to them. So the situation with regards to criticisms of, for example, self-centredness ends up as Catch-22 whereby, as reported above, 'the seekers' dilemma is how to continue to develop autonomous authority *and* to get help from someone who has a greater degree of truly autonomous authority than does the seeker ... without opening themselves up to manipulation and exploitation'.[129]

This problem may be very real for New Age participants, the majority of whom claim not to follow any one particular teacher or teaching and who appear to be comfortable learning from a variety of sources while using their intuition and experience as their primary tools for evaluating what seems right for them. Some of the criticisms made appear to have a basis in truth, although the suggestion of greater reliance on external and perhaps more visible forms of authority, which may go towards reducing the perceived individualistic nature of the New Age, appears to go against its basic ideas. In the end, there may not be a meeting point between participants and their critics because those involved are likely to respond with the argument that, as indicated above, through a connectedness to a Universal Energy, the Higher Self is not necessarily experienced in the terms expressed by the critics.

127   Op. cit.: 9.
128   Ibid.
129   Ibid.

12. Transforming the World

ours is the only culture since the world began which has not in some way held that life began in a great unity and that life on our earth plane is held by a great and living organism of spiritual being. Our arrogant age has abandoned this world-view, writing off earlier thinkers as victims of superstition. Now it begins to reawaken.

Sir George Trevelyan[1]

In concluding this study, firstly a brief review of participant involvement in the New Age is given, and this is followed by an analysis of consistencies and inconsistencies which have been found to exist between those involved and the numerous commentators and critics. Finally, I present a short overview of what the New Age embodies which is, in essence, a demand for a transformation not just of the self but of the whole world.

Recapitulation

The findings of my survey have provided a detailed account of a substantial number of New Age participants both in terms of establishing their social and demographic characteristics, their views on the New Age, and in reporting their practices. The survey did not set out to record all activities undertaken by these participants; it concentrated instead on revealing the principal aspects of their spirituality, the nature of their healing activities, and, to a lesser extent, their community activities. What has been shown is that in social and demographic

1   Sir George Trevelyan, 1997: 52.

terms those involved in the New Age, whether in North America or Britain, are broadly middle class and middle aged. The majority of participants grew up at the time of the campus-based counter-culture movement or before, and have now become an ageing generation – in fact, some of the leading counter-culturalists are becoming elderly or have died. Participants demonstrate that the turn to the New Age did not happen to any great degree during their youth but occurs more towards their early middle age, although they may have been active in areas of interest to the New Age prior to this – the prime example being concern for environmental issues. Certainly, younger participants demonstrate that they are less active in core spiritual activities of the New Age in comparison with older groups. This situation may be no different from characteristics of the total population, where certain people have a propensity for some form of spiritual content to their lives.

Participants can be found in most middle-class walks of life and cannot be clearly separated out by social and demographic methods of analysis from the general middle-class profile. Many participants are married and it must be assumed that the majority have families, yet there is also a large number of single participants – in fact, proportionally much more so than can be found generally. It is not known what kind of education participants received, although a large number of the middle-classes as a whole are university- or college- educated. There is no particular income level among which participants are most likely to be found, which means that there are both rich and poor in the New Age. Participants on the whole tend to live in mainstream society and have regular jobs, although the type of occupation they have includes many forms of service to the community, for example in health and education. Furthermore, there are many more women who claim to be involved in the New Age than men, and there appears to be a concentration of women in those activities which are to do with healing and bodywork.

Following on from this description, it becomes apparent that while many seemingly radical and unconventional practices are undertaken, participants, on the whole, do not appear to be fanatical, extremist, or eccentric in the manner in which they carry out their lives. While many are optimistic about the future, those involved demonstrate little overt political activity, as is illustrated by the low affiliation with organizations dedicated to social change; and although there appears to be a desire for greater local involvement in community concerns, action to achieve this is not particularly great. In fact, the greatest concern with regard to community activities is in terms of environmental and animal-welfare issues and not so much in social ones.

The key to an individual's approach to the New Age appears to be through personal transformation which is claimed to be established by means of a heightened awareness of an inner potentiality often, it appears, brought about by a dissatisfaction with their life, especially its spiritual content, coupled with a growing need to create change within themselves. Methods used to enact such change include teachings given in books and cassette tapes together with attendance at workshops, and networking is primarily associated with education and information-gathering.

The spirituality that participants demonstrate appears to have no fixed path in comparison to the more formalized paths of religious traditions. Yet, a great many New Age participants claim that their spiritual practice is a deeply religious experience, one which frequently draws upon both Western and Eastern traditions. However, actual membership of religious traditions and groups appears to be low and no one spiritual path suffices to satisfy participants' spiritual requirements. Christianity has been an important influence – either positively or, more likely, negatively – in most participants' lives, especially at the formative stages. Among other such influences, the turn to New Age spirituality for some is reported to have been a more psychically-oriented occurrence often approached through channelled teachings, of which there are increasing numbers. A substantial number of participants claimed multiple experience of paranormal phenomena, and many individuals claim to have contact with their own personal spirit guide or guides.

Influence of the spiritual sphere of the New Age appears to be of overall prime significance to participants, although other influences are claimed to exist and the most mentioned of these is healing. Healing for repair, which often uses techniques that can be included among New Age 'tools', has not been claimed to any great degree by participants. The situation is entirely different with regards to healing as a form of nurture. In this area, therapies for healing are reported as being widely used in participants' transformatory processes and many claim these have unblocked their 'pathways' to personal and spiritual empowerment. In healing activities alone, participants claim to have used an average of 15 such therapies and psychotechnologies. Here, creative visualization is the practice which is most used and, moreover, its use has been established in a number of ways. Community activity is also important, although less so than spiritual empowerment and healing. Relationships with other people are not significantly found in the separate communities, which are seen to perpetuate disunity. Environmental issues, as in mainstream society, appear more important than those which are principally political or economic, although these are increasingly seen to be interconnected. Those involved place greater emphasis in sorting out their private world, and we have yet to see if that effort will extend into the more public sphere to any significant degree or whether, in fact, such efforts will percolate up into mainstream society as it further adopts various New Age practices.

Consistencies and inconsistencies

a. Consistencies

1. The overall conclusion which can be drawn by comparing the views of survey participants with those expressed by many of the various commentators is that, in the main, there is remarkably little difference or conflict between the two. Through my survey findings and other field research, many of the assertions made by the commentators have been substantiated – that is, from both outside observers and from those writing from within the New Age itself. Among participants, considerable accord has been registered in many instances both in the types of activities which are undertaken and with regards to how they

view the New Age and their spirituality. Those involved concur with most, if not all, of William Bloom's six basic New Age ideas – which were themselves found to be similar to other commentators' interpretations of the New Age – and, importantly, no additions were suggested by participants. It is not productive to retrace here all of the consistencies which have been found, although points of particular interest are now raised.

2. The importance of the notion of personal transformative occurrences in the New Age cannot be overstated. Participants and many of the various commentators from David Spangler[2] to Michael York[3] alike see that transformation is a basic and significant entry point to – and an ongoing characteristic of – an individual's association with the New Age and that participation in its ideas and activities do not appear to have much substance unless such change is experienced. Transformation is more often described as involving an individual's consciousness and frequently entails an increase in the spiritual content of that person's life.

3. A particular influence on, or result of, transformative occurrences relates to how mainstream society is viewed. Here, both survey respondents and New Age writers alike appear to believe that this substantial change involves individuals coming to the view that 'old' age's capitalistic materialism lacks sufficient spiritual content, and is found to be both divisive and counterproductive in relation to developing new, more harmonious and sustainable alternatives. To many participants, the New Age represents a move towards new (or renewed) ways of approaching money, the environment, education, and the like, as described, for example, by William Bloom[4] or Jonathon Porritt.[5]

4. There also appears to be significant consistency among survey participants with regard to meeting the difficulties involved in their transformative occurrences. These events are seen to produce surmountable, yet ongoing, problems of conflict in participants' lives with regard to how New Age values can be put into practice while

2   David Spangler, 1984: 80f.
3   Michael York, 1995: 39.
4   William Bloom, 1995b.
5   Jonathon Porritt, 1996.

living in (and generally abiding by the rules of) 'old'-age society. Most participants tend to stay living within the parameters of existing society, and most New Age teachings do not advocate withdrawal from it. Each individual relies almost entirely on their own devices to cultivate a particular path by which they can live in a transformed manner within their existing society, albeit locating various elements of scaffolding (as William Bloom described) which contain and support their individualized 'journey'. This situation is described by Marilyn Ferguson, who suggests that 'when people become autonomous, their values become *internal*. Their purchases and their choice of work begin to reflect their own authentic needs and desires rather than the values imposed by advertisers, family, peers, media.'[6] Following on from Ferguson, it can be argued that because those involved tend to want to establish their own paths and values, the need for the New Age itself to have structure and institutions is diminished – in fact, most would agree that such structures appear to be counter to its overall ethos.

5. The heightened spiritual content of a participant's life incorporates a form of motivating authority which drives individuals along their chosen paths. A consistent factor expressed both by those involved and by the various commentators is that, as a result of transformation, New Age individuals are able to maintain an environment where they can develop their spirituality independent of religious traditions (although not necessarily excluding the practice of any religious tradition). This activity, if sustained, could have significant implications for religions as a whole. For example, William Bloom believes that in the future 'the great thought structures and organizations of the contemporary world religions will melt away.'[7] Bloom does not see that spirituality will diminish; far from it, he suggests that removal of structures will unblock the way to many new or renewed spiritual paths and, in the end, create a more fertile environment for spirituality to flourish.

6. The existence of three core domains of activities – spirituality, healing practices, and community activity – has not been disputed,

6   Marilyn Ferguson, 1982: 359.
7   William Bloom, 1990: 7.

although priorities of these three among individuals and commentators has been seen to vary. No commentator has proposed an alternative combination,[8] and the participants' activities which have been recorded do not generally appear to stretch beyond the parameters of the three proposed domains.

7. Finally, there appear to be consistencies in how participants have described their practices in comparison with the measures of levels and categories of association. With regard to levels of association, those surveyed seem to fall primarily into the upper segment of partial association and some into the full level of association. There exists little evidence of association among these participants at the unwitting or lower segment of partial levels (what David Spangler describes as 'glamorous' association) – in fact, the majority of participants and the various commentators appear to agree that a great deal of association with the New Age is undertaken with deliberate intent. With regard to the spectrum of categories of association proposed by Paul Heelas, participants appear to be drawn from the upper segments of harmonial categories – that is, from the mainstream-transformers and counter-culturalists – and from the world-rejecting category (interpreting world-rejection as rejection of the capitalistic mainstream), although more will be said below. Moreover, commentators such as John Drane[9] and Ben Fong-Torres[10] believe that the majority of participants are ex-counter-culturalists.

b. Inconsistencies

I. General inconsistencies

1. Christian critics and some, but not all, more objective commentators such as Robert Basil[11] and James Lewis,[12] view the New Age as

---

8   William Bloom and Mary Farrell Bednarowski both suggested a fourth domain, that of New Science, which has been stated to be beyond the remit of this study.
9   John Drane: 1991: 62.
10   Ben Fong-Torres, 1988: B5.
11   Robert Basil, 1988: 28.
12   James Lewis, 1992: 6.

an amorphous hodgepodge of activities and appear not to believe that there is much in the way of continuity or direction in its ideas and activities. This view conflicts with survey participants and New Age writers, who claim to perceive defining principles which undergird the majority of its ideas and activities and which have been encapsulated in William Bloom and David Spangler's writings. Some academics, too, believe there to be a degree of continuity in the New Age even though, as Mary Farrell Bednarowski points out, its characteristics are eclectic.[13]

2. Again from academe, Paul Heelas has suggested that two broad types of people become engaged with the New Age – those who reject the capitalistic mainstream and those who wish to make capitalism work at its optimum potential. It would appear that the latter type of person is not represented to any degree in the genre. Only one in five participants reported incomes of above £20,000 (US$32,000), and of these only one-third claimed their incomes were in excess of £30,000 (US$48,000). A large number of those involved gave their reasons for the rise of the New Age at this time to be a reaction against the institutions of capitalism and the Christian Church. Heelas's latter group of New Age participants may be drawn from what he describes as self-enhancers or self-empowerers who may be more involved with worldly personal development than with spiritual empowerment. In fact, the spirituality experienced by these groups is described by Heelas as humanistic. This view, in turn, raises a further inconsistency – related to (1) above – among commentators in their definitions of what might be considered New Age and what might not.

3. Some of the literature and descriptions of what might be contained within the New Age give the impression that a great deal of visible activity is taking place although, in practice, this is not the case. For example, less than half of participants surveyed recycle their waste or are vegetarians, few are active in political or environmental concerns, and large numbers had not attended New Age events (workshops, festivals, and the like) in the previous twelve months. In contrast, what I have found is that the vast majority of participants claim they are actively pursuing a spiritual and healing path, and currently

13   Mary Farrell Bednarowski, 1991: 215.

used on average seven activities (out of a list of 32) that can be described as New Age, and most of which can be used in the home. This suggests that New Age participation as a whole is not so much carried out in the public sphere of social engagement but privately, and primarily with regard to spiritual practices and self-healing.

II. Demographic inconsistencies

4. The research has shown that a very much larger volume of participation in the New Age is undertaken by women than by men, although this evidence is not reflected in many of the commentaries. Notable exceptions to this view are recorded in the findings of Marilyn Ferguson's 1982 survey, and by Lowell Streiker who suggests that the 'New Age [...] is largely of, by, and for women'.[14] Streiker's conclusions incorporate some, but not all, of the principal reasons that women gave for becoming involved, together with some which were not given. It can be remembered, for example, that they reported dissatisfaction with what mainstream society has to offer and claimed to find greater spiritual fulfilment in New Age ideas and activities. Streiker draws support for his views from Robert Ellwood, who has pointed out that 'The predominance of women in ecstatic, possession, mystical, and healing cults is a world-wide fact. It is as evident in Haitian voodoo, the ancient Greek Dionysiacs, and the Japanese new religions, as in the somewhat more decorous Shakers, Spiritualists, Theosophists, and Pentecostalists of America.'[15] The current numbers of women in the New Age can, at least in part, therefore be seen to be incorporated in a wider spectrum of activities and traditions to do with spirituality and healing as a whole and with which, historically, women have been more involved.

5. Following on from the inconsistency with regard to gender differences, it is further found that the characteristics of New Age practices differ between the genders; and, again, this has not been identified to any great degree prior to my survey. It is possible that the gender issues – in relation to the volume of participation and the char-

14   Lowell Streiker, 1991: 50.
15   Robert Ellwood, 1979: 68.

acteristic differences in practices – may have a major influence on the composition and direction of the New Age in total. Men do not appear to be as involved as women in healing ideas and activities, which, because such activities form a substantial part of the New Age as a whole, goes some way to explain the different volumes of participation which were recorded. Moreover, the significantly lower number of men involved may be a cause of the previously noted inconsistency involving the apparent low levels of social engagement by participants in comparison to the more private spiritual and healing practices they reportedly undertake.

These gender inconsistencies also give rise to several questions relating to what the current and longer-term consequences for the New Age might be. For example, is the spiritual content of women's and men's activities in any way comparable? Will more men take up bodywork healing practices, or will women become more involved in social concerns? To answer these questions qualitative research needs to be undertaken although, regarding the latter, the indications are (though difficult to confirm statistically) that, in a limited way, men are slowly becoming more interested in bodywork, especially where this relates directly to spiritual practice – for example, there is little current gender difference among those participants who claim to practice t'ai chi or yoga.

6. Also noted in the demographic study of those involved (and not noted by the various commentators) are the differences in the practice of New Age ideas and activities between participants of different ages. However, it is not possible to conclude from a single survey whether or not the three age/practice characteristics represent in any way a model of the progression through the types of activities a participant could be expected to engage with during the progress of her or his life. What has been shown is that New Age practices develop or change according to a participant's age – that is, unlike traditional religious practices, for example, life-long continuity of activities may be seen as another form of blockage to unrestricted spiritual development.

7. There is inconsistency in the description of the age and income of participants. In this respect, media commentators generally consider participants of the New Age to be in their youth and they are often

portrayed as New Age travellers or hippies. Taking a different view, one academic observer believes they are primarily 'young upwardly mobile urban adults'.[16] I have shown that, proportionately, there are very few young people – that is, persons under 25 years of age – active in the New Age. However, a number of commentators' views regarding the age of participants concur with my findings in that those involved are seen to be predominantly comprised of the middle-aged middle class.[17] Several of these and other commentators also imply that participants are, as another commentator suggests, 'economically comfortable'.[18] Here, I have shown that 60% of participants have incomes of under £15,000 (US$24,000), which demonstrates that a much wider spectrum of economic status exists. In fact, those involved appear to be biased, in volume terms, towards the lower income levels. From this evidence, it would seem logical to suggest that participants, in the main, follow the dictums of basic New Age ideas by reducing their materialistic pursuits. It can be remembered that when asked to mention any negative results of association with the New Age, some participants claimed to have less money; but this was, in the end, thought to be a good thing.

8. The New Age is often portrayed as a drug-oriented culture, but survey findings prove this now to be generally false. With regard to psychedelic drugs, current usage was confined to 14 out of over 900 individuals. A number of commentators[19] have given the view that they believe the influence of drug use in the New Age of the late 1980s and the 1990s has diminished. These commentators point out that, as another suggests, drug use in the New Age is 'a part of the mythology of the past'.[20] The current findings are remarkably different from similar questions asked by Marilyn Ferguson in 1977 regarding the use of psychedelic drugs. At this time, she found that over a quarter of her respondents in America were occasionally using these

---

16   Gordon Melton, 1988: 51; J. Gordon Melton *et al.*, 1990: xxx.
17   For example, Robert Basil, 1988: 10; Susan Love Brown, 1992: 90; John Drane, 1991: 62; Lowell Streiker, 1991: 46; and Ben Fong-Torres, 1988: B5.
18   Andrew Ross, 1991: 66.
19   Including Robert Basil, 1988: 27 and John Drane, 1991: 63.
20   Susan Love Brown, 1992: 95.

drugs.[21] It would appear, therefore, that the use of drugs in spiritual empowerment may have substantially declined.

III. Healing

9. It is becoming increasingly difficult to clearly delineate between what can be termed as New Age healing practices and those of the Western medical mainstream because the mainstream seems to be rapidly adopting complementary and alternative ideas and activities. One inconsistency still appears to remain between the two, however, and this is the reasons for the use of healing practices. The mainstream and some commentators remain fixed in the notion that the use of complementary practices is for repair of the body's malfunctions, yet there is little evidence to demonstrate that this is why New Age participants use the practices they do. In the New Age, healing is seen to be holistic in that its therapies are predominantly used to nurture the whole person, and it primarily approaches the causes of dis-ease rather than its symptoms or effects. Overall, it must be pointed out that there seems to be very little in the way of inconsistencies between participants and New Age writers in this regard; and Christian critics (with notable conservative exceptions) are almost silent on the matter of the role of healing in the New Age.

IV. Spirituality

10. According to many academic and Christian critics, each individual in the New Age believes they have an outer personality and a Higher Self, and these are often described as if they represent separate entities. Yet a core philosophy of the New Age seems to be that everything is interconnected, that there are no divisions. If this is the case, then it represents a substantial inconsistency between those in the New Age and their critics. Moreover, it has not been possible to arrive at a clear view of whether or to what degree participants themselves might see a separation between the two. William Bloom, in his six basic

---

21 Marilyn Ferguson, 1982: 462. It has to be remembered that the respondent's 'cultural' characteristics cannot be compared.

New Age ideas, considers what he calls the multi-dimensional inner being and the outer personality to be two aspects of a single 'invisible, inner and causal reality',[22] yet other writers regard the two as being more separate. If a basic principle of the New Age is that everything is interconnected, it would make little sense to then suggest that consciousness itself is in some way divided.

11. Continuing with the possible inconsistencies regarding the interconnected nature of the New Age, again, critics regard its spirituality to be monistic.[23] Monistic spirituality, it can be noted, is in itself divided in that what has been called the Higher Self is thought to be immanently connected with God, although the outer personality is separate. However, if the above-described argument given by Bloom is representative of the New Age, then, fundamentally, New Age spirituality need not necessarily be considered as monistic but as non-dualistic. This is also the ultimate view of Ken Wilber,[24] and of David Spangler.[25] However, the general view of several commentators who are not themselves participants in the New Age[26] is that New Age spirituality is monistic.

12. A final point of inconsistency regarding the nature of spirituality in the New Age has been raised by Matthew Fox. Fox suggests that such spirituality is not pantheistic as some Christian commentators suggest,[27] but that it is panentheistic. Fox[28] describes the difference as being that, on the one hand, pantheism relates to the notion that everything is God. In this regard, some New Age writers and participants imply their spirituality is pantheistic in that they have stated that they believe they are God, or that God is knowable. Shirley MacLaine's earlier and widely reported claims can be seen as being pantheistic although (as noted in an earlier chapter) she appears to

22   William Bloom, 1990: 13.
23   For example, Ted Peters, 1991: 59ff; James Lewis, 1992: 7. Lewis also cites Robert Ellwood as having a similar view.
24   Ken Wilber, 1990: 307ff.
25   David Spangler, 1984: 81.
26   Including Peters, Lewis and Ellwood, together with Paul Heelas, 1996a: 37; Michael Perry, 1992: 24; Michael York, 1995: 167f.
27   For example, Michael Perry, 1992: 149.
28   Matthew Fox, 1983.

have amended this view. On the other hand, Fox describes panentheism as being where God is seen to be in everything and everything can be seen to be in God. This notion is markedly different from pantheism primarily because God (or what other term is used) is seen to be very much more expansive and, therefore, also unknowable.

Following on from the above points regarding the nature of spirituality in the New Age as a whole, some academics[29] suggest that New Age spirituality is wholly immanent, which suggests a strong humanistic content. This view, by implication, does not incorporate notions of spiritual transcendence. However, New Age writers and participants alike, in the main, have described their spirituality in terms of being *both* immanent and transcendent – a notion which can be seen to go hand in hand with that of non-dualism and panentheism noted above.

Transforming the World

The New Age has been shown to have different levels of participation, and the focus of this study has been upon individuals who appear to be spiritually engaged with New Age ideas and activities and who participate in its healing practices. It is among these people that a rejection of the bases of capitalist ideology has been found. This rejection seems to be universal in the New Age. Those involved report such ideologies to be spiritually inadequate as well as divisive and exploitive, and in their place have developed a more sacral and harmonial content in their lives. The nature of this sacred content does not appear to be primarily based on a humanistic self-sacralization[30] but upon one which also incorporates the notion of connection to one Universal Energy or Divine Spirit.

The New Age has little in the way of formal structure, no institutions, and no single tradition, and there is broad agreement among par-

29 For example, Paul Heelas, 1996a: 2; Michael York, 1995: 145.
30 As Paul Heelas suggests (1996a: 160ff; also 1996b).

ticipants with the basic ideas outlined by William Bloom. Moreover, it may be said that the New Age marks a transition from one period to the next (often expressed as from the Piscean to the Aquarian Age).

In sum, many report that their current life is but one incarnation among many, occurring in an ongoing spiritual evolution or development. They suggest that by awakening to a heightened spiritual consciousness a deeper quality of love and compassion will fill their lives and eventually bring about what William Bloom calls 'a completely new planetary culture'[31] or, as David Spangler believes, 'a deeper state of communion with God'.[32]

Some critics will not agree with this description, which returns us to the difficult problem of arriving at an agreed view of what the New Age is. At its most inclusive, we can see that the New Age represents a religiously-oriented spiritual momentum which voices discontents with Western religious traditions while apparently not being wholly able or willing completely to adopt Eastern traditions, or ancient wisdoms, or new teachers in their place. Individualized, eclectic mixtures selected from all that is available are thus produced: these spiritualities are not static but continue to develop. The ideas involved affect practically all areas of life in society for participants. What is more, there appears to be very little that is completely new in the New Age, whereas there is a great deal that is renewed, albeit assisted by what is claimed to be the much stronger influx of Cosmic (God-given) energies at this present time.

It seems highly unlikely, for the present at least, that adoption of the New Age as described here will become widespread because such change requires significant upheaval – New Age activities are reported to entail concerted endeavour requiring regular and even disciplined practice. As a consequence, they are not without their problems, especially where the forces of capitalism are strong. It seems not to be the case, as has been suggested,[33] that all a person has to do to engage with the New Age is participate, because a greater commitment is required of those who wish to become fully involved: nor, however,

---

31   William Bloom, 1990: 14.
32   David Spangler, 1984: 84.
33   See Paul Heelas, 1996a: 173.

does joining involve a form of religious conversion. There is a middle path between the two in the form of a transformation of consciousness, often described as an awakening, which incorporates both the immanent and the transcendent – not just the former. Individuals claim to undergo this transformation on their own and are not necessarily supported by any particular sets of beliefs or external authority: although such institutional influences can play a substantial part in the transformation, they may not be essential to it. Healing practices (particularly spiritual and psychological), however, seem to play an intrinsic part.

It may well be the case that this transformation is existential, although this is not an existentiality which creates a fearful anguish because, through the notion of interconnectedness, participants claim not to experience isolation.[34]

The New Age individual is said to be led and healed by the Higher Self, which is believed to be intimately connected with – if not a part of or the same as – God. The evident difference between New Age spirituality and Western religious traditions, therefore, mostly centres on the source of spiritual authority. In the New Age, ultimately there is little sense of separation from God – God is not Other.

Turning to the relationship between the New Age and the Western world at large, mainstream – that is, primarily capitalist – culture is viewed as picking over what has been developing in the counterculture and the New Age and absorbing those practices which best suit its purposes in terms of profitability or profit-potential. The majority of the cherry-picking revolves around humanistic psychotechnologies that have been successful in increasing *managed* human potential and which contain little in the way of spirituality. Environmental and health concerns have been only grudgingly accepted by the mainstream, which sees such changes as unnecessary and costly. It appears certain that, given free reign, capitalist society would remain competitive and mechanistic in terms of its use of the planet and its view of health.

---

34   This notion may be similar to some existential theistic beliefs, for instance those of Søren Kierkegaard, 1941.

On a more positive note, an element of the core New Age values of harmony and cooperation may have penetrated the capitalistic mainstream. Moreover, with regards to environmental concerns, there appears to be only a narrow ideological gap between notions for deep ecology – seen by many as the balance and harmony of human and non-human life – with that of a sacred interconnected energy which is claimed to exist in the New Age; there is cooperation and harmony, not competitiveness and division between the two schools of thought.

And finally, while many New Age ideas and activities have penetrated to the heart of Western society, it is not possible to predict whether the New Age represents a generational occurrence which will naturally decline or a perennial phenomenon which will, after decreasing in influence, reappear at another time. It is the New Age hope, however that its core values will be sustained, if not snowball, without any such decline. Pre-eminent among these values is that of love, as it is love that participants see to be the driving force behind all other values.

Clearly many problems face those involved in their attempts to establish what exactly they can accept as being valuable and what they might discard from all that is contained within the 'old' age. In the end, however, participants demonstrate that the New Age represents a new, or renewed, way of life – a means for transformation of the self and, as the ideas and activities penetrate upwards, of the world – which they believe marks a significant improvement on what the mainstream has to offer.

Appendix: Survey Questions

Q1. Do you believe we are entering a new era, or do you think the existing era is still continuing to develop? Q2. Do you see New Age activities as new, ancient, or a mixture of both? Q3. In a few words please describe what you think the New Age is. Q4. Do you believe there has been a rise in New Age ideas and activities in the last few years? If your answer is yes, please give your views on what might be causing this rise.

Q5. To what degree do you see the New Age is involved with: spiritual affairs, holism, feeling good, healing, personal transformation, and ecology? Q6. Do you consider that all New Age ideas and activities always include at least some notion of God or an Eternal/Divine Spirit? Q7. Do you believe that there can exist the concept of a separate theistic God – as in Christianity, Judaism, and Islam – in New Age ideas and activities? Q8. Would you agree or disagree with the statement: 'Without a heightened degree of love there would be no New Age'? Q9. In a few words, describe what you mean when you use the word 'spirituality'. Q10. In your opinion, are there varying types of spirituality – e.g. New Age spirituality, Christian spirituality – or is spirituality universally the same?

Q11. Would you consider yourself to be a spiritual person? Q12. Are you actively pursuing a spiritual path? Q13. Do you meditate? If so, how often? Q14. What spiritual discipline(s) or teaching has had the greatest influence on your life? Q15. Can spirituality be described as a human experience and, if so, is it a human emotion? Please give the reason for your answer. Q16. Would you describe spirituality as the highest human emotion? Q17. Do you believe that spirituality can be experienced without love, or is love always present in spirituality?

Q18. Have you ever participated in or used any of the following? Also, what of the following are you currently engaged in?: Acupuncture/Shiatsu, Alexander Technique, Aromatherapy, Buddhism, Channelling, Colour Therapy, Creative Visualization, Crystals, Dance

Therapy, Earth Mysteries, Ethical Investing, Flower Remedies, Green Politics, Healing Workshops, Herbalism, Homoeopathy, Hypnotherapy, Massage, Neurolinguistic Programming, Past Life Therapy, Psychotherapy, Rebirthing, Reflexology, Recycling, Shaman/Pagan Rituals, Sound Therapy, Spiritualism, T'ai Chi Ch'uan/Yoga, Transactional Analysis, Veganism, Vegetarianism, Women's Studies Groups. Q19. Have you participated in or used any other New Age activities or products not listed above?

Q20. Have you ever had a psychic or astrological reading? If yes, what type(s) of reading have you had? At what frequency do you have a reading? Q21. Why have you had these readings? Q22. Have you experienced any forms of Psi (paranormal phenomena)? If so, have you experienced: Clairvoyance, Cosmic Intelligence, Past Life, Precognition, Psychokinesis, Clairaudience, Synchronicity, or Telepathy? Have you experienced any other forms of Psi?

Q23. Have you ever attended a New Age type workshop, lecture, exhibition/festival, or retreat? How many of each have you attended in the past 12 months? Q24. What amount in total would you estimate that you have spent on activities and treatments which can broadly be called New Age in the last 12 months?

Q25. Do you follow a particular New Age teacher or teaching? If yes, which is this? Q26. Do you follow more than one teaching at the same time? Q27. Describe what in particular made you adopt the New Age ideas or practices which you have? Q28. In what way would you say that adopting New Age ideas and practices might have positively changed your life, was there no change, or has it become more spiritual, more self-empowered, happier, more meaningful, more pleasurable, more responsible, more playful, more healed, or more fulfilled? Have there been any other positive changes? Q29. Describe any negative changes there have been.

Q30. If you have adopted New Age ideas or practices, how long has this been for? Q31. On a scale of 0 to 9, to what extent do you consider yourself to be 'green'? Q32. Are you optimistic or pessimistic about the future of humankind on this planet? Q33. Is the move to a sustainable society desirable or not desirable? Q34. Do you believe it will be possible to achieve a fully sustainable society within the existing social and political system? Q35. Which is a better political system, representative democracy or a democratic system in which more people participate? Q36. Do you believe PR (proportional representation) is the fairest system? Is it the best system? If no, what do you think is the best system? Q37. Are you a member of, or do you contribute to, any pressure group or alternative political organization? State which. Q38. Have you ever taken, or do you currently use, cannabis or psychedelic drugs?

Q39. Do you share your values and interests with others or do you keep them more to yourself? Q40. Name individuals whose ideas have had an important influence on your life, firstly by contact with them and, secondly, through their writings. Q41. Approximately how many books have you read on New Age or related subjects? Q42. Do you read any New Age magazines? If yes, which ones? Q43. How many people read your copy of *Kindred Spirit*?

Are you male or female, partnered or single? What is your age group? What is the first part of your postcode? What is your approximate annual income? What is your occupation?

Bibliography

Adler, Margot. 1986 *Drawing Down the Moon*. Boston, Mass.: Beacon Press.

Ahern, Geoffrey. 1990 'Spiritual/Religious Experience in Modern Society' in *Religion Today* 6.1, 4–6.

Akong, Rinpoche Dharma-Arya. 1987 *Taming the Tiger*. Eskdalemuir, Scotland: Dzalendara.

Albanese, Catherine L. 1990 *Nature Religion in America: From the Algonkian Indians to the New Age*. Chicago: University of Chicago Press.

——1992 'The Magical Staff: Quantum Healing in the New Age' in *Perspectives on the New Age*. (eds) James R. Lewis and J. Gordon Melton. New York: State University of New York Press, 68–84.

Alexander, Kay. 1992 'Roots of the New Age' in *Perspectives on the New Age*. (eds) James R. Lewis and J. Gordon Melton. New York: State University of New York Press, 30–47.

Anthony, Dick and Ecker, Bruce. 1987 'The Anthony Typology: A Framework for Assessing Spiritual and Consciousness Groups' in *Spiritual Choices: The Problems of Recognizing Authentic Paths to Inner Transformation*. (eds) Dick Anthony, Bruce Ecker, and Ken Wilber. New York: Paragon House, 35–105.

Anthony, Honor M. 1987 'Some Methodological Problems in the Assessment of Complementary Therapy' in *Statistics in Medicine* 6, 761–771.

Assagioli, Roberto. 1980 *Psychosynthesis: A Manual of Principles and Techniques*. Wellingborough, Northants: Turnstone.

Bach, Richard. 1994 *Jonathan Livingstone Seagull*. London: Harper Collins.

Badiner, Allan (ed.). 1990 *Dhamma Gaia: A Harvest of Essays in Buddhism and Ecology*. Berkeley, California: Paralax Press.

Barker, Eileen. 1989 *New Religious Movements: A Practical Introduction*. London: HMSO.

Basil, Robert (ed.). 1988 *Not Necessarily the New Age: Critical Essays*. New York: Prometheus Books.

Bastick, Tony. 1982 *Intuition: How we think and act*. Chichester: Wiley.

Bednarowski, Mary Farrell. 1991 'Literature of the New Age: A Review of Representative Sources' in *Religious Studies Review* 17.3, 209–216.

——1992 'The New Age Movement and Feminist Spirituality' in *Perspectives on the New Age*. (eds) James R. Lewis and J. Gordon Melton. New York: State University of New York, 167–178.

——1995 *New Religions and the Theological Imagination in America*. Bloomington, Indiana: Indiana University Press.

Belk, R. W., Wallendorf, M. W., and Sherry, J. F., jr. 1989 'The Sacred and the Profane in Consumer Behaviour: Theodicy on the Odyssey' in *Journal of Consumer Research* 16, 1–38.

Benner, David G. 1989 'Towards a Psychology of Spirituality: Implications for Personality and Psychotherapy' in *Journal of Psychology and Christianity* 8, 19–30.

Bennett, T. S. 1994 'Brain Laterality' in *Encyclopaedia of Psychology*. Ed. R. J. Corsini. New York: John Wiley, *s. v.*

Benor, Daniel J. 1995 'Spiritual Healing: A Unifying Influence in Complementary Therapies' in *Complementary Therapies in Medicine* 3, 234–238.

Berry, Wendell. 1991 'Out of your Car, off your Horse' in *The Atlantic Monthly* February 1991, 61–63.

Bloom, William. 1990 *Sacred Times: A New Approach to Festivals.* Forres, Scotland: Findhorn Press.

——(ed.) 1991 *The New Age: An Anthology of Essential Writings.* London: Rider.

——1995a *The Christ Sparks: The Inner Dynamics of Group Consciousness.* Forres, Scotland: Findhorn Press.

——1995b *Money, Heart and Mind: Financial Well-Being for People and Planet.* London: Viking.

——(ed.) 2000 *Holistic Revolution: The Essential Reader.* London: Allen Lane.

Bookchin, Murray. 1985 'Radical Social Ecology: A Basic Overview' in *Harbinger* 1.3, 26–38.

——1990 *Remaking Society: Pathways to a Green Future.* Boston, Mass.: South End Press.

Brady, Kate and Considine, Mike. 1990 *Holistic London.* London: Brainwave.

Bramwell, Anna. 1994 *The Fading of the Greens: The Decline of Environmental Politics in the West.* London: Yale University Press.

Brierley, Peter and Hiscock, Val, (eds) 1993 *UK Christian Handbook 1994/95.* London: Christian Research Association.

British Medical Association. 1993 *Complementary Medicine: New Approaches to Good Practice.* Oxford: Oxford Paperbacks.

Bro, Harmon Hartzell. 1993 'New Age Spirituality: A Critical Appraisal' in *New Age Spirituality: An Assessment.* (ed.) Duncan S. Ferguson. Louisville, Kentucky: John Knox Press, 169–195.

Brown, David Jay and Novick, Rebecca McClen. 1993 *Mavericks of the Mind: Conversations for the New Millennium.* Freedom, California: The Crossing Press.

Brown, Michael F. 1997 *The Chaneling Zone: American Spirituality in an Anxious Age.* Cambridge, Mass.: Harvard University Press.

Brown, Susan Love. 1992 'Baby Boomers, American Character, and the New Age: A Synthesis' in *Perspectives on the New Age*. (eds) James R. Lewis and J. Gordon Melton. New York: State University of New York Press, 87–96.

Bruce, Steve (ed.). 1992 *Religion and Modernization*. Oxford: Clarendon Press.

——1995 *Religion in Modern Britain*. Oxford: Oxford University Press.

——1996 *Religion in the Modern World: From Cathedrals to Cults*. Oxford: Oxford University Press.

——1998 'Good Intentions and Bad Sociology: New Age Authenticity and Social Roles' in *Journal of Contemporary Religion* 13.1, 23–35.

Bush, Clive. 1996 '"Why do we always say angel?": Herbert Huncke and Neal Cassidy' in *The Beat Generation Writers*. (ed.) A. Robert Lee. London: Pluto, 129.

Butterfield, Stephen T. 1994 *The Double Mirror: A Skeptical Journey into Buddhist Tantra*. Berkeley, California: North Atlantic Books.

Button, John. 1990 *Green Pages: A Directory of Natural Products, Services, Resources and Ideas*. London: Optima.

Button, John and Bloom, William. 1992 *The Seeker's Guide: A New Age Resource Book*. London: Aquarian.

Campbell, Colin. 1999 'The Easternization of the West' in *New Religious Movements: Challenge and Response*. (eds) Wilson, Bryan and Cresswell, Jamie. Routledge: London, 34–48.

Campbell, Eileen and Brennan, J. H. 1990 *The Aquarian Guide to the New Age*. Wellingborough, Northants: Aquarian Press.

Cant, Sarah L. and Sharma, Ursula. 1996 'Professionalization of Complementary Medicine in the United Kingdom' in *Complementary Therapies in Medicine* 4, 157–162.

Capra, Fritjof. 1984 *The Turning Point: Science, Society, and the Rising Culture*. London: Flamingo.

——1988 *The Tao of Physics*. London: Flamingo.

——1993 'A Systems Approach to the Emerging Paradigm' in *The New Paradigm in Business: Emerging Strategies for Leadership and Organizational Change*. (eds) Michael Ray and Alan Rinzer. New York: Jeremy P. Tarcher, 230–237.

——1997 *The Web of Life: A New Synthesis of Mind and Matter*. London: Flamingo.

Cave, David. 1993 *Mircea Eliade's Vision for a New Humanism*. New York: Oxford University Press.

Chandler, Cynthia K., J. M. Holden, and C. A. Kolander. 1992 'Counseling for Spiritual Wellness: Theory and Practice' in *Journal of Counseling and Development* 71.2, 168–175.

Chistie, Hakim G. M. 1988 *The Traditional Healer: A Comprehensive Guide to the Principles and Practices of Unani Herbal Medicine.* Wellingborough: Thorsons.

Chopra, Deepak. 1996 *The Seven Spiritual Laws of Success: A Practical Guide to the Fulfilment of your Dreams.* London: Bantam.

——1997 *The Path to Love: Spiritual Lessons for Creating the Love You Need.* London: Rider.

Chow, Effie Poy Yew. 1985 'Traditional Chinese Medicine: A Holistic System' in *Alternative Medicines: Popular and Policy Perspectives.* (ed.) Salmon, J. Warren. New York: Tavistock, 114–137.

Clark, David K. and Geisler, Norman L. 1992 *Apologetics in the New Age: A Christian Critique of Pantheism.* Grand Rapids, Michigan: Baker Book House.

Clark, John. 1986 *The Anarchist Movement: Reflections on Culture, Nature, and Power.* Montreal: Black Rose Books.

Clecak, Peter. 1983 *America's Quest for the Ideal Self: Dissent and Fulfilment in the 60s and 70s.* New York: Oxford University Press.

Coulter, Harris L. 1985 'Homoeopathy' in *Alternative Medicines: Popular and Policy Perspectives.* (ed.) Salmon, J. Warren. New York: Tavistock, 57–79.

Course in Miracles, A. 1985 London: Arkana.

Coward, Rosalind. 1989 *The Whole Truth: The Myth of Alternative Health.* London: Faber & Faber.

Craig, Erik. 1992 'Self as Spirit, Self as Miracle, Self as Other' in *The Humanist Psychologist* 20.1, 18–32.

Creedon, Jeremiah. 1998 'God with a Million Faces' in *Utne Reader* 88, 42–48.

Crowley, Vivianne. 1994 *Phoenix from the Flame: Pagan Spirituality in the Western World.* London: Aquarian.

Cumbey, Constance E. 1983 *The Hidden Dangers of the Rainbow.* Shreveport, Louisiana: Huntington House.

Cupitt, Don. 1984 *The Sea of Faith.* London: BBC.

——1993 'From Dogma to Therapy' in *Resurgence.* 157, 4–7.

Curtis, Jim. 1993 *Rock Eras: Interpretations of Music and Society 1954–1984.* Bowling Green, Ohio: Bowling Green State University Popular Press.

Dass, Ram. 1971 *Be Here Now.* San Cristobel, New Mexico: Lama Foundation.

——1979 *Miracle of Love: Stories about Neem Keroli Baba.* New York: Dutton.

Dass, Ram and Bush, Mirabai. 1992 *Compassion in Action: Social and Spiritual Growth and Healing on the Path of Service.* London: Rider.

Dass, Ram and Gorman, Paul. 1994 *How can I help?: Emotional support and spiritual inspiration for those who care for others*. London: Rider.

Davie, Douglas G. (comp.) 2000 *Signposts to Sathya Sai Speaks Vols 1–6* Prashanthi Nilayam, India: Sri Sathya Sai Baba Books and Publications Trust.

Devall, Bill and Sessions, George. 1985 *Deep Ecology: Living as if Nature Mattered*. Salt Lake City, Utah: Peregrine Smith.

Dossey, Larry. 1989 *Recovering the Soul: A Scientific and Spiritual Search*. New York: Bantam.

——1993 'Science and Healing' in *Resurgence* 161, 21–25.

——1994 'God in the Laboratory' in *Caduceus* 24.

Douthwaite, Richard. 1992 *The Growth Illusion*. Dublin: Lilliput Press.

Drane, John. 1991 *What is the New Age saying to the Church?* London: Marshall Pickering.

Drury, Nevill. 1989 *The Elements of Human Potential*. Dorset: Element Books.

——1994 *Echoes from the Void*. Bridport, Dorset: Prison.

Durkheim, Emile. 1947 *The Division of Labour in Society*. Trans. G. Simpson. New York: Macmillan.

——1951 *Suicide. A Study in Sociology*. Trans. J. A. Spaulding and G. Simpson. Free Press of Glencoe.

——1953 *Sociology and Philosophy*. Trans. D. F. Pocock. Free Press of Glencoe.

Edwards, Gill. 1991 *Living Magically – A New Vision of Reality*. London: Piatkus.

Elkins, D. N. *et al.* 1984 'Towards a Humanistic-Phenomenological Spirituality: Definitions, Description, and Measurement' in *Journal of Humanistic Psychology* 28.4, 5–18.

Ellwood, Robert. 1979 *Alternative Altars: Unconventional and Eastern Spirituality in America*. Chicago: University of Chicago Press.

——1992 'How New is the New Age?' in *Perspectives on the New Age*. (eds) James R. Lewis and J. Gordon Melton. New York: State University of New York Press, 59–67.

Emslie, Margaret, Campbell, Marion, and Walker, Kim. 1996 'Complementary therapies in a local healthcare setting. Part 1: Is there really public demand?' in *Complementary Therapies in Medicine* 4, 39–42.

English-Lueck, June Anee. 1990 *Health in the New Age: A Study in California Holistic Practices*. Albuquerque: University of New Mexico Press.

Ferguson, Andrew. 1992 *Creating Abundance: How to bring Wealth and Fulfilment into your Life*. London: Piatkus.

Ferguson, Duncan S. (ed.) 1993 *New Age Spirituality: An Assessment*. Louisville, Kentucky: John Knox Press.

Ferguson, Marianne. 1995 *Women and Religion*. Englewood Cliffs, NJ: Prentice Hall.

Ferguson, Marilyn. 1982 *The Aquarian Conspiracy: Personal and Social Transformation in the 1980s*. London: Routledge & Keegan Paul.

——1994 'What ever happened to the Age of Aquarius?' in *Kindred Spirit* 3.4, 14–16.

Feuerstein, Georg. 1990 *Encyclopedic Dictionary of Yoga*. London: Unwin.

——1992 *Holy Madness: The Shock Tactics and Radical Teachings of Crazy-Wise Adepts, Holy Fools, and Rascal Gurus*. New York: Arkana.

——1997 'To light a candle in a dark age' in *What is Enlightenment?* 12 at http://wie.org/s12/feuerstein.asp.

Fong-Torres, Ben. 1988 'Journey into the New Age' in *San Francisco Chronicle* 24/4/88.

Foster, Edward Halsey. 1992 *Understanding the Beats*. University of South Carolina Press.

Fox, Matthew. 1979 *A Spirituality Named Compassion and the Healing of the Global Village, Humpty Dumpty and Us*. Minneapolis, Minnesota: Winston Press.

——1983 *Original Blessings: A Primer in Creation Spirituality*. Santa Fe, New Mexico: Bear.

——1988 *The Coming of the Cosmic Christ*. San Francisco: Harper & Row.

——1991 *Creation Spirituality: Liberating Gifts for the People of the Earth*. San Francisco: Harper & Row.

——1992 'Creation Spirituality' in *Resurgence* 154, 24–28.

——1993 'Spirituality for a New Age' in *New Age Spirituality: An Assessment*. (ed.) Duncan S. Ferguson. Louisville, Kentucky: John Knox Press, 196–219.

Freud, Sigmund. 1970 'Civilization and its Discontents' in *The Standard Edition of the Complete Psychological Works of Sigmund Freud*. Trans. J Strachey *et al*. London: Hogarth Press.

Fulder, Stephen J. and Munro, Robin E. 1985 'Complementary Medicine in the United Kingdom: Patients, Practitioners, and Consultations' in *The Lancet* 7/9/85, 542–545.

Fuller, Robert C. 1989 *Alternative Medicine and American Religious Life*. New York: Oxford University Press.

Gallup Political and Economic Index. 1989, 352.

—— 1993, 391.

—— 1995, 415.

Gallup, George jr and Castelli, Jim. 1989 *The People's Religion: American Faith in the 1990s*. New York: Macmillan.

Gandhi, Mohandas K. 1993 *An Autobiography - The Story of My Experiments with Truth*. Trans. Mahadev Desai. Boston: Beacon Press.

Gawain, Shakti. 1985 *Creative Visualization*. New York: Bantam.

——1993 *The Path of Transformation: How Healing Ourselves Can Change The World.* Mill Valley, California: Nataraj.

Gerber, Richard. 1988 *Vibrational Medicine.* Santa Fe, New Mexico: Bear.

Gerlach, Luther P. and Hine, Virginia H. 1973 *Lifeway Leap: The Dynamics of Change in America.* Minneapolis: University of Minnesota Press.

——1979 *People, Power, Change: Movements of Social Transformation.* Indianapolis: Bobbs-Merrill Educational Publishing.

Gettings, Fred. 1990 *The Arkana Dictionary of Astrology.* London: Arkana.

Gillman, Harvey. 1994 *A Light That Is Shining.* London: Quaker Home Service.

Ginsberg, Allen. 1996 *Indian Journals March 1962–May 1963.* New York: Grove Press.

Godman, David (ed.). 1985 *Be As You Are: The Teachings of Sri Ramana Maharshi.* London: Arkana.

Gordon-Brown, Ian and Sommers, Barbara. 1988 'Transpersonal Psychotherapy' in *Innovative Therapy in Britain.* (eds) John Rowan and Windy Dryden. Milton Keynes: Open University Press, 227–249.

Graham, H. 1990 *Time, Energy, and the Psychology of Healing.* London: Jessica Kingsley.

Graham, Helen. 1991 'The Return of the Shaman: the Emergence of a Bio-psychosocial Approach to Health and Healing' in *Complementary Medical Research* 5.3, 165–171.

Griffiths, Bede. 1982 *The Marriage of East and West.* London: Collins.

Grof, Christina and Grof, Stanislav. 1991 *The Stormy Search for the Self: Understanding and Living with Spiritual Emergency.* London: Mandala.

Groothuis, Douglas. 1988 *Confronting the New Age: How to Resist a Growing Religious Movement.* Illinois: InterVarsity Press.

Grossinger, Richard. 1990 *Planet Medicines: From Stone Age Shamanism to Post-Industrial Healing.* Berkeley, California: North Atlantic Books.

——1995 *Planet Medicine: Origins.* Berkeley, California: North Atlantic Books.

Guiley, Rosemary Ellen. 1991 *Encyclopaedia of Mystical and Paranormal Experience.* London: Grange.

Haga, Manabu and Kisala, Robert J. 1995 'The New Age in Japan' in *Japanese Journal of Religious Studies* 22.3–4, 235–241.

Hanegraaf, Wouter J. 1996 *New Age Religion and Western Culture: Esotericism in the Mirror of Secular Thought.* Leiden, The Netherlands: E. J. Brill.

Hardy, Alister. 1979 *The Spiritual Nature of Man.* Oxford: Clarendon Press.

Harman, Willis, W. 1991 'Metanoia' in *The New Age: An Anthology of Essential Writings.* (ed.) William Bloom. London: Rider, 18–19.

——1993 'Approaching the Millennium: Business as a vehicle for Global Transformation' in *The New Paradigm in Business: Emerging Strate-*

gies for Leadership and Organizational Change. (eds) Michael Ray and Alan Rinzer New York: Jeremy P. Tarcher/Perigee Books, 281–288.

Harner, Michael. 1990 *The Way of the Shaman.* San Francisco: Harper.

Harper, Clifford. 1987 *Anarchy: A Graphic Guide.* London: Camden Press.

Harris, Marvin. 1981 *America Now: The Anthropology of a Changing Culture.* New York: Touchstone.

Harris, Melvin. 1988 'Past-Life Regression: The Grand Illusion' in *Not Necessarily the New Age: Critical Essays.* (ed.) Robert Basil. New York: Prometheus Books, 130–144.

Harris, R. 1988 *Language, Saussure and Wittgenstein: How to play Games with Words.* London: Routledge.

Harvey, Graham. 1993 *'Gods Within: A Critical Guide to the New Age,* Michael Perry' (review) in *Theology* 96, 240–241.

Hawken, Paul. 1994 'Ecology is a Serious Business' in *Resurgence* 163, 16–19.

Hay, Louise L. 1988 *You Can Heal Your Life.* London: Eden Grove.

Heelas, Paul. 1996a *The New Age Movement: The Celebration of the Self and the Sacralization of Modernity.* Oxford: Blackwell.

——1996b 'On Things Not being Worse, and the Ethics of Humanity' in *Detraditionalization.* (eds) Paul Heelas, Scott Lash and Paul Morris. Oxford: Blackwell, 200–222.

——1999 'Prosperity and the New Age Movement: The Efficacy of Spiritual Economics' in *New Religious Movements: Challenge and Response.* (eds) Bryan Wilson and Jamie Cresswell. London: Routledge, 51–77.

Hewitt, James. 1983 *The Complete Yoga Book.* London: Leopard Books.

Hexham, Irving. 1992 'The Evangelic Response to the New Age' in *Perspectives on the New Age.* (eds) James R. Lewis and J. Gordon Melton. New York: State University of New York Press, 152–164.

Issel, William. 1985 *Social Change in the United States 1945–1983.* Basingstoke, Hants.: Macmillan.

Jacobs, Michael. 1996 *The Politics of the Real World: Meeting the New Century.* London: Earthscan.

Jacoby, Russell. 1995 'Christopher Lasch (1932–1994)' in *Telos.* No. 97, 121–123.

James, William. 1952 *The Varieties of Religious Experience: A Study in Human Nature.* London: Longmans, Green & Co.

John Paul II, Pope. 1994 *Crossing the Threshold of Hope.* London: Cape.

Jung, Carl G. 1921 *Psychological Types.* Vol. 6 of *The Collected Works of Carl G. Jung.* Trans. R. F. C. Hull. Bollingen Series, XX. NJ: Princeton University Press.

——1971 *Memories, Dreams, Reflections.* London: Fontana.

——1976 *The Portable Jung.* (ed.) Joseph Campbell. New York: Penguin.

Kane, Pat. 1996 'The Company We Keep' in *The Guardian Weekend.* 25 May 1996.

Kaplan, E. Ann. 1987 *Rocking Around the Clock: Music Television, Postmodernism, and Consumer Culture.* London: Routledge.

Karl, Frederick R. and Hamalian, Leo (eds). 1973 *The Existential Imagination.* London: Picador.

Kerouac, Jack. 1971 'The Origins of the Beat Generation' in *A Casebook on the Beat.* (ed.) Thomas Parkinson. New York: T. Y. Crowell, 68–76.

Kierkegaard, Søren. 1941 *Concluding Unscientific Postscript.* Trans. D. F. Swanson. New Jersey: Princeton University Press.

King, Ursula. 1980 *Towards a New Mysticism: Teilhard de Chardin and Eastern Religions.* London: Collins.

Kinney, Jay. 1998 'The New Age Trajectory' in *Gnosis* 49, 15–16.

Kinsley, David. 1995 *Ecology and Religion: Ecological Spirituality in Cross-Cultural Perspective.* Englewood Cliffs, NJ: Prentice Hall.

Kovel, Joel. 1978 *A Complete Guide to Therapy.* London: Penguin.

——1990 'Human Nature, Freedom, and Spirit' in *Renewing the Earth: The Promise of Social Ecology.* (ed.) J. Clark. London: Green Print, 137–152.

——1991 *History and Spirit: An Enquiry into the Philosophy of Liberation.* Boston: Beacon Press.

Koziell, Sophie Poklewski. 1999 'Two Women of the Soil' in *Resurgence* 195, 36–38.

Krippner, Stanley. 1988 'Shamans: The First Healers' in *Shaman's Path: Healing, Personal Growth, and Empowerment.* (ed.) G. Doore. Boston, Mass.: Shambhala, n.p.

Krishnamurti, Jiddu. 1974 *The Penguin Krishnamurti Reader.* (comp.) M. Lutyens. London: Penguin.

——1987 *Krishnamurti to Himself: His Last Journal.* London: Gollancz.

——1995 'Out of Silence Look and Listen' in *Krishnamurti Foundation Trust Bulletin* 69, 2–16.

Krus, David J. and Harold S. Blackman. 1980 'Contributions to Psychohistory: V. East–West Dimensions of Ideology Measured by Transtemporal Cognitive Matching' in *Psychological Reports* No. 47, 947-55.

Laquey, Tracy. 1994 *The Internet Companion: A Beginner's Guide to Global Networking* (2nd Edition). Reading, Mass.: Editorial Inc.

Lao Tsu. 1976 *Tao Te Ching.* Trans. Gia-Fu Feng and Jane English. London: Wildwood House.

Lasch, Christopher. 1979 *The Culture of Narcissism.* London: Abacus.

——1985 *The Minimal Self: Psychic Survival in Troubled Times.* London: Pan.

——1987 'Soul of a New Age' in *Omni* 10.1, 73–85, 180.

———1995 *The Revolt of the Elites and the Betrayal of Democracy.* New York: W. W. Norton.

Lawrence, Ethel (ed.). 1985 *Annual Abstract of Statistics No. 121.* London: HMSO.

Lazenby, Gina. 1994 'Firewalking: The Ultimate Motivator' in *Changing Times* Launch Issue, 9.

Lee, A. Robert. (ed). 1996 *The Beat Generation Writers.* London: Pluto.

Levine, Frederick E. 1989 'Results of the Body, Mind and Spirit Spirituality Survey' in *Body, Mind and Spirit* May/June, 83, 111–112.

Lewis, James R. 1992 'Approaches to the Study of the New Age Movement' in *Perspectives on the New Age.* (eds). James R. Lewis and J. Gordon Melton. New York: State University of New York Press, 1–12.

Lewis, James R. and Melton, J. Gordon (eds). 1992 *Perspectives on the New Age.* New York: State University of New York Press.

Linn, Denise. 1994 *Past Lives, Present Dreams: How to Use Reincarnation for Personal Growth.* London: Piatkus.

Lipnack, Jessica and Stamps, Jeffrey. 1982 *Networking: The First Report and Directory.* New York: Dolphin.

Long, J. Bruce. 1987 'Love' in *Encyclopaedia of Religion.* Ed. Mircea Eliade. New York: Macmillan, *s. v.*

Lovelock, James. 1991 *Gaia: The Practical Science of Planetary Medicine.* London: Gaia Books.

Lovins, Amory. 2000 'Natural Capitalism' in *Resurgence* 198, 8–13.

Lowry, Katherine. 1987 'Channelers' in *Omni* 10.1, 47–50, 146–150.

Lucas, Phillip C. 1992 'The New Age Movement and the Pentecostal/Charismatic Revival: Distinct Yet Parallel Phases of a Fourth Great Awakening?' in *Perspectives on the New Age.* (eds) James R. Lewis and J. Gordon Melton. New York: State University of New York Press, 189–212.

Luckmann, Thomas. 1967 *The Invisible Religion: The Transformation of Symbols in Industrial Society.* New York: Macmillan.

MacLaine, Shirley. 1991 *Going Within.* London: Bantam.

McCullough, Bob. 1994 'The New Spin is Spirituality' in *Publishers Weekly* 241, 38–43.

McGuire, Meredith B. 1988 *Ritual Healing in Suburban America.* New Brunswick: Rutgers University Press.

———1993 'Health and Spirituality as Contemporary Concerns' in *The Annals of the American Academy of Political and Social Sciences.* 527, 153.

McNeil, Helen. 1996 'The Archaeology of Gender in the Beat Movement' in *The Beat Generation Writers.* (ed.) A. Robert Lee. London: Pluto, 189.

Macy, Joanna. 1998 'The Great Turning' in *Resurgence* 186, 28–29.

Mahony, William K. 1987 'Spiritual Discipline' in *Encyclopaedia of Religion.* (ed.) M. Eliade New York: Macmillan, *s. v.*

354

Mann, J. H. 1994 'Human Potential' in *Encyclopaedia of Psychology*. (ed.) R. J. Corsini. New York: John Wiley, *s. v.*

Margulis, Lynn and Dorion Sagan. 1995 *What is life?* New York: Simon and Schuster.

Marshall, Peter. 1993 *Demanding the Impossible: A History of Anarchism*. London: Harper Collins.

Martin, James Alfred, jr. 1987 'Religious Experience' in *The Encyclopaedia of Religion*. (ed.) M. Eliade. New York: Macmillan, *s. v.*

Maslow, Abraham H. 1964 *Religions, Values, and Peak Experiences*. Columbus, Ohio: Ohio State University Press.

——1970 *Motivations and Personality* (second edition). New York: Harper & Row.

Matrisciana, Caryl. 1985 *Gods of the New Age*. Eugene, Oregon: Harvest House.

Matthews, Caitlin. 1991 *The Elements of the Goddess*. Shaftesbury, Dorset: Element Books.

Matthews, Eric. 1991 *The Challenge of Secular Humanism*. Kilmarnock, Ayrshire: Humanist Society of Scotland.

Meadows, Kenneth. 1995 *The Medicine Way: A Shamanic Path to Self Mastery*. Shaftesbury, Dorset: Element

Meera, Mother. 1994 *Answers*. London: Rider.

Mehl, Lewis E. 1988 'Modern Shamanism: Integration of Biomedicine with Traditional World Views' in *Shaman's Path: Healing, Personal Growth, and Empowerment*. (ed.) Gary Doore. Boston, Mass.: Shambhala, 129–133.

Melton, J. Gordon. 1988 'A History of the New Age' in *Not Necessarily the New Age: Critical Essays*. (ed.) Robert Basil. New York: Prometheus Books, 35–53.

Melton, J. Gordon, Clark, Jerome, and Kelly, Aidan A. 1990 *New Age Encyclopaedia*. Detroit: Gale Research Inc.

——1991 *New Age Almanac*. Detroit: Visible Ink Press.

Miller, Eliot. 1990 *A Crash Course on the New Age Movement*. Eastbourne: Monarch.

Mills, Simon. 1993 'The Development of the Complementary Medical Professions' in *Complementary Therapies in Medicine* 1, 24–29.

——1995 'What are Complementary Practitioners Competent to Do?' in *Complementary Therapies in Medicine* 3, 3–4.

Mithers, Carol Lynn. 1994 *Therapy Gone Mad: The True Story of Hundreds of Patients and a Generation Betrayed*. Reading, Mass.: Addison-Wesley.

Monk, Donald. 1970 *Social Grading on the National Readership Survey*. London: JICNARS.

Naess, Arne. 1988 'The Basics of Deep Ecology' in *Resurgence* 126, 5–7.

——1989 *Ecology, Community and Lifestyle.* Cambridge: Cambridge University Press.

——1995 'Self-Realization: An Ecological Approach to Being in the World' in *Deep Ecology for the Twenty-First Century: Readings on the Philosophy and Practice of the New Environmentalism.* (ed.) George Sessions. Boston: Shambhala, 225–239.

Naisbitt, John and Aburdene, Patricia. 1990 *Megatrends 2000: the Next Ten Years ... Major Changes in Your Life and World.* London: Sidgwick & Jackson.

Nation, Ihla F. 1998 'Notes of a New Age Survivor' in *Gnosis* 49, 18–22.

Needleman, Jacob. 1970 *The New Religions.* New York: Doubleday.

——1998 *On Love: Is the Meaning of Life to be Found in Love?* London: Arkana.

Newport, John P. 1998 *The New Age Movement and the Biblical Worldview: Conflict and Dialogue.* Grand Rapids, Michigan: Wm. B. Eerdman Press.

Noll, Richard. 1994 *The Jung Cult: Origins of the Charismatic Movement.* Princeton, New Jersey: Princeton University Press.

Olds, Glenn A. 1993 'The New Age: Historical and Metaphysical Foundations' in *New Age Spirituality: An Assessment.* (ed.) D. S. Ferguson. Louisville, Kentucky: John Knox Press, 59–78.

O'Neil, Paul. 1971 'The Only Rebellion Around' in *A Casebook on the Beat.* (ed.) Thomas Parkinson. New York: T. Y. Crowell, 232–246.

Orr, Leonard and Ray, Sondra. 1983 *Rebirthing in the New Age.* Berkeley, California: Celestial Arts.

Osborne, Arthur. 1978 *Ramana Maharshi and the Path of Self-Knowledge.* London: Rider.

Osho. 1995 *Meditation: The First and Last Freedom.* London: Boxtree.

Palmer, Martin. 1993 *Coming of Age: An Exploration of Christianity and the New Age.* London: Aquarian.

Parkinson, Thomas. 1971 'Phenomenon or Generation' in *A Casebook on the Beat.* (ed.) Thomas Parkinson. New York: T. Y. Crowell, 276ff.

Peale, Norman Vincent. 1996 *The Power of Positive Thinking.* London: Cedar.

Peck, M. Scott. 1993 *The Road Less Travelled: A New Psychology of Love, Traditional Values and Spiritual Growth.* London: Hutchinson.

Perry, Michael. 1992 *Gods Within: A Critical Guide to the New Age.* London: SPCK.

Peters, Ted. 1991 *The Cosmic Self: A Penetrating Look at Today's New Age Movements.* San Francisco: Harper.

Pfäfflin, F. 1977 *Herman Hesse 1877–1977: Stationen seines Lebens, des Werkes und seiner Wirkung.* Munich: Kosël.

Plato. 1980 Extract from Book 10 of the *Republic* cited in Richard Lamerton *Care of the Dying*. London: Penguin, 210.

Poggi, Isotta. 1992 'Alternative Spirituality in Italy' in *Perspectives on the New Age*. (eds) James R. Lewis and J. Gordon Melton. New York: State University of New York Press, 271–286.

Porritt, Jonathon. 1988 'Let the Green Spirit Live' in *Resurgence* 127, 4–12.

——1996 'Real World' in *Resurgence* 177, 18–19.

Porritt, Jonathan and Winner, David. 1988 *The Coming of the Greens*. London: Fontana.

Prince, Ruth, and Riches, David. 2000 *The New Age in Glastonbury: The Construction of Religious Movements*. New York: Berghahn Books.

Quakers. 1995 *Quaker Faith and Practice*. Britain: Religious Society of Friends.

Rael, Joseph. 1992 *Beautiful Painted Arrow: Stories and Teachings from the North American Tradition*. Shaftesbury, Dorset: Element.

——1993 *Being and Vibration*. Tulsa, Oklahoma: Council Oak Books.

Rajneesh, Bhagwan Shree. 1970 *On Loving Yourself and Others*. Poona, India: Osho Commune International (tape Cassette).

——1983 *The Orange Book*. Oregon: Rajneesh Foundation International.

——1995 (see Osho).

Ramana, Sri Maharshi. 1969 *Who am I?* Tiruvannamalai, India: Sri Ramanashramam.

Raschke, Carl A. 1980 *The Interruption of Eternity: Modern Gnosticism and the Origins of the New Religious Consciousness*. Chicago: Nelson-Hall.

Ray, Paul H. 1996 'The Rise of Integral Culture' in *Noetic Sciences Review* Spring Edition, 4–15.

Redfield, James. 1994 *The Celestine Prophesy*. London: Bantam.

Reeves, Donald. 1990 *1990 – 2000: A Vision for Ten Years*. London: St James's Church.

Riddell, Carol. 1990 *The Findhorn Community: Creating a Human Identity for the Twenty-First Century*. Forres, Scotland: Findhorn Press.

Rietveld, Hillegonda. 1993 'Living the Dream' in *Rave Off: Politics and Deviance in Contemporary Youth Culture*. (ed.) Steve Redhead. Aldershot, Hants.: Avebury, 68f.

Riordan, Suzanne. 1992 'Channeling: A New Revelation?' in *Perspectives on the New Age*. (eds) James R. Lewis and J. Gordon Melton. New York: State University of New York Press, 105–126.

Robbins, Thomas. 1989 'Not Necessarily the New Age: Critical Essays' in *Journal for the Scientific Study of Religion* 28, 375–376.

Roberts, David E. 1968 *Existentialism and Religious Belief*. New York: Oxford University Press.

Roland, Paul. 2000 *New Age Living: A Guide to Principles, Practices and Beliefs*. London: Hamlyn.

Roof, Wade Clark. 1993 *A Generation of Seekers: The Spiritual Journeys of the Baby Boom Generation.* San Francisco: Harper.

——1999 *Spiritual Marketplace: Baby Boomers and the Remaking of American Religion.* Princeton, NJ: Princeton University Press.

Rose, Stuart. 1998 'An Examination of the New Age Movement: Who is Involved and What Constitutes its Spirituality' in *Journal of Contemporary Religion* 13.1, 5–22.

——2001a 'New Age Women: Spearheading the Movement?' in *Women's Studies: An Interdisciplinary Journal* 30, 329–350.

——2001b 'Is the Term "Spirituality" a Word that Everyone Uses but Nobody Knows What Anyone Means by it?' in *Journal of Contemporary Religion* 16.2, 193–207.

——2004 'Spiritual Love: Questioning the Unquestionable' in *Journal of Contemporary Religion* 19.2, 205–217.

Ross, Andrew. 1991 *Strange Weather: Culture, Science, and Technology in the Age of Limits.* New York: Verso.

Roszak, Theodore. 1970 *The Making of a Counter Culture: Reflections on the Technocratic Society and its Youthful Opposition.* London: Faber & Faber.

——1993 *The Voice of the Earth: An Exploration of Ecopsychology.* London: Bantam.

——1994 *The Cult of Information: A Neo-Luddite Treatise on High-Tech, Artificial Intelligence, and the True Art of Thinking.* Berkeley, California: University of California Press.

Rushkoff, Douglas. 1994 *Cyberia: Life in the Trenches of Hyperspace.* London: Flamingo.

Russell, Peter. 1979 *The TM Technique – A Skeptics' Guide to the TM Program.* Boston, Mass.: Routledge & Keegan Paul.

——1982 *The Awakening Earth: Our Next Evolutionary Leap.* London: Routledge & Keegan Paul.

Sathya Sai Baba, Bhagavan Sri. 1991 *Yoga of Action: Significance of Selfless Service.* Prashanthi Nilayam, India: Sri Sathya Sai Books & Publications Trust.

Satin, Mark. 1978 *New Age Politics: Healing Self and Society.* West Vancouver, Canada: Whitecap Books.

Saunders, Nicholas. 1995 *Ecstasy and the Dance Culture.* London: Turnabout.

Saussure, Ferdinand de. 1964 *Course in General Linguistics.* (eds) Charles Bailey and Albert Sechehaye, Trans. Wade Baskin. London: Peter Owen.

Schur, Edwin. 1977 *The Awareness Trap: Self-Absorption Instead of Social Change.* New York: McGraw-Hill.

Schwarz, Walter. 1994 'Interview with Anita Roddick' in *Resurgence* 164, 44–45.

Seigel, Jerrold. 1986 *Bohemian Paris: Culture, Politics and the Boundaries of Bourgeois Life, 1830–1930.* New York: Viking.

Sharma, Ursula. 1992 *Complementary Medicine Today: Practitioners and Patients.* London: Tavistock.

Sheldrake, Rupert. 1988 *A New Science of Life: The Hypothesis of Formative Causation.* London: Paladin.

——1990 *The Rebirthing of Nature: The Greening of Science and God.* London: Century.

——1994 *Seven Experiments that could Change the World.* London: Fourth Estate.

Sire, James W. 1988 *Shirley MacLaine and the New Age Movement.* Donners Grove, Illinois: InterVarsity Press.

Sjoo, Monica. 1994 'New Age and Patriarchy' in *Religion Today* 9, 22–28.

Slee, Colin. 1999 'New Religious Movements and the Churches' in *New Religious Movements: Challenge and Response.* (eds) Bryan Wilson and Jamie Cresswell. London: Routledge, 165–180.

Slocombe, Jeremy. 1998 'Creating Sustainable Community' in *Living Lightly* 5, 22.

Sorokin, Pitirim. 1941 *The Crisis of Our Age.* N.p.: E. P. Dutton.

Spangler, David. 1971 *Revelation: The Birth of a New Age.* Forres, Scotland: Findhorn Foundation.

——1984 *Emergence: The Rebirth of the Sacred.* New York: Dell.

Spangler, David and Thompson, William Irwin. 1991 *Reimagination of the World.* Santa Fe, New Mexico: Bear & Co.

Spink, Peter. 1983 *The End of an Age.* Winford, Avon: Omega Trust.

——1990 'Introduction' in *The Universal Christ.* Bede Griffiths. London: Darton, Longman and Todd, x–xvii.

——1991 *A Christian in the New Age.* London: Darton, Longman and Todd.

Spretnak, Charlene. 1986 'The Spiritual Dimension of Green Politics' in *Green Politics: The Global Promise.* (eds) Charlene Spretnak and Fritjof Capra. London: Paladin, 230–258.

Stanway, A. 1982 *Alternative Medicine.* London: Penguin.

Starhawk. 1989 *The Spiral Dance* (10th anniversary edition). San Francisco: Harper Collins.

——1991 'The Rebirth of the Goddess' in *The New Age: An Anthology of Essential Writings.* (ed.) William Bloom. London: Rider, 33–40.

Steyn, Chrissie. 1995 *Worldviews in Transition: An Investigation into the New Age Movement in South Africa.* Pretoria: University of South Africa.

Storm, Rachel. 1992 *In Search of Heaven on Earth.* London: Aquarian.

Streiker, Lowell D. 1991 *New Age Comes to Main Street: A Non-Hysterical Survey of the New Age Movement.* Nashville: Abingdon Press.

Sutcliffe, Steven. 2002 *Children of the New Age: A History of Alternative Spirituality.* London: Routledge.

Sutcliffe, Steven and Marion Bowman (eds). 2000 *Beyond the New Age: Exploring Alternative Spirituality.* Edinburgh: Edinburgh University Press.

Sutich, Anthony J. 1976 'The Emergence of the Transpersonal Orientation: A Personal Account' in *Journal of Transpersonal Psychology* 8.1, 5–14.

Tarnas, Richard. 1996 *The Passion of the Western Mind: Understanding the Ideas that Have Shaped Our World View.* London: Pimlico.

Tart, Charles. 1975 *Transpersonal Psychologies.* London: Routledge & Keegan Paul.

Teilhard de Chardin, Pierre. 1959 *The Phenomenon of Man.* London: Collins.

——1978 *The Heart of the Matter.* London: Collins.

Temerlin, Maurice K. and Temerlin, Jane W. 1982 'Psychotherapy Cults: An Iatrogenic Perversion' in *Psychotherapy: Theory, Research and Practice* 19, 131–141.

Thompson, Gerry Maguire. 1999 *Encyclopaedia of the New Age.* London: Time Life Books.

Timpe, E. F. 1977 'Hermann Hesse in the United States' in *Hermann Hesse: A Collection of Criticism.* (ed.) J. Liebmann. New York: McGraw-Hill, 136–142.

Tipton, Steven M. 1984 *Getting Saved from the Sixties: Moral Meaning in Conversion and Cultural Change.* Berkeley, California: University of California Press.

Trevelyan, Sir George. 1997 'Shakespeare and the Vision of Wholeness' in *The Mountain Path* 34.1,2, 51–7.

Trungpa, Chogyam. 1987 *Cutting Through Spiritual Materialism.* Boston: Shambhala.

Turner, Steve. 1995 *Hungry for Heaven: Rock and Roll and the Search for Redemption.* London: Hodder & Stoughton.

Van de Weyer, Robert. 1991 *The Health of Nations: Political Morality for the Twenty-First Century.* Bideford, Devon: Green Books.

Vitz, Paul. 1983 *Psychology as Religion: The Cult of Self Worship.* Grand Rapids, Michigan: W. B. Eerdmans.

Walker, Martin J. 1993 *Dirty Medicine: Science, Big Business, and the Assault on Natural Health Care.* London: Slingshot.

Wallis, Roy and Bruce, Steve. 1986 *Sociological Theory, Religion and Collective Action.* Belfast: Queen's University Press.

Walters, Tony. 1992 'Why are most churchgoers women?' in *Vox Evangelica* 20, 73–90.

Waterson, M. J. 1993 *Marketing Pocket Book 1994*. Henley-on-Thames: NTC/Advertising Association.

Watts, Alan. 1973 *This is IT and Other Essays on Zen and Spiritual Experience*. New York: Vintage Books.

Watts, Janet. 1995 *The Observer* 'Life' Magazine, 5 November.

Weir, Michael. 1993 'Bristol Cancer Help Centre: Success and Setbacks but the Journey Continues' in *Complementary Therapies in Medicine* 1, 42–45.

West, John Anthony. 1991 *The Case for Astrology*. London: Viking.

Whole Earth Catalog. 1971 *The Last Whole Earth Catalog*. San Francisco: Portola Institute.

Wilber, Ken. 1977 *The Spectrum of Consciousness*. Weaton, Illinois: Theosophical Publishing House.

——1981 *No Boundary: Eastern and Western Approaches to Personal Growth*. Boston, Mass.: Shambhala.

——1983 *A Sociable God: A Brief Introduction to a Transcendental Sociology*. New York: McGraw-Hill.

——1987 'Baby-Boomers, Narcissism, and the New Age' in *Vajradhatu Sun* Oct/Nov issue, 11–13.

——1990 *Eye to Eye: The Quest for the New Paradigm*. Boston, Mass.: Shambhala.

——1993 *Grace and Grit: Spirituality and Healing in the Life and Death of Treya Killam Wilber*. Boston, Mass.: Shambhala.

——1995a *Sex, Ecology, Spirituality: The Spirit of Evolution*. Boston, Mass.: Shambhala.

——1995b 'Ken Wilber on the New Age' in *Kindred Spirit* 3.10, 45–47.

——1996 *A Brief History of Everything*. Boston: Shambhala.

——1998 'Up Close and Transpersonal with Ken Wilber'. Interviewer Mark Matousek. In *Utne Reader* 88, 51–55, 106–7.

Wild, K. W. 1938 *Intuition*. Cambridge: Cambridge University Press.

Williamson, Marianne. 1992 *A Return to Love: Reflections on the Principles of 'A Course of Miracles'*. London: Aquarian.

Wilson, Roy I. 1994 *Medicine Wheels: Ancient Teachings for Modern Times*. New York: Crossroads.

Wilson, Stuart. 1989 *A Guide to the New Age*. Newton Abbot, Devon: Wayseeker Books.

Witmer, J. M. and Sweeney, T. J. 1992 'A Holistic Model for Wellness and Prevention Over the Life Span' in *Journal of Counseling and Development* 71.2, 140–148.

Wittgenstein, Ludwig J. J. 1967 *Philosophical Investigations* (3rd edition). Trans. G. E. M. Anscombe. Oxford: Blackwell.

Woodham, Anne. 1994 *HEA Guide to Complementary Medicine and Therapies*. London: Health Education Authority.

Woodhead, Lesley. 1994 *Children of Woodstock*. London: Twenty Twenty Vision (TV programme).
Woodhead, Linda. 1993 'Post-Christian Spiritualities' in *Religion* 23, 167–181.
Woodside, Lisa N. 1993 'New Age Spirituality: A Positive Contribution' in *New Age Spirituality: An Assessment*. (ed.) Duncan S. Ferguson. Louisville, Kentucky: John Knox Press, 145–168.
Wuthnow, Robert. 1998 *After Heaven: Spirituality in America Since the 1950s*. Berkeley, California: University of California Press.
Yankelovich, Daniel. 1981 *New Rules: Searching for Self-Fulfilment in a World Turned Upside Down*. New York: Random House.
Yogananda, Paramahansa. 1994 *Autobiography of a Yogi*. London: Rider.
York, Michael. 1994 'New Age Britain: An Overview' in *Religion Today* 9, 14–22.
——1995 *The Emerging Network: A Sociology of the New Age and Neo-Pagan Movements*. Lanham, Maryland: Rowman & Littlefield.
Zappone, Catherine. 1991 *The Hope for Wholeness: A Spirituality for Feminists*. Mystic, Conn.: Twenty-Third Publications.

Index

acupuncture 18, 21, 47, 67, 96, 112,
  145, 188, 191, 193f, 197, 210
Adler, Margot 90
Age of Aquarius 22
age of New Age participants 85
Akashic Records 111
Alternatives 31, 88, 99, 119, 120f,
  170, 284, 315
Amnesty International 98, 226
amorphous 9, 15, 24, 26, 38, 41, 81,
  119, 130, 160, 281, 330
anarchism 25
Anthony, Dick 124
anthropocentrism 289
Aquarian Conspiracy, The 10, 18, 25,
  83, 139, 176
aromatherapy 67, 96f, 186, 189, 194,
  196, 234, 310
astrology 19, 20f, 34, 83, 93, 110
Auroville 52
Ayurveda 188

Bach, Richard 137
Barker, Eileen 61, 286
Basil, Robert 19, 329, 333
Beat Generation 51f, 54ff
Bednarowski, Mary Farrell 41, 82,
  140, 159, 161, 329f
Bellah, Robert 299
Ben & Jerry's 224
Berry, Wendell 229
Blake, William 37
Bloom, William 18f, 31ff, 39, 41, 70,
  100, 119, 121, 129, 131, 143,
  145, 150, 152, 155, 159ff, 180f,
  214ff, 220, 279, 283, 294, 303f,
  315, 316, 319, 327ff, 334ff

Boddhi Tree 114
Body Shop 224
Bohemians 51
Bristol Cancer Help Centre 202, 208
Brown, Michael 70
Bruce, Steve 27, 36, 69, 76, 114,
  124, 126, 147, 217, 292f
Buddhism 48, 55, 73, 77, 79, 96,
  147, 172, 198, 227, 285, 302,
  304

Caddy, Peter and Eileen 217
California 23, 46, 48, 52, 61, 66, 70,
  114, 118, 120, 123, 179, 287
Campbell, Colin 46f
Campbell, Eileen 19, 72
capitalism 28, 45, 123, 220f, 229,
  291, 314, 330, 337
Capra, Fritjof 110, 142, 177, 186,
  197, 218f, 228, 296
Casteneda, Carlos 55
categories of involvement 123ff
cause of the New Age 27ff
Cayce, Edgar 18, 46, 49, 68, 94, 177,
  204, 284
Celestine Prophecy, The 119, 180
central ideas of the New Age 30ff
chakras 254f
channelling 19, 29, 61, 68ff, 74, 78,
  96, 100, 110, 134, 144, 203,
  235, 254, 316
Chopra, Deepak 178, 206, 215f
Christian acceptance 282ff
Christian response 266ff
Christian view of New Age ideas
  277ff
cleansing ceremony 237

Clecak, Peter 308
communes 218
complementary health and medicine
    21, 26, 34, 66, 118, 185ff, 199,
    207ff
connectedness 142ff
consumerism 310
Co-operative Bank 224
core domains of the New Age 159
Cosmic Christ 29, 153, 179, 286
counter-culture 49ff, 61, 78, 86, 200,
    210, 263, 298, 307ff, 320, 324,
    338
Course in Miracles, A 18, 69f, 172,
    183, 268
Creation-Centred Spirituality 228
Crowley, Vivianne 188, 273
Cumbey, Constance 266ff, 272ff
Cupitt, Don 285

deep ecology 228
demonism 267
dis-ease 186
DIY religion 274
Dossey, Larry 203,
Douthwaite, Richard 222
drugs 18, 52, 60, 71, 81, 93, 99ff,
    104, 210, 236, 333
Drury, Nevill 18, 64, 66, 141, 180,
    188
Durkheim, Emile 134

Earth First! 225
Earth Summit 231
Easternization 47
ecology 16, 22ff, 38, 87, 142, 159,
    228, 276
Edwards, Gill 316
efficacy 207ff, 291f, 296, 303, 321
Ellwood, Robert 45, 331, 335
Esalen 52, 61, 64
Essenes 172, 271
est 18, 63f, 312

etheric plane 255
evil 280
existentialism 57

Ferguson, Andrew 316
Ferguson, Duncan S. 19
Ferguson, Marianne 66
Ferguson, Marilyn 10, 25, 52, 62, 78,
    83, 99, 101, 109f, 127, 135,
    139f, 150ff, 161ff, 173, 176,
    179ff, 214ff, 293f, 297, 309,
    314, 328, 331, 333f
Feuerstein, Georg 21, 65, 149, 152,
    173, 190, 269, 296f
Findhorn 18, 52, 159, 218f, 224, 318
flower power 51
forms of involvement 122ff
Fortune, Dion 49, 154, 178
Fox, Matthew 120, 147f, 153, 172,
    228, 237, 268, 287f, 314, 335
frequency of activities 94ff
Freud, Sigmund 194
Friends of the Earth 97, 122, 222,
    225, 229
Fulder, Stephen J. 199, 205f, 209f
fundamentalist 266ff, 273

Gaia 19, 116, 120, 136, 143, 228
Gandhi, Mohandas K 161, 229
Gawain, Shakti 139, 177ff, 200ff,
    206
gender 82ff
Ginsberg, Allen 50, 54f, 317
Gnosticism 45, 74, 270, 306f
God and the New Age 151, 168
Goddess spirituality 67, 135
going within 108ff
Green politics 96ff, 225f
Greenpeace 52, 74, 97, 225, 229
Greer, Germaine 65
Griffiths, Bede 265, 286
Grof, Stanislav 63, 71ff, 154, 167
Groothuis, Douglas 268ff, 278, 281

Guiley, Rosemary Ellen 35f, 69, 71, 101, 110, 145, 188, 190, 200, 235, 254f
Gurdjieff, G. I. 48, 293

Hanegraaff, Wouter J. 21, 27, 100, 220
Harman, Willis W. 141, 150, 178, 221
Harper, Clifford 25
Hay, Louise L. 34, 81, 177, 179, 200, 202, 206, 216, 297
healing 15, 18ff, 30, 38ff, 66, 71, 76f, 78, 83, 87, 90, 93, 96, 113f, 118, 127, 131, 136, 138, 145f, 153, 159, 160ff, 172, 176, 179f, 183–212, 232ff, 243, 249ff, 259, 265, 278f, 282, 285, 289, 310, 313, 318f, 323ff, 328ff, 332, 334
healing and the paranormal 202f
Healing Circle workshop 234
Heelas, Paul 26f, 32, 34, 39, 87f, 114, 122ff, 131ff, 169, 174, 218, 280f, 286, 291ff, 303, 310ff, 317ff, 329f, 335ff
Hesse, Hermann 48, 56f, 178
Higher Self 33, 35, 73, 92, 129, 132, 149ff, 166, 174, 181, 188, 192, 194, 234, 268, 277ff, 293, 310, 320f, 334f, 338
holism 25, 38f, 142, 189, 195
homoeopathy 93, 96, 191, 194, 208ff
Human Potential Movement 61f

identifying varieties of spiritual empowerment 171ff
income levels 90f
inner child 243
inner voices 111, 293
Inter Faith Network 282f
interconnectedness 32

International Humanist and Ethical Union 24
intuition 25, 31, 35, 47, 71, 103, 108ff, 140, 174, 211, 230, 251, 294, 306, 321
ISKCON 52
Isle of Avalon Foundation 120

John F. Kennedy University 118
Jung, Carl 45, 49, 85, 94, 108, 144, 159, 177f, 297

karma 35, 134, 189, 216
Kerouac, Jack 54
Kierkegaard, Søren 57, 338
Kindred Spirit 8, 10, 20, 76, 115ff
kinship 214
Kohlberg test 123
Kovel, Joel 32, 63, 132, 152, 188, 298
Krishnamurti, Jiddu 73f, 94, 140, 145f, 152, 172f, 177f

Lasch, Christopher 18, 49, 278, 291f, 305ff
Leary, Timothy 55, 121
length of association 88f
LETS 120, 224
levels of involvement 126ff
Levine, Frederick E. 46, 82, 86, 90, 100, 168
Lewis, James R. 15, 19, 23, 27, 34, 142, 146f, 329, 335
Linn, Denise 176, 178, 201, 206, 247
literary Influences on the New Age 54ff
love 16f, 29, 33, 37, 39, 41, 70, 81, 111, 132f, 136, 145ff, 153f, 161, 164ff, 180, 189, 194, 215, 222, 230, 236, 240, 242, 244, 248, 256, 296, 310, 315f, 319, 337, 339
Lovelock, James 143, 228
Luckmann, Thomas 46

MacLaine, Shirley 18, 32, 69, 139, 150, 178, 254, 269, 335
Macy, Joanna 230, 231
main qualities of the New Age 37ff
manifestation of Spirit 31
marital status 84f
Maslow, Abraham 62f, 71, 177ff
McGuire, Meredith 184, 192, 203, 210
'me decade' 303
medicine wheel 235
Medicine Wheel Blessing Ceremony 257
Meera, Mother 152, 170, 176, 178
Megatripolis 75
Melton, J. Gordon 19, 23, 27, 30, 34, 44, 114, 118, 138, 152f, 333
Mesmer, Franz 44
metanoia 141
middle-class 52, 192, 198, 324
millennium 21, 43, 74, 78f
Millet, Kate 65
Movement 24ff, 123, 228, 266
Mysteries 114

Naess, Arne 213, 228
narcissism 149, 291, 305ff, 321
Natural Law Party 190
Nazi 267
Needleman, Jacob 52, 77
negative change 102ff
networking 112ff, 325
new economics 16, 220
New Economics Foundation 120, 224
new paradigm/paradigm shift 25, 41, 47, 126, 219ff, 314
New Thought 307
newness of the New Age 15f, 54
Newport, John P. 272f
Nietzsche, Friedrich 45
non-duality 73, 84, 304

Paganism 34, 60, 75, 188, 198, 227
panentheism 287, 335
pantheism 44, 268, 272, 280, 335
paranormal 18f, 34, 36, 61, 74, 78, 83, 92, 100f, 104, 110, 144, 190, 202ff, 272, 325
participatory democracy (PR) 226
past lives 34, 83, 181, 246ff
Pax World 224
Peale, Norman Vincent 34
Peck, M. Scott 148, 178, 206, 275f
Pentecostalists 279
Perry, Michael 266, 274f, 278ff, 288, 335
Peters, Ted 25, 45, 62, 150f, 169, 271ff, 335
physical access to the New Age 112
Plain Truth, The 269
Porritt, Jonathon 132, 222, 229, 298, 327
positive change 101
power animal 237
prosperity 313ff
Psychosynthesis 64, 74, 110, 218
psychotechnologies 62ff, 77, 99, 109, 127, 134, 138f, 180, 188, 196, 198, 218, 263, 268, 300f, 311ff, 326, 338
psychotherapy cult mentality 303

Rael, Joseph 233ff
Rajneesh, Bhagwan Shree (Osho) 146, 178, 202, 285, 291, 321
Ram Dass 55, 99, 147f, 161, 173, 176, 178, 311, 321
Ramana Maharshi 163, 304
Rampa, T. Lobsang 55
Raschke, Carl A. 45
Ray, Paul H. 22, 27, 76, 138
Real World Coalition 122, 222
reasons for association 92ff
rebirthing 64, 74, 97, 138, 192
reincarnation 29, 33ff, 134, 247, 272

Religious Society of Friends
    (Quakers) 285
Robbins, Thomas 312
Roddick, Anita 224
Romanticism 36, 44f
Roof, Wade Clark 88, 135, 211, 272,
    294, 311f
Rose, Stuart 11, 132, 147, 193, 298
Rosicrucians 48
Roszak, Theodore 50, 55, 75, 121,
    216, 291, 308
Russell, Peter 295f, 304f, 311, 319f

Sai Baba 48, 94, 161, 170f, 176, 178
satanic 272
Satin, Mark 221, 222
Saunders, Nicholas 87
Saussure, Ferdinand de 131
Schumacher College 120
scope of the New Age 11, 15, 18ff,
    30, 159, 183, 185, 187, 292
self-centredness of participants 318
service 160ff
Shamanism 19f, 74, 93, 96, 116, 135,
    142, 146, 188, 200, 227, 235,
    237, 251, 258
Sheldrake, Rupert 101, 144, 229f,
    295
Skyros 89, 120
Slee, Colin 276
social status 89ff
soul retrieval 251
Spangler, David 19, 30, 46, 69ff,
    107ff, 122, 126ff, 135, 153f,
    167, 216, 222, 297f, 327ff, 335,
    337
specialist magazines 115
spectrum of consciousness 299
Spink, Peter 285ff
spiritual love 17, 145ff
spiritual materialism 317
spirituality 132ff, 159–178, passim
Spretnak, Charlene 132, 298

St James's Church 119, 170, 284
Starhawk 67
Steiner, Rudolf 46, 49, 177
Steyn, Crissie 23
Storm, Rachel 319
Streiker, Lowell D. 30, 75, 272, 331,
    333
Subud 48
Sustainable living 219ff
Swedenborg, Emanuel 44, 48
synchronicity 30, 100, 144, 204

t'ai chi ch'uan 96, 190, 193, 285
'talking' bear 248
Tarnas, Richard 44f
Tart, Charles 110
Teilhard de Chardin, Pierre 49, 143,
    147, 153, 177ff
The Farm 218
Theosophical Society 44, 46, 48
therapists in the New Age 204ff
Tibb 189
Transcendental Meditation (TM) 190
transformation 11, 33, 38ff, 62, 78,
    102, 105, 108, 112, 127ff, 132f,
    137ff, 149, 153f, 159, 163, 172,
    184, 191f, 197, 212ff, 218, 220,
    223, 225f, 230, 268, 274f, 282,
    301, 323, 325ff, 338f
transmodernism 22
transpersonal 18, 22f, 43, 61ff, 71ff,
    78, 110f, 123, 132f, 138, 141,
    167, 218, 230, 263, 299ff, 307
travellers 26, 75, 333
Trevelyan, Sir George 176, 178, 323
Triodos Bank 224
trivialization 298, 302, 317, 321
Trungpa, Chogyam 52, 122, 317
Turner, Steve 51, 60, 75

Unitarians 286
unity in diversity 37, 214, 273

Van de Weyer, Robert 223
Vatican 270
Vedanta 73, 304
Vietnam War 50
visualization 199
Vivekananda, Swami 49

Walker, Martin J. 208
Wallis, Roy 124, 292, 293
Watts, Alan 50, 55, 89, 178
White Eagle 48, 116, 177, 204
Wilber, Ken 18, 36, 64f, 72f, 79, 88,
    122ff, 132, 137f, 141, 143, 147,
    149, 152, 154, 167, 291, 296ff,
    307, 317, 320, 335

Wittgenstein, Ludwig J. J. 131
women in the New Age 65ff
Women's Environment Network
    (WEN) 227
Woodhead, Linda 58, 82, 277, 288
Woodstock 51, 58
World Congress of Faiths 282
Wuthnow, Robert 27, 293

Yoga 115, 189, 190
Yogananda, Paramahansa 48, 131,
    178
York, Michael 24, 27, 34, 87, 120,
    270, 286, 327, 335f